Current Research on Dermatology: Pathology, Clinical Manifestation, Investigation and Therapy

Current Research on Dermatology: Pathology, Clinical Manifestation, Investigation and Therapy

Editor

Alin Laurentiu Tatu

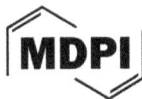

Basel • Beijing • Wuhan • Barcelona • Belgrade • Novi Sad • Cluj • Manchester

Editor
Alin Laurentiu Tatu
Clinical Medical Department,
Dermatology, Faculty of
Medicine and Pharmacy
Dunarea de Jos University
Galati
Romania

Editorial Office
MDPI
St. Alban-Anlage 66
4052 Basel, Switzerland

This is a reprint of articles from the Special Issue published online in the open access journal *Life* (ISSN 2075-1729) (available at: https://www.mdpi.com/journal/life/special_issues/Dermatology_research).

For citation purposes, cite each article independently as indicated on the article page online and as indicated below:

Lastname, A.A.; Lastname, B.B. Article Title. *Journal Name* **Year**, *Volume Number*, Page Range.

ISBN 978-3-7258-0847-2 (Hbk)
ISBN 978-3-7258-0848-9 (PDF)
doi.org/10.3390/books978-3-7258-0848-9

Cover image courtesy of Alin Laurentiu Tatu

© 2024 by the authors. Articles in this book are Open Access and distributed under the Creative Commons Attribution (CC BY) license. The book as a whole is distributed by MDPI under the terms and conditions of the Creative Commons Attribution-NonCommercial-NoDerivs (CC BY-NC-ND) license.

Contents

About the Editor vii

Preface ix

Fabiola Sârbu, Violeta Diana Oprea, Alin Laurențiu Tatu, Eduard Polea Drima,
Violeta Claudia Bojincă and Aurelia Romila
Hereditary Hemorrhagic Telangiectasia Associating Neuropsychiatric Manifestations with a
Significant Impact on Disease Management—Case Report and Literature Review
Reprinted from: Life 2022, 12, 1059, doi:10.3390/life12071059 1

Ana Fulga, Doriana Cristea Ene, Laura Bujoreanu Bezman, Oana Maria Dragostin,
Iuliu Fulga, Elena Stamate, et al.
Pharyngeal-Esophageal Malignancies with Dermatologic Paraneoplastic Syndrome
Reprinted from: Life 2022, 12, 1705, doi:10.3390/life12111705 11

Caterina Foti, Paolo Romita, Francesca Ambrogio, Carlo Manno, Raffaele Filotico,
Nicoletta Cassano, et al.
Treatment of Severe Atopic Dermatitis with Dupilumab in Three Patients with Renal Diseases
Reprinted from: Life 2022, 12, 2002, doi:10.3390/life12122002 23

Alin Codrut Nicolescu, Marius-Anton Ionescu, Maria Magdalena Constantin, Ioan Ancuta,
Sinziana Ionescu, Elena Niculet, et al.
Psoriasis Management Challenges Regarding Difficult-to-Treat Areas: Therapeutic Decision
and Effectiveness
Reprinted from: Life 2022, 12, 2050, doi:10.3390/life12122050 28

Doriana Sorina Chilom, Simona Sorina Farcaș and Nicoleta Ioana Andreescu
Primary Cutaneous B-Cell Lymphoma Co-Existing with Mycosis Fungoides—A Case Report
and Overview of the Literature
Reprinted from: Life 2022, 12, 2067, doi:10.3390/life12122067 43

Shashank Bhargava, Sara Yumeen, Esther Henebeng and George Kroumpouzos
Erosive Pustular Dermatosis: Delving into Etiopathogenesis and Management
Reprinted from: Life 2022, 12, 2097, doi:10.3390/life12122097 53

Cristina-Raluca (Jitian) Mihulecea and Maria Rotaru
Review: The Key Factors to Melanomagenesis
Reprinted from: Life 2023, 13, 181, doi:10.3390/life13010181 76

Cristina-Raluca (Jitian) Mihulecea, Gabriela Mariana Iancu, Mihaela Leventer and
Maria Rotaru
The Many Roles of Dermoscopy in Melanoma Detection
Reprinted from: Life 2023, 13, 477, doi:10.3390/life13020477 92

Carmen Giuglea, Andrei Marin, Iulia Gavrila, Alexandra Paunescu, Nicoleta Amalia Dobrete
and Silviu Adrian Marinescu
Basal Cell Carcinoma—A Retrospective Descriptive Study Integrated in Current Literature
Reprinted from: Life 2023, 13, 832, doi:10.3390/life13030832 104

Sandra Marinović Kulišić, Marta Takahashi, Marta Himelreich Perić, Vedrana Mužić Radović and Ružica Jurakić Tončić
Immunohistochemical Analysis of Adhesion Molecules E-Selectin, Intercellular Adhesion Molecule-1, and Vascular Cell Adhesion Molecule-1 in Inflammatory Lesions of Atopic Dermatitis
Reprinted from: *Life* **2023**, *13*, 933, doi:10.3390/life13040933 . . . . **116**

Hanieh Kolahdooz, Vahid Khori, Vahid Erfani-Moghadam, Fatemeh Livani, Saeed Mohammadi and Ali Memarian
Niosomal Curcumin Suppresses IL17/IL23 Immunopathogenic Axis in Skin Lesions of Psoriatic Patients: A Pilot Randomized Controlled Trial
Reprinted from: *Life* **2023**, *13*, 1076, doi:10.3390/life13051076 . . . . **126**

Nicolas Kluger
Annular Erythemas and Purpuras
Reprinted from: *Life* **2023**, *13*, 1245, doi:10.3390/life13061245 . . . . **140**

Monika Słowińska, Iwona Czarnecka, Robert Czarnecki, Paulina Tatara, Anna Nasierowska-Guttmejer, Małgorzata Lorent, et al.
Clinical, Dermoscopic, and Histological Characteristics of Melanoma Patients According to the Age Groups: A Retrospective Observational Study
Reprinted from: *Life* **2023**, *13*, 1369, doi:10.3390/life13061369 . . . . **154**

About the Editor

Alin Laurentiu Tatu

In 1994, Alin Laurentiu Tatu graduated at the Carol Davila University of Medicine and Pharmacy, Bucharest, Romania, where he also obtained a PhD degree. Since 2007, he has been affiliated with the Clinical Department of Dermatology, Faculty of Medicine and Pharmacy, Dunarea de Jos University, Galati, Romania. Since 2019, he has been the Head of the Dermatology Department at the Saint Parascheva Clinical Hospital of Infectious Diseases, Galati, and, since 2022, he has been involved with the Multidisciplinary Integrated Center of Dermatological Interface Research (MICDIR), Galati, Romania. His general interests include the following: demodex; endosymbionts; cutaneous microbiome; integrative medicine; optical coherence tomography; dermoscopy; confocal microscopy; cutaneous comorbidities; and skin cancer. He is currently focused on projects on the multimodal imaging monitoring of skin diseases, such as RCM, OCT, dermoscopy, and clinical monitoring during biological treatments. He is an Editor/Associate Editor for 17 Clarivate/PubMed-indexed journals and has received 33 awards, 2 of which have paramount personal value. The first of these is the award received for the "Steroid-induced facial dermatitis—a dermoscopic point of view oral presentation" at the 23rd World Congress of Dermatology, 8–13 June 2015, Vancouver, Canada. The second one is the award received for session FC03 on Dermoscopy and Skin Imaging, Vancouver Convention Center East, 8:15—the Prize from the International Leagues of Dermatology Societies (ILDS). He has also received a Diploma of appreciation and gratitude from the American Academy of Dermatology, in 2018.

Preface

This collection is the result of the joint creation, editing, and publishing efforts of not only the authors involved but also those of MDPI and the personal efforts of the editor Crystal Ma, whom I thank for her continuous efforts and involvement in this project. This collection of representative articles, published in Edition 1 of the Special Issue of *Life*, represents invaluable material both for readers and researchers involved in the study of skin along with related specialties. This material can form the basis of future research, possibly followed by new perspectives on the recognition, diagnosis, and treatment of skin diseases. I dedicate this collection of articles to my mother Sofia and also to Simona, David, and Iacob.

Acknowledgment: This collection was academically supported by the Dunarea de Jos University of Galati through the Multidisciplinary Integrated Center of Dermatological Interface Research Center (MICDIR), "Dunărea de Jos" University of Galați, Galati, Romania.

Alin Laurentiu Tatu
Editor

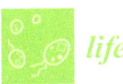 life

Case Report

Hereditary Hemorrhagic Telangiectasia Associating Neuropsychiatric Manifestations with a Significant Impact on Disease Management—Case Report and Literature Review

Fabiola Sârbu [1,2,†], Violeta Diana Oprea [1,3,*], Alin Laurențiu Tatu [4,5,*,‡], Eduard Polea Drima [1,2], Violeta Claudia Bojincă [6,7,†] and Aurelia Romila [1,3]

1. Medical Department, Faculty of Medicine and Pharmacy, "Dunărea de Jos" University of Galati, 800216 Galati, Romania; sarbu_fabiola@yahoo.co.uk (F.S.); drima_edi1963@yahoo.com (E.P.D.); aurelia.romila@yahoo.com (A.R.)
2. "Elisabeta Doamna" Psychiatric Hospital, 800179 Galati, Romania
3. "St. Apostle Andrei" Clinical Emergency County Hospital Galati, 800578 Galati, Romania
4. Clinical, Medical Department, Dermatology, ReForm UDJ, Faculty of Medicine and Pharmacy, "Dunărea de Jos" University of Galati, 800216 Galati, Romania
5. Dermatology Department, Clinical Hospital of Infectious Diseases Saint Parascheva, 800179 Galati, Romania
6. Internal Medicine Department, Faculty of Medicine, "Carol Davila" University of Medicine and Pharmacy in Bucharest, 020021 Bucharest, Romania; vmbojinca@yahoo.com
7. Department of Internal Medicine and Rheumatology, "Sf. Maria" Hospital, 011172 Bucharest, Romania
* Correspondence: diana.v.oprea@gmail.com (V.D.O.); dralin_tatu@yahoo.com (A.L.T.)
† These authors contributed equally to this work.
‡ Multidisciplinary Integrated Center of Dermatological Interface Research MIC-DIR, "Dunărea de Jos" University of Galati, 800008 Galati, Romania.

Citation: Sârbu, F.; Oprea, V.D.; Tatu, A.L.; Polea Drima, E.; Bojincă, V.C.; Romila, A. Hereditary Hemorrhagic Telangiectasia Associating Neuropsychiatric Manifestations with a Significant Impact on Disease Management—Case Report and Literature Review. *Life* 2022, *12*, 1059. https://doi.org/10.3390/life12071059

Academic Editor: Alfredo De Giorgi

Received: 23 June 2022
Accepted: 12 July 2022
Published: 15 July 2022

Publisher's Note: MDPI stays neutral with regard to jurisdictional claims in published maps and institutional affiliations.

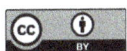

Copyright: © 2022 by the authors. Licensee MDPI, Basel, Switzerland. This article is an open access article distributed under the terms and conditions of the Creative Commons Attribution (CC BY) license (https:// creativecommons.org/licenses/by/ 4.0/).

Abstract: (1) Background: Genetic hereditary hemorrhagic telangiectasia (HHT) is clinically diagnosed. The clinical manifestations and lack of curative therapeutic interventions may lead to mental illnesses, mainly from the depression–anxiety spectrum. (2) Methods: We report the case of a 69-year-old patient diagnosed with HHT and associated psychiatric disorders; a comprehensive literature review was performed based on relevant keywords. (3) Results: Curaçao diagnostic criteria based the HHT diagnosis in our patient case at 63 years old around the surgical interventions for a basal cell carcinoma, after multiple episodes of epistaxis beginning in childhood, but with a long symptom-free period between 20 and 45 years of age. The anxiety–depressive disorder associated with nosocomephobia resulted in a delayed diagnosis and low adherence to medical monitoring. A comprehensive literature review revealed the scarcity of publications analyzing the impact of psychiatric disorders linked to this rare condition, frequently associating behavioral disengagement as a coping strategy, psychological distress, anxiety, depression, and hopelessness. (4) Conclusions: As patients with HHT face traumatic experiences from disease-related causes as well as recurring emergency hospital visits, active monitoring for mental illnesses and psychological support should be considered as part of the initial medical approach and throughout the continuum of care.

Keywords: hereditary hemorrhagic telangiectasia; Rendu–Osler–Weber syndrome; arteriovenous malformations; epistaxis; mental illness; neuropsychiatric; depression; anxiety

1. Introduction

Patients suffering from Rendu–Osler–Weber syndrome or hereditary hemorrhagic telangiectasia (HHT) are frequently diagnosed very late, as the manifestations require knowledge of this rare disease affecting 1 in 5000–8000 individuals globally [1,2]. HHT is an autosomal dominant genetic disorder, with ~90% of the patients associated with heterozygous mutations of ACVRL1 or ENG genes, while ~10% of cases also affect genes that encode components of the BMP9/ALK1 signaling pathway [2–4].

The mutations in HHT alter TGF-beta-mediated pathways in vascular endothelial cells, resulting in the manifestation of aberrant blood vessel development with extreme fragility and arteriovenous malformations (AVMs) [3–5]. The most prevalent clinical symptoms include epistaxis, which can be severe or even lethal in rare cases; telangiectasia (cutaneous blood vessels dilatations); and manifestations induced by AVMs or telangiectasia at the pulmonary, gastrointestinal hepatic, or cerebral level. These may lead to hemorrhages and anemia as well as other serious complications. Studies report that ~50% of HHT patients experience disabling or life-threatening complications, such as stroke or transient ischemic attacks, cerebral abscess, or heart failure [5,6].

A positive diagnosis of HHT is almost always clinical, based on the Curaçao diagnostic criteria established in 1999 [3,7,8], requiring at least three out of these four criteria to be met: spontaneous recurrent epistaxis, multiple telangiectasias, visceral involvement, and a relevant family history. If only two characteristics are present, the diagnosis is probable, and further tests or follow-up are necessary. The genetic tests are also available in some centers.

Concerning the alarming manifestations and scarce therapy options, and in relation to intrinsic pathophysiology, these patients may develop mental illnesses like anxiety, post-traumatic stress disorder, and depression [8,9]. Moreover, the presence of cerebral AVMs—although less frequent, identified in 10–20% of HHT cases [8,10,11]—could induce psychiatric manifestations depending on their localization, although these are very rarely mentioned in the available publications [6,7,11].

2. Materials and Methods

We report the case of a 69-year-old female patient suffering from HHT and associated severe depression, with episodes of anxiety significantly impacting her quality of life. A comprehensive literature review was performed based on relevant keywords, using PubMed and Google Scholar databases.

3. Results

The patient has been under clinical monitoring by an ad-hoc multidisciplinary medical team since February 2021. She recalls multiple episodes of epistaxis during childhood, spontaneously remitting at around 10 years old. She was symptom-free until 45 years of age, when she started to observe cutaneous telangiectasias and reported occasional nose bleeds, for which she rarely consulted her family physician. A severe epistaxis occurred in 2020, requiring emergency intervention; anemic syndrome was diagnosed and the medical team suspected HHT, recommending additional specialty examinations. She is highly anxious and refuses further investigations, and she presents herself to outpatient psychiatry complaining of unrest and depressive symptomatology, sleep disturbances, attention deficits, and emotional lability. She was diagnosed with mixed anxiety and depressive disorder (ICD-10 code F41.2 [12]), receiving a prescription for an antidepressant (sertraline 50 mg/day) and anxiolytic (alprazolam 0.25 mg/day), and it was also recommended that she undergo psychotherapy. The patient uses the medication intermittently upon symptom amelioration, and has been missing the advised periodic follow-ups.

At 63 years old, a nasal cutaneous ulcerative lesion brought the patient to a dermatologist, who identified a basocellular carcinoma, but also insisted on identifying diagnostic criteria for HHT, asking about hereditary background. In the presence of multiple telangiectasias, anamnesis of recurrent epistaxis, and a relevant family history (mother with similar cutaneous telangiectasias and retinal arteriovenous malformations, resulting in retinal scars with consequent decreased visual acuity; a sister with similar ocular manifestations; and father deceased at a young age after four successive strokes), the patient was diagnosed with HHT.

Mohs surgery was performed for the basocellular carcinoma, and further investigations related to HHT revealed a mild anemia (hemoglobin (Hb)—10.9 mg/dL, mean corpuscular volume (MCV)—76 fL with a normal interval of 80–96 fL, and iron deficit at 28 mg/dL). The results of an abdominal ultrasound were normal, except for a few renal cortical microcysts in her left kidney. Upon receiving detailed information on her newly diagnosed genetic disease, the anxiety symptoms reoccurred and the patient refused to undergo further imaging, fearing what it may discover.

Over the last 6 years, the patient presented several aggravated episodes of epistaxis (2–5 times/year) requiring medical assistance, which were treated for chemical/surgical cautery and/or hemostatic sponges; chronic anemia; hypertension (systolic blood pressure increased up to 180 mmHg); and other cardiac-related symptoms like palpitations and dyspnea, urinary symptoms due to a urethral polyp, three severe episodes of depression requiring hospitalization (10 to 21 days' admittance), and recurrent headache associated with dizziness.

In February 2021, after another severe epistaxis that was treated at the emergency room by Merocel nasal packing, the patient was referred to our psychiatry clinic and agreed to a complex medical evaluation, which revealed the following:

1. Psychiatric evaluation:
   - Severe depression (scoring 22 when evaluated by Hamilton Depression Rating Scale (HAM-D) [13–15] and 23 by Geriatric Depression Scale (GDS) [16]);
   - Associated anxiety manifestations (evaluated by Hamilton Anxiety Rating Scale (HRSA)—score 27 [17,18];
   - Autolytic ideation, dysphoria, tendency to negative thinking with focus on self and the genetic disease, insomia, nosocomephobia, somatization;
   - Score of Global Assessment of Functioning Scale (GAFS) [19–21] of 40, corresponding to impairment in communication and reality testing, significant impact regarding family relations, thinking, and mood;
   - Amnestic Mild Cognitive Impairment (MCI) was determined using Mini Mental State Examination scale (MMSE [21–26])—score 23, Montreal Cognitive Assessment (MoCA) [21,24,27]—score 22.4, Clock Drawing Test [26,27], and Clinical Dementia Rating-Sum of Boxes (CDR-SOB) [22,23,27–30]—score 2.1.

2. Clinical check-up:
   - Moderate hypertension (154/85 mmHg) with a low patient adherence to recommended chronic therapy (candesartan 8 m twice daily, metoprolol 50 mg/day, and lacidipine 4 mg/day);
   - Blood tests: microcytic anemia (Hb 10.4 mg/dL, MCV 72 fL, iron deficit 29 μg/dL), hypercholesterolemia 338.9 mg/dL, with LDL cholesterol (low density lipoprotein) 263.77 mg/dL and HDL cholesterol (high density lipoprotein) 53.5 mg/dL, and normal hepatic and renal profile.
   - Epistaxis Severity Score (ESS) [31,32] of 4.13—moderate.
   - Severe generalized atherosclerosis, indicated by Doppler ultrasound of carotids, vertebral, and subclavian arteries showing 40–76% obstructions.

3. Dermatological exam: multiple mucocutaneous telangiectasias, especially on the hands, face, nostrils, and tongue (see Figures 1 and 2), with seborrheic keratosis on her thorax, and a nasal postoperative scar without any regional sign of recurrence from the previous basocellular carcinoma.

4. Urologic evaluation: microscopic hematuria due to urethral mucosal ectropion, overactive bladder syndrome, ultrasound showing few bilateral renal cortical microcysts, and minimal bladder post-void residue (see Figures 3 and 4).

5. Gastroenterology exam: normal function, lack of gastrointestinal bleeding, and no hepatic AVM identified.

6. Pneumology assessment: normal lung function and normal image in chest CT.

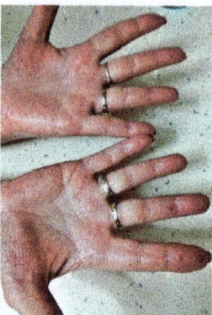

Figure 1. Multiple cutaneous telangiectasias on both hands—clinical presentation in February 2021.

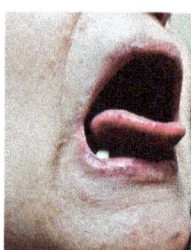

Figure 2. Mucosal telangiectasias at tongue and lips level—clinical presentation in February 2021.

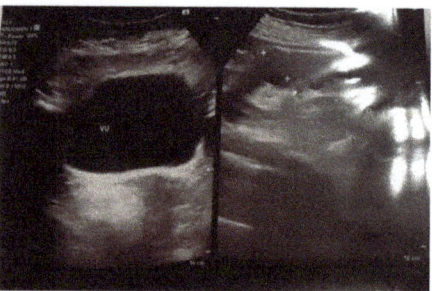

Figure 3. Ultrasound image of bladder, with minimal post-void residue—February 2021 (VU = urinary bladder).

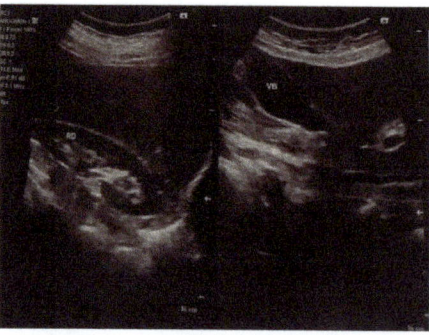

Figure 4. Ultrasound image of renal microcysts in the right kidney and normal image of biliary bladder—February 2021 (RD = right kidney; VB = gallbladder).

The patient became progressively anxious despite specific anxiolytic medication, refusing cerebral imaging and further assessment, so she was discharged after 6 days with a prescription and a recommended 6-month follow-up scheduled.

Because of COVID-19 pandemic restrictions and her own fear of hospital/medical care, the patient missed the routine check-ups, but more strictly followed the medical advice on therapy, especially as she observed an improvement in her mental state and sleep. Medication used for 13 months: tianeptine 12.5 mg three times daily, alprazolam 0.5 mg/day, zopiclone 7.5 mg/day, candesartan 8 m twice daily, bisoprolol 5 mg/day, lacidipine 4 mg/day, atorvastatin 20 mg/day, combination of rutoside 20 mg + ascorbic acid 50 mg three times/day plus supplementary vitamin C 1000 mg/day.

She presented in March 2022 with improved clinical and paraclinical parameters:

- Improved symptomatology and scoring for depression and anxiety (Hamilton Depression Rating Scale (HRSD) score 17, Geriatric Depression Scale (GDS) score 15, Hamilton Anxiety Rating Scale (HRSA) score 18, Global Assesment of Functioning Scale (GAFS) score 52);
- Lack of severe episodes of epistaxis (thus no emergency room visits);
- Epistaxis Severity Score (ESS) 2.14 (mild);
- no anemia and normal blood tests, except for persistent hypercholesterolemia [33] (total cholesterolemia 224 mg/dL, HDL cholesterol 164 mg/dL).

Again, the patient declined brain imaging, which is necessary in order to identify any possible cerebral AVMs, claiming that she would rather not know and fearing the certitude of a brain impairment. She admitted that the last 2 years during the COVID-19 pandemic added to her anxiety and distress of potential difficulties to receive emergency medical care if needed. As no AVMs were identified by the imaging, the patient could not be offered a therapy targeting the underlying pro-angiogenic pathophysiologic mechanism, as per current local protocols [34–39].

4. Discussion

Mental illness associated with hereditary hemorrhagic telangiectasia is not frequently reported in the literature, but patients often present with a significant impact on their health-related quality of life [1,6,7,40,41]. There are many possible reasons for a high prevalence of depression (88.7%), post-traumatic stress disorder (28.1%), and anxiety (43.9%) in individuals living with HHT [40–42].

One reason is related to the fear of death and frequent visits to the hospital emergency room, as well as the presence of recurrent bleeding. HHT is associated with a significant morbidity and mortality—some studies indicate a double versus normal mortality rate in patients aged <60 years [1,6,8,42,43]. There are reports of a bimodal distribution of mortality, age-related, with peaks at 50 years old and then from 60 to 80 years old. Generally, the mortality of HHT is generated by complications of AVMs, particularly in the brain, lungs, and gastrointestinal area. In our case, each bleeding episode and even the chronic anemia associated with recurrent hemorrhaging added to the anxiety and fear of hospital care [6,7,40–42].

Another problem with depressive symptomatology is the rarity of the disease and limited information available for patients, as well as the lack of curative or event-preventative therapies. Some HHT individuals have difficulties in social or working life, have troubles maintaining normal family relationships, and may become either obsessed with or otherwise reluctant to anything regarding their disease [6,40,43,44].

Patients with HHT may exhibit abnormal language development, learning difficulties, disinhibited behavior, or schizophrenia-like symptoms at younger ages [44,45], and later life reports include various psychiatric manifestations such as depressive or manic episodes, delusions, incoherence of speech, euphoric mood, inhibited behavior, poor social judgment, extreme anxiety, or impairment of different cognitive processes [45–47].

Neuropsychiatric symptomatology associated with HHT diagnosis could be a pathogenic feature resulting from the mechanism of the disease. Hypo-oxygenation of the neurons or microscopic cerebral embolism may occur from silent pulmonary arteriovenous malformations. The disturbed angiogenesis with the fragility of small vessels could generate brain dysfunction and different psychiatric manifestations depending on the location of these disturbances [3,5,9,45]. A recent report presents the positive outcomes of psychiatric pharmacotherapy combined with counseling and psychological interventions in a case of HHT with associated symptoms of depression and anxiety—the benefit of this patient-centered approach was evident [48].

For our patient, mental issues prevented a complete medical evaluation and caused a poor adherence to any recommended medical schedule. It is likely that some of the epistaxis episodes were related to poorly managed high blood pressure, in the context of her vessel frailty. A lack of evidence regarding brain AVMs is a problem in itself, excluding a possible surgical removal, not supporting anti-vascular endothelial growth factor (VEGF) therapy, and maintaining constant fear of a lethal hemorrhagic stroke [34–39].

Scientific evidence has connected chronic anemia to mental illnesses (such as depression, mood, or affectivity disorders), but also to a higher degree of impaired cognition as an age-related phenomenon [49–53] through various or concurrent mechanisms: cerebral hypoxia; iron deficiency with subsequent impaired myelin integrity; or deficient synthesis processes of some neurotransmitters—dopamine, serotonin, norepinephrine, or even genetic alterations found in hemoglobin deficiencies associated with certain mental disorders [51–53]. These correlations were not consistently reported by all prospective trials, but for HHT, such a connection between chronic anemia following frequent bleeding and neuropsychiatric manifestations cannot be ignored.

Some researchers indicated that the neurovascular manifestations show an age-related penetrance with an increased prevalence of cerebral manifestations over the lifespan [41,45]. A large number of patients suffering from HHT are able to identify one or more traumatic events related to their disease that caused psychological distress; therefore, the longer they live and the more bleeding episodes they experience, the more mentally affected they may be [47,54–59]. Our patient has a long history of hypertension and a poor therapy adherence; therefore, the causality connection between high blood pressure and anxiety, depression, or even an evolution towards dementia cannot be excluded [54,55].

Patients should receive updated information concerning their disease, and diagnostic as well as therapeutic options, so that they understand that access to a more efficient management of the disease would significantly improve their life expectancy and quality of life [60–62]. Patient support groups/patient associations are proven to be very effective in helping all rare disease patients, in general, to better cope with their illness; unfortunately, in our case, the patient did not agree to be referred to a rare disease organization and no specific HHT patient group was locally available. The current guidelines for the approach to HHT [10,63] and research evidence show a broadening spectrum of therapeutic solutions like well-known or repurposed drugs (including bevacizumab, propranolol, pazopanib, tacrolimus, and antithrombotic drugs) and new surgical techniques [64–69]. These would require more supporting evidence on efficacy and standardized algorithms for clinical use.

As for other chronic conditions, the COVID-19 pandemic has also impacted HHT patients and in particular the case presented here. Nevertheless, we noted the paucity of publications related to HHT care during the COVID-19 pandemic. A PubMed search using both "hereditary hemorrhagic telangiectasia/Rendu–Osler–Weber syndrome" and "COVID-19/coronavirus/SARS-CoV2" returned only 11 publications (search performed on 17 May 2022); a positive counterbalancing is constituted by the quality of these articles, including frameworks from The European Rare Disease Network for HHT, recommending approaches that augment the health and safety of HHT patients [63]. It was demonstrated that HHT individuals may develop paradoxical thromboembolic stroke from pulmonary AVMs, but also possess an inherent prothrombotic state because of disturbances in the regulation of coagulation at the endothelial surface [3,9]. They present higher levels of coagulation factor VIII (FVIII) than the general population, which correlates with thrombotic risk. Although subjects suffering from COVID-19 are at increased risk of thrombosis, and we have strong evidence that subjects with HHT often suffer from medical conditions that may negatively influence the clinical course of COVID-19 (like chronic anemia, heart failure, and pulmonary AVMs), recent data suggest that, actually, HHT patients may generally present milder forms of SARS-CoV2 infection [70–76]. Some preliminary data show a significant decrease in inflammatory cytokines detected in the HHT population—with differences lower than 50% for some cytokines like interleukines (ILs: IL-6, IL-1β, and IL12p40) and around 50% for Chemokine (C-C motif) ligand 20 (CCL20), Thrombospondin-1 (TSP-1), and Activin A [70–76]. If confirmed by larger studies, these HHT characteristics may explain some sort of protection against developing severe forms of COVID-19 [70–73]. Our patient does not recall presenting with specific COVID-19 symptoms, but she opted for SARS-CoV2 vaccination in complete schedule as soon as it became available (March 2021).

5. Conclusions

The presented case is highly relevant to illustrate the neuropsychiatric profile of Rendu–Osler–Weber syndrome and the significant impact that associated depression and anxiety may have on the management of the disease. These mental issues could prevent the patient from complete investigations and adherence to recommended therapeutic approaches—in our case, early signs of a ruptured cerebral AVM could possibly have been ignored, resulting in severe or lethal consequences.

Early identification and even active screening for neuropsychiatric manifestations in HHT could help patients better manage their symptoms and avoid developing PTSD after severe hemorrhagic episodes. Moreover, continuous education regarding their disease and recent advances in medicine could help them overcome depression and anxiety and allow them to adhere to medical recommendations and even therapy for associated comorbidities. An improved health-related quality of life would enable HHT patients to enjoy a fulfilled life and act more effectively when acute events occur.

Author Contributions: Conceptualization, F.S., V.D.O. and A.R.; methodology, V.D.O. and V.C.B.; validation, A.L.T., V.C.B. and A.R.; formal analysis, F.S. and E.P.D.; investigation, F.S.; resources, A.L.T. and A.R.; data curation, F.S. and E.P.D.; writing—original draft preparation, F.S. and V.D.O.; writing—review and editing, V.C.B. and A.R.; visualization, V.D.O.; supervision, A.L.T. and A.R.; project administration, F.S. All authors have read and agreed to the published version of the manuscript.

Funding: The article publishing charge was paid by the "Dunărea de Jos" University of Galati, Romania.

Institutional Review Board Statement: Approved by the Ethics Committee of the "Elisabeta Doamna" Psychiatric Hospital Galati, Romania.

Informed Consent Statement: Written informed consent was obtained from the patient to publish this paper.

Data Availability Statement: Data supporting the reported results can be obtained from the main authors upon reasonable request.

Acknowledgments: The authors wish to acknowledge that the present study was academically supported by the "Dunărea de Jos" University of Galati, Romania, through the research center Multidisciplinary Integrated Center of Dermatological Interface Research MIC-DIR (Centrul Integrat Multidisciplinar de Cercetare de Interfata Dermatologica—CIM-CID).

Conflicts of Interest: The authors declare no conflict of interest.

References

1. Kjeldsen, A.D.; Vase, P.; Green, A. Hereditary haemorrhagic telangiectasia: A population-based study of prevalence and mortality in Danish patients. *J. Intern. Med.* **1999**, *83*, 45–351. [CrossRef] [PubMed]
2. Govani, F.S.; Shovlin, C.L. Hereditary haemorrhagic telangiectasia: A clinical and scientific review. *Eur. J. Hum. Genet.* **2009**, *178*, 60–871. [CrossRef] [PubMed]
3. Dupuis-Girod, S.; Bailly, S.; Plauchu, H. Hereditary hemorrhagic telangiectasia: From molecular biology to patient care. *J. Thromb. Haemost.* **2010**, *81*, 447–1456. [CrossRef] [PubMed]

4. Saito, T.; Bokhove, M.; Croci, R.; Zamora-Caballero, S.; Han, L.; Letarte, M.; de Sanctis, D.; Jovine, L. Structural basis of the human Endoglin-BMP9 interaction: Insights into BMP signaling and HHT1. *Cell Rep.* **2017**, *191*, 917–1928. [CrossRef]
5. Gaetani, E.; Peppucci, E.; Agostini, F.; Di Martino, L.; Lucci Cordisco, E.; Sturiale, C.L.; Puca, A.; Porfidia, A.; Alexandre, A.; Pedicelli, A.; et al. Distribution of Cerebrovascular Phenotypes According to Variants of the ENG and ACVRL1 Genes in Subjects with Hereditary Hemorrhagic Telangiectasia. *J. Clin. Med.* **2022**, *11*, 2685. [CrossRef]
6. Higa, L.A.; McDonald, J.; Himes, D.O.; Rothwell, E. Life experiences of individuals with hereditary hemorrhagic telangiectasia and disclosing outside the family: A qualitative analysis. *J. Community Genet.* **2016**, *7*, 81–89. [CrossRef]
7. Floria, M.; Năfureanu, E.D.; Iov, D.-E.; Sîrbu, O.; Dranga, M.; Ouatu, A.; Tănase, D.M.; Bărboi, O.B.; Drug, V.L.; Cobzeanu, M.D. Hereditary Hemorrhagic Telangiectasia and Arterio-Venous Malformations—From Diagnosis to Therapeutic Challenges. *J. Clin. Med.* **2022**, *11*, 2634. [CrossRef]
8. Macri, A.; Wilson, A.M.; Shafaat, O.; Sharma, S. *Osler-Weber-Rendu Disease (Hereditary Hemorrhagic Telangiectasia, HHT)*; StatPearls Publishing: Treasure Island, FL, USA, 2020. Available online: https://www.ncbi.nlm.nih.gov/books/NBK482361/ (accessed on 17 May 2022).
9. Sharathkumar, A.A.; Shapiro, A. Hereditary haemorrhagic telangiectasia. *Haemophilia* **2008**, *14*, 1269–1280. [CrossRef]
10. Faughnan, M.E.; Palda, V.A.; Garcia-Tsao, G.; Geisthoff, U.W.; McDonald, J.; Proctor, D.D.; Spears, J.; Brown, D.H.; Buscarini, E.; Chesnutt, M.S.; et al. International guidelines for the diagnosis and management of hereditary haemorrhagic telangiectasia. *J. Med. Genet.* **2011**, *48*, 73–87. [CrossRef]
11. Jackson, S.B.; Villano, N.P.; Benhammou, J.N.; Lewis, M.; Pisegna, J.R.; Padua, D. Gastrointestinal Manifestations of Hereditary Hemorrhagic Telangiectasia (HHT): A Systematic Review of the Literature. *Dig. Dis. Sci.* **2017**, *62*, 2623–2630. [CrossRef]
12. World Health Organization (WHO). The ICD-10 Classification of Mental and Behavioural Disorders. 1993. Available online: https://www.who.int/standards/classifications/classification-of-diseases (accessed on 17 May 2022).
13. Carrozzino, D.; Patierno, C.; Fava, G.A.; Guidi, J. The Hamilton Rating Scales for Depression: A Critical Review of Clinimetric Properties of Different Versions. *Psychother. Psychosom.* **2020**, *891*, 33–150. [CrossRef] [PubMed]
14. Hamilton, M. Development of a rating scale for primary depressive illness. *Br. J. Soc. Clin. Psychol.* **1967**, *6*, 278–296. [CrossRef] [PubMed]
15. Bech, P.; Wilson, P.; Wessel, T.; Lunde, M.; Fava, M. A validation analysis of two self-reported HAM-D6 versions. *Acta Psychiatr. Scand.* **2009**, *119*, 298–303. [CrossRef] [PubMed]
16. Kørner, A.; Lauritzen, L.; Abelskov, K.; Gulmann, N.; Marie Brodersen, A.; Wedervang-Jensen, T.; Marie Kjeldgaard, K. The Geriatric Depression Scale and the Cornell Scale for Depression in Dementia. A validity study. *Nord. J. Psychiatry* **2006**, *60*, 360–364. [CrossRef] [PubMed]
17. Maier, W.; Buller, R.; Philipp, M.; Heuser, I. The Hamilton Anxiety Scale: Reliability, validity and sensitivity to change in anxiety and depressive disorders. *J. Affect. Disord.* **1988**, *14*, 61–68. [CrossRef]
18. Vaccarino, A.L.; Evans, K.R.; Sills, T.L.; Kalali, A.H. Symptoms of anxiety in depression: Assessment of item performance of the Hamilton Anxiety Rating Scale in patients with depression. *Depress. Anxiety* **2008**, *25*, 1006–1013. [CrossRef]
19. Aas, I.H. Global Assessment of Functioning (GAF): Properties and frontier of current knowledge. *Ann. Gen. Psychiatry* **2010**, *9*, 20. [CrossRef]
20. Aas, I.H. Guidelines for rating global assessment of functioning (GAF). *Ann. Gen. Psychiatry* **2011**, *10*, 2. [CrossRef]
21. Ismail, Z.; Rajji, T.K.; Shulman, K.I. Brief cognitive screening instruments: An update. *Int. J. Geriatr. Psychiatry* **2010**, *251*, 11–20. [CrossRef]
22. Petersen, R.C. Mild cognitive impairment. *N. Engl. J. Med.* **2011**, *3642*, 227–234. [CrossRef]
23. Kim, J.; Na, H.K.; Byun, J.; Shin, J.; Kim, S.; Lee, B.H.; Na, D.L. Tracking Cognitive Decline in Amnestic Mild Cognitive Impairment and Early-Stage Alzheimer Dementia: Mini-Mental State Examination versus Neuropsychological Battery. *Dement. Geriatr. Cogn. Disord.* **2017**, *44*, 105–117. [CrossRef] [PubMed]
24. Trzepacz, P.T.; Hochstetler, H.; Wang, S.; Walker, B.; Saykin, A.J. Alzheimer's Disease Neuroimaging Initiative: Relationship between the Montreal Cognitive Assessment and Mini-Mental State Examination for assessment of mild cognitive impairment in older adults. *BMC Geriatr.* **2015**, *15*, 107. [CrossRef] [PubMed]
25. Marioni, R.E.; Chatfield, M.; Brayne, C.; Matthews, F.E. Medical Research Council Cognitive Function and Ageing Study Group: The reliability of assigning individuals to cognitive states using the Mini Mental-State Examination: A population-based prospective cohort study. *BMC Med. Res. Methodol.* **2011**, *111*, 27. [CrossRef]
26. Palsetia, D.; Rao, G.P.; Tiwari, S.C.; Lodha, P.; de Sousa, A. The Clock Drawing Test versus Mini-mental Status Examination as a Screening Tool for Dementia: A Clinical Comparison. *Indian J. Psychol. Med.* **2018**, *40*, 1–10. [CrossRef]
27. Perneczky, R.; Wagenpfeil, S.; Komossa, K.; Grimmer, T.; Diehl, J.; Kurz, A. Mapping scores onto stages: Mini-Mental State Examination and Clinical Dementia Rating. *Am. J. Geriar. Psychiatry* **2006**, *14*, 139–144. [CrossRef] [PubMed]
28. Griffith, H.R.; Netson, K.L.; Harrell, L.E.; Zamrini, E.Y.; Brockington, J.C.; Marson, D.C. Amnestic mild cognitive impairment: Diagnostic outcomes and clinical prediction over a two-year time period. *J. Int. Neuropsychol. Soc.* **2006**, *12*, 166–175. [CrossRef]
29. O'Bryant, S.E.; Waring, S.C.; Cullum, C.M.; Hall, J.; Lacritz, L.; Massman, P.J.; Lupo, P.J.; Reisch, J.S.; Doody, R.; Texas Alzheimer's Research Consortium. Staging dementia using Clinical Dementia Rating Scale Sum of Boxes scores: A Texas Alzheimer's research consortium study. *Arch. Neurol.* **2008**, *65*, 1091–1095. [CrossRef]

30. Lynch, C.A.; Walsh, C.; Blanco, A.; Moran, M.; Coen, R.F.; Walsh, J.B.; Lawlor, B.A. The clinical dementia rating sum of box score in mild dementia. *Dement. Geriatr. Cogn. Disord.* **2006**, *21*, 40–43. [CrossRef]
31. Hoag, J.B.; Terry, P.; Mitchell, S.; Reh, D.; Merlo, C.A. An epistaxis severity score for hereditary hemorrhagic telangiectasia. *Laryngoscope* **2010**, *120*, 838–843. [CrossRef]
32. Peterson, A.M.; Kallogjeri, D.; Spitznagel, E.; Chakinala, M.M.; Schneider, J.S.; Piccirillo, J.F. Development and Validation of the Nasal Outcome Score for Epistaxis in Hereditary Hemorrhagic Telangiectasia (NOSE HHT). *JAMA Otolaryngol. Head Neck Surg.* **2020**, *146*, 999–1005. [CrossRef]
33. Nwabudike, L.C.; Elisei, A.M.; Buzia, O.D.; Miulescu, M.; Tatu, A.L. Statins. A review on structural perspectives, adverse reactions and relations with non-melanoma skin cancer. *Rev. Chim.* **2018**, *692*, 557–2562. [CrossRef]
34. Al-Samkari, H.; Kasthuri, R.S.; Parambil, J.G.; Albitar, H.A.; Almodallal, Y.A.; Vázquez, C.; Serra, M.M.; Dupuis-Girod, S.; Wilsen, C.B.; McWilliams, J.P.; et al. An international, multicenter study of intravenous bevacizumab for bleeding in hereditary hemorrhagic telangiectasia: The InHIBIT-Bleed study. *Haematologica* **2021**, *106*, 2161–2169. [CrossRef] [PubMed]
35. Epperla, N.; Hocking, W. Blessing for the bleeder: Bevacizumab in hereditary hemorrhagic telangiectasia. *Clin. Med. Res.* **2015**, *13*, 32–35. [CrossRef] [PubMed]
36. Iyer, V.N.; Apala, D.R.; Pannu, B.S.; Kotecha, A.; Brinjikji, W.; Leise, M.D.; Kamath, P.S.; Misra, S.; Begna, K.H.; Cartin-Ceba, R.; et al. Intravenous bevacizumab for refractory hereditary hemorrhagic telangiectasia–related epistaxis and gastrointestinal bleeding. *Mayo Clin. Proc.* **2018**, *93*, 155–166. [CrossRef] [PubMed]
37. Flieger, D.; Hainke, S.; Fischbach, W. Dramatic improvement in hereditary hemorrhagic telangiectasia after treatment with the vascular endothelial growth factor (VEGF) antagonist bevacizumab. *Ann. Hematol.* **2006**, *85*, 631–632. [CrossRef]
38. Kanellopoulou, T.; Alexopoulou, A. Bevacizumab in the treatment of hereditary hemorrhagic telangiectasia. *Expert Opin. Biol. Ther.* **2013**, *13*, 1315–1323. [CrossRef]
39. Guilhem, A.; Fargeton, A.E.; Simon, A.C.; Duffau, P.; Harle, J.R.; Lavigne, C.; Carette, M.F.; Bletry, O.; Kaminsky, P.; Leguy, V.; et al. Intra-venous bevacizumab in hereditary hemorrhagic telangiectasia (HHT): A retrospective study of 46 patients. *PLoS ONE* **2017**, *12*, e0188943. [CrossRef]
40. ORPHA774. Available online: https://www.orpha.net/consor/cgi-bin/index.php?lng=EN (accessed on 10 May 2022).
41. Krings, T.; Ozanne, A.; Chng, S.M.; Alvarez, H.; Rodesch, G.; Lasjaunias, P.L. Neurovascular phenotypes in hereditary haemorrhagic telangiectasia patients according to age: Review of 50 consecutive patients aged 1 day–60 years. *Neuroradiology* **2005**, *477*, 11–720. [CrossRef]
42. Chaturvedi, S.; Clancy, M.; Schaefer, N.; Oluwole, O.; McCrae, K.R. Depression and post-traumatic stress disorder in individuals with hereditary hemorrhagic telangiectasia: A cross-sectional survey. *Thromb. Res.* **2017**, *1531*, 4–18. [CrossRef]
43. Seebauer, C.T.; Freigang, V.; Schwan, F.E.; Fischer, R.; Bohr, C.; Kühnel, T.S.; Andorfer, K.E.C. Hereditary Hemorrhagic Telangiectasia: Success of the Osler Calendar for Documentation of Treatment and Course of Disease. *J. Clin. Med.* **2021**, *10*, 4720. [CrossRef]
44. Geisthoff, U.W.; Heckmann, K.; D'Amelio, R.; Grünewald, S.; Knöbber, D.; Falkai, P.; König, J. Health-related quality of life in hereditary hemorrhagic telangiectasia. *Otolaryngol. Head Neck Surg.* **2007**, *1367*, 26–733, discussion 725–734. [CrossRef]
45. Kuijpers, H.J.; van der Heijden FM, M.A.; Tuinier, S.; Verhoeven WM, A. Hereditary hemorrhagic telangiectasia and psychopathology. *J. Neuropsychiatry Clin. Neurosci.* **2007**, *19*, 199–200. [CrossRef]
46. Geirdal, A.Ø.; Dheyauldeen, S.; Bachmann-Harildstad, G.; Heimdal, K. Quality of life in patients with hereditary hemorrhagic telangiectasia in Norway: A population based study. *Am. J. Med. Genet. Part A* **2012**, *158*, 1269–1278. [CrossRef]
47. Pasculli, G.; Resta, F.; Guastamacchia, E.; Suppressa, P.; Sabbà, C. Health-related quality of life in a rare disease: Hereditary hemorrhagic telangiectasia (HHT) or Rendu-Osler-Weber disease. *Qual. Life Res.* **2004**, *131*, 715–1723. [CrossRef]
48. Marano, G.; Mazza, M.; Di Martino, L.; Agostini, F.; Cesare Passali, G.; Sani, G.; Pola, R.; Gaetani, E. Treatment of a Patient with a Diagnosis of HHT with a Combined Psychological and Physical Approach. *Psychiatr. Danub.* **2022**, *34*, 304–305. [CrossRef]
49. Shafi, M.; Taufiq, F.; Mehmood, H.; Afsar, S.; Badar, A. Relation between Depressive Disorder and Iron Deficiency Anemia among Adults Reporting to a Secondary Healthcare Facility: A Hospital-Based Case Control Study. *J. Coll. Physicians Surg. Pak.* **2018**, *28*, 456–559. [CrossRef] [PubMed]
50. Stewart, R.; Hirani, V. Relationship between depressive symptoms, anemia, and iron status in older residents from a national survey population. *Psychosom. Med.* **2012**, *74*, 208–213. [CrossRef]
51. Lee, H.S.; Chao, H.H.; Huang, W.T.; Chen, S.C.; Yang, H.Y. Psychiatric disorders risk in patients with iron deficiency anemia and association with iron supplementation medications: A nationwide database analysis. *BMC Psychiatry* **2020**, *20*, 216. [CrossRef]
52. Hidese, S.; Saito, K.; Asano, S.; Kunugi, H. Association between iron-deficiency anemia and depression: A web-based Japanese investigation. *Psychiatry Clin. Neurosci.* **2018**, *72*, 513–521. [CrossRef]
53. Altinoz, M.A.; Ince, B. Hemoglobins emerging roles in mental disorders. Metabolical, genetical and immunological aspects. *Int J. Dev. Neurosci.* **2017**, *617*, 3–85. [CrossRef]
54. Nemcsik-Bencze, Z.; Kőrösi, B.; Gyöngyösi, H.; Batta, D.; László, A.; Torzsa, P.; Kovács, I.; Rihmer, Z.; Gonda, X.; Nemcsik, J. Depression and anxiety in different hypertension phenotypes: A cross-sectional study. *Ann. Gen. Psychiatry* **2022**, *21*, 23. [CrossRef]
55. Shahimi, N.H.; Lim, R.; Mat, S.; Goh, C.H.; Tan, M.P.; Lim, E. Association between mental illness and blood pressure variability: A systematic review. *Biomed. Eng. Online* **2022**, *21*, 19. [CrossRef]

56. Merlo, C.A.; Yin, L.X.; Hoag, J.B.; Mitchell, S.E.; Reh, D.D. The effects of epistaxis on health-related quality of life in patients with hereditary hemorrhagic telangiectasia. *Int. Forum Allergy Rhinol.* **2014**, *49*, 21–925. [CrossRef]
57. Tedstone, J.E.; Tarrier, N. Posttraumatic stress disorder following medical illness and treatment. *Clin. Psychol. Rev.* **2003**, *234*, 409–448. [CrossRef]
58. Kronish, I.M.; Edmondson, D.; Goldfinger, J.Z.; Fei, K.; Horowitz, C.R. Posttraumatic stress disorder and adherence to medications in survivors of strokes and transient ischemic attacks. *Stroke* **2012**, *432*, 192–2197. [CrossRef] [PubMed]
59. Jones, C.; Griffiths, R.D.; Humphris, G.; Skirrow, P.M. Memory, delusions, and the development of acute posttraumatic stress disorder-related symptoms after intensive care. *Crit. Care Med.* **2001**, *295*, 73–580. [CrossRef]
60. Rapaport, M.H.; Clary, C.; Fayyad, R.; Endicott, J. Quality-of-life impairment in depressive and anxiety disorders. *Am. J. Psychiatry* **2005**, *1621*, 171–1178. [CrossRef] [PubMed]
61. Rae, C.; Furlong, W.; Horsman, J.; Pullenayegum, E.; Demers, C.; St-Louis, J.; Lillicrap, D.; Barr, R. Bleeding disorders, menorrhagia and iron deficiency: Impacts on health-related quality of life. *Haemoph. Off. J. World Fed. Hemoph.* **2013**, *193*, 85–391. [CrossRef] [PubMed]
62. Zarrabeitia, R.; Fariñas-Álvarez, C.; Santibáñez, M.; Señaris, B.; Fontalba, A.; Botella, L.M.; Parra, J.A. Quality of life in patients with hereditary haemorrhagic telangiectasia (HHT). *Health Qual. Life Outcomes* **2017**, *15*, 19. [CrossRef] [PubMed]
63. Shovlin, C.L.; Buscarini, E.; Sabbà, C.; Mager, H.J.; Kjeldsen, A.D.; Pagella, F.; Sure, U.; Ugolini, S.; Torring, P.M.; Suppressa, P.; et al. The European Rare Disease Network for HHT Frameworks for management of hereditary haemorrhagic telangiectasia in general and speciality care. *Eur. J. Med. Genet.* **2022**, *65*, 104370. [CrossRef]
64. Mei-Zahav, M.; Gendler, Y.; Bruckheimer, E.; Prais, D.; Birk, E.; Watad, M.; Goldschmidt, N.; Soudry, E. Topical Propranolol Improves Epistaxis Control in Hereditary Hemorrhagic Telangiectasia (HHT): A Randomized Double-Blind Placebo-Controlled Trial. *J. Clin. Med.* **2020**, *9*, 3130. [CrossRef]
65. Albiñana, V.; Cuesta, A.M.; de Rojas, P.I.; Gallardo-Vara, E.; Recio-Poveda, L.; Bernabéu, C.; Botella, L.M. Review of Pharmacological Strategies with Repurposed Drugs for Hereditary Hemorrhagic Telangiectasia Related Bleeding. *J. Clin. Med.* **2020**, *9*, 1766. [CrossRef]
66. Gaetani, E.; Agostini, F.; Giarretta, I.; Porfidia, A.; Di Martino, L.; Gasbarrini, A.; Pola, R.; on behalf of the Multidisciplinary Gemelli Hospital Group for HHT. Antithrombotic Therapy in Hereditary Hemorrhagic Telangiectasia: Real-World Data from the Gemelli Hospital HHT Registry. *J. Clin. Med.* **2020**, *9*, 1699. [CrossRef]
67. Mora-Luján, J.M.; Iriarte, A.; Alba, E.; Sánchez-Corral, M.Á.; Berrozpe, A.; Cerdà, P.; Cruellas, F.; Ribas, J.; Castellote, J.; Riera-Mestre, A. Gastrointestinal Bleeding in Patients with Hereditary Hemorrhagic Telangiectasia: Risk Factors and Endoscopic Findings. *J. Clin. Med.* **2020**, *9*, 82. [CrossRef]
68. Dupuis-Girod, S.; Fargeton, A.-E.; Grobost, V.; Rivière, S.; Beaudoin, M.; Decullier, E.; Bernard, L.; Bréant, V.; Colombet, B.; Philouze, P.; et al. Efficacy and Safety of a 0.1% Tacrolimus Nasal Ointment as a Treatment for Epistaxis in Hereditary Hemorrhagic Telangiectasia: A Double-Blind, Randomized, Placebo-Controlled, Multicenter Trial. *J. Clin. Med.* **2020**, *9*, 1262. [CrossRef]
69. Sadick, H.; Schäfer, E.; Weiss, C.; Rotter, N.; Müller, C.E.; Birk, R.; Sadick, M.; Häussler, D. An in vitro study on the effect of bevacizumab on endothelial cell proliferation and VEGF concentration level in patients with hereditary hemorrhagic telangiectasia. *Exp. Ther. Med.* **2022**, *24*, 555. [CrossRef]
70. Baroiu, L.; Lese, A.C.; Stefanopol, I.A.; Iancu, A.; Dumitru, C.; Ciubara, A.B.; Bujoreanu, F.C.; Baroiu, N.; Ciubara, A.; Nechifor, A.; et al. The Role of D-Dimers in the Initial Evaluation of COVID-19. *Ther. Clin. Risk Manag.* **2022**, *18*, 323–335. [CrossRef] [PubMed]
71. Tatu, A.L.; Nadasdy, T.; Bujoreanu, F.C. Familial clustering of COVID-19 skin manifestations. *Derm. Ther.* **2020**, *33*, e14181. [CrossRef]
72. Marcos, S.; Albiñana, V.; Recio-Poveda, L.; Tarazona, B.; Verde-González, M.P.; Ojeda-Fernández, L.; Botella, L.M. SARS-CoV-2 Infection in Hereditary Hemorrhagic Telangiectasia Patients Suggests Less Clinical Impact Than in the General Population. *J. Clin. Med.* **2021**, *10*, 1884. [CrossRef]
73. Niculet, E.; Chioncel, V.; Elisei, A.M.; Miulescu, M.; Buzia, O.D.; Nwabudike, L.C.; Craescu, M.; Draganescu, M.; Bujoreanu, F.; Marinescu, E.; et al. Multifactorial expression of IL-6 with update on COVID-19 and the therapeutic strategies of its blockade (Review). *Exp. Ther Med.* **2021**, *21*, 263. [CrossRef]
74. Marano, G.; Gaetani, E.; Gasbarrini, A.; Janiri, L.; Sani, G.; Mazza, M.; Multidisciplinary Gemelli Group for HHT. Mental health and counseling intervention for hereditary hemorrhagic telangiectasia (HHT) during the COVID-19 pandemic: Perspectives from Italy. *Eur. Rev. Med. Pharmacol. Sci.* **2020**, *24*, 10225–10227. [CrossRef] [PubMed]
75. Sârbu, F.; Oprea, V.D.; Tatu, A.L.; Drima, E.P.; Ștefănescu, C.; Nechita, A.; Onose, G.; Romila, A. COVID-19-related psychiatric manifestations requiring hospitalization: Analysis in older vs. younger patients. *Exp. Ther. Med.* **2022**, *24*, 497. [CrossRef]
76. Gaetani, E.; Cesare Passali, G.; Elena Riccioni, M.; Tortora, A.; Pola, R.; Costamagna, G.; Gasbarrini, A. Hereditary haemorrhagic telangiectasia: A disease not to be forgotten during the COVID-19 pandemic. *J. Thromb. Haemost.* **2020**, *18*, 1799–1801. [CrossRef] [PubMed]

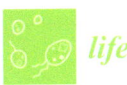

Article

Pharyngeal-Esophageal Malignancies with Dermatologic Paraneoplastic Syndrome

Ana Fulga [1,2,†], Doriana Cristea Ene [2,†], Laura Bujoreanu Bezman [1,2], Oana Maria Dragostin [1,2], Iuliu Fulga [1,2,*], Elena Stamate [1,3,†], Alin Ionut Piraianu [1,2,*], Florin Bujoreanu [1,4,†] and Alin Laurentiu Tatu [1,4]

1. Faculty of Medicine and Pharmacy, Dunarea de Jos University of Galati, 35 AI Cuza st, 800010 Galati, Romania
2. Saint Apostle Andrew Emergency County Clinical Hospital, 177 Brailei st, 800578 Galati, Romania
3. Cardiology Department, University Emergency Hospital Bucharest, 169 Independence Square st, 050098 Bucharest, Romania
4. Saint Parascheva Clinical Hospital of Infectious Diseases, 393 Traian st, 800179 Galati, Romania
* Correspondence: iuliu.fulga@ugal.ro (I.F.); alin.piraianu@ugal.ro (A.I.P.)
† These authors contributed equally to this work.

Abstract: Systemic changes often send signals to the skin, and certain neoplastic diseases of the internal organs can also trigger skin manifestations. In this article, the authors make clinical photography presentations of the patients seen at our clinic with dermatologic paraneoplastic syndromes within pharyngeal–esophageal malignancies, describe several paraneoplastic dermatoses, and also review high-quality scientific literature in order to be able to highlight the dermatological signs of pharyngoesophageal malignant tumors. The majority of our patients with paraneoplastic dermatoses, filtering for pharyngoesophageal malignancies, had esophageal neoplasms, out of whom seven were female and two were male, making esophageal cancer more common within the paraneoplastic dermatoses within pharyngoesophageal malignancies. An early recognition of paraneoplastic dermatoses can diagnose neoplasms and sequentially contribute to a better prognosis for the patient. This matter is also useful for front-line medical personnel in order to improve early diagnosis of the underlying malignancy, curative interventions with prompt therapy administration and good prognosis.

Keywords: paraneoplastic syndrome; skin manifestations; neoplasm; pharynx; esophagus

Citation: Fulga, A.; Cristea Ene, D.; Bezman, L.B.; Dragostin, O.M.; Fulga, I.; Stamate, E.; Piraianu, A.I.; Bujoreanu, F.; Tatu, A.L. Pharyngeal-Esophageal Malignancies with Dermatologic Paraneoplastic Syndrome. *Life* **2022**, *12*, 1705. https://doi.org/10.3390/life12111705

Academic Editor: Teresa Macarulla

Received: 19 September 2022
Accepted: 21 October 2022
Published: 26 October 2022

Publisher's Note: MDPI stays neutral with regard to jurisdictional claims in published maps and institutional affiliations.

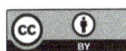

Copyright: © 2022 by the authors. Licensee MDPI, Basel, Switzerland. This article is an open access article distributed under the terms and conditions of the Creative Commons Attribution (CC BY) license (https://creativecommons.org/licenses/by/4.0/).

1. Introduction

Paraneoplastic diseases are disorders of hematological, endocrine, or nervous system as well as clinical and biochemical imbalances that are related to the existence of malignant tumors but are not directly linked to the tumor invasion or the metastasis of the original tumor [1]. The skin may also provide a clinician with signs that are suggestive of systemic diseases, thus contributing to the diagnosis of many diseases, including malignant tumors [2,3].

Globally, esophageal cancer is one of the leading causes of cancer mortality, being responsible, together with other gastrointestinal cancers, for about 1/3 of all disability adjusted life-years (DALYs) from cancer [4,5]. In the last almost 20 years, the incidence of this pathology has increased for the new cases by 52.3%, from 310,000 to 473,000, the number of deaths increased by 40%, from 311,000 to 436,000, and the total DALYs increased by 27.4%, from 7,680,000 to 9,780,000 [6]. If we refer to esophageal adenoma, in the last 30 years, its incidence has increased faster than of any other solid tumor in the Western world, with an increase of 500% [7], and the five-year survival rates remain unacceptably low, at only 10%, reflecting late addressability for esophageal tumors [8].

The low survival rate of patients with esophageal carcinoma and the disabling nature of the specific paraneoplastic syndrome obliges the scientific community to a prompt systemic response to combat the phenomenon, which requires major efforts regarding early identification and reduction of risk factors, focusing on the problem through the appropriate allocation of material and human resources, as well as the development of effective methods of prediction and prophylaxis by monitoring the categories of patients with predisposing factors [9].

In this article, the authors present clinical photographs of patients with dermatologic paraneoplastic syndromes within pharyngeal–esophageal malignancies, describe several of these paraneoplastic dermatoses, and review high-quality scientific literature to be able to highlight the dermatological signs of pharyngoesophageal malignant tumors useful for front-line medical personnel in order to improve the early diagnosis of the underlying malignancy, curative interventions with prompt therapy administration and good prognosis.

2. Methods

A literature search was conducted for articles published in the English language in the ScienceDirect, SpringerLink and PubMed electronic database. The keywords used for our research purposes were "paraneoplastic syndrome", "skin manifestations", "neoplasm", "pharynx". Furthermore, we analyzed clinical photographs of nine patients with paraneoplastic dermatoses and pharyngeal–esophageal malignancies over a period of 10 years dating 2012–2022 from the Saint Parascheva Clinical Hospital of Infectious Diseases and the Saint Apostle Andrew Emergency County Clinical Hospital from Galati, Romania, with the patient consent forms containing patient details and/or images signed by all the patients.

3. Relevant Literature

The original articles written in English were found in Web of Science, Science Direct, and Springer Link using the following keywords: paraneoplastic, skin manifestations, neoplasm, pharynx, esophagus. In the database, 13 papers regarding skin manifestations in pharyngoesophageal neoplasms were identified [2,3,10–22], which are all shown in Table 1.

Table 1. Skin manifestations in pharyngoesophageal malignancies.

Author	Dermatological Manifestation	Neoplastic Topography
Thiers et al., 2009 [10] Lee, 2009 [15] Dourmishev and Draganov, 2009 [11] Bologna et al., 1991 [14] Bazex et al., 1965 [23] Ljubenovic et al., 2009 [24]	Bazex paraneoplastic acrokeratosis/ Bazex syndrome	Upper aerodigestive tract/ pharynx/esophagus
Pipkin et al., 2008 [3] Ehst et al., 2010 [12] Edgin et al., 2008 [16] Boyce and Harper, 2002 [17] Dourmishev and Draganov, 2009 [11] Kartan et al., 2017 [25] Helm et al., 1993 [26] Kimyai-Asadi et al., 2001 [27] Choi et al., 2012 [28]	Paraneoplastic pemphigus	Hypopharynx/esophagus
Ramos-E-Silva et al., 2011 [2] Pipkin et al., 2008 [3] Dourmishev and Draganov, 2009 [11] De La Torre et al., 2011 [29] Serrao et al., 2008 [30]	Erythema gyratum repens	Esophagus
Pipkin et al., 2008 [3] Dourmishev and Draganov, 2009 [11]	Pityriasis rotunda	Esophagus

Table 1. *Cont.*

Author	Dermatological Manifestation	Neoplastic Topography
Thiers et al., 2009 [10] Ehst et al., 2010 [12] McLean, 1987 [13] Dourmishev and Draganov, 2009 [11]	Palmoplantar keratoderma	Esophagus
Leow and Goh, 1997 [18] Wakata et al., 2002 [19] Joly et al., 2000 [20] Anhalt, 2004 [21] Dourmishev and Draganov, 2009 [11]	Paraneoplastic dermatomyositis	Pharynx
Tutakne et al., 1983 [22] Leser et al., 1901 [31] Swartz et al., 1991 [32] Yeh et al., 2000 [33] Kameya et al., 1988 [34] Cohn et al., 1993 [35] Hodak et al., 1987 [36] Liddell et al., 1975 [37] Heng et al., 1988 [38] Brauer et al., 1992 [39] Ginarte et al., 2001 [40] Klimopoulus et al., 2001 [41] Ohashio et al., 1997 [42] Kocygit et al., 2007 [43] Tajima et al., 1991 [44]	Leser–Trelat sign	Esophagus

4. Discussion

The pharyngoesophageal junction, also called "the mouth of the esophagus" [45], represents the passage from the hypopharynx to the cervical esophagus (C5–C6 vertebral interspace, inferior cricoid cartilage border) and is a high intraluminal pressure area that serves as a barrier between the pharynx and the cervical esophagus. Three responses are implied by this definition: tone generation, phasic response activity, and sphincter opening. During swallowing, the pharyngoesophageal junction relaxes and opens, allowing foods and liquids to pass into the esophagus while acting as a barrier to retrograde flow. By doing so, it performs an important protective function, preventing aspiration of acidic gastric content into the respiratory tract on the one hand, and on the other—entry of air into the esophagus. The pharyngoesophageal junction also allows retrograde flow of material during belching and vomiting due to physiologic relaxation.

Not only anatomy but the treatment and prognosis of these tumors are intermediate between hypopharyngeal and esophageal tumors [45]. The diagnosis of this type of neoplasms varies depending on the circumstances of emergence and the neoplastic growth in this region. Pharyngeal–esophageal tumor symptoms are primarily characterized by selective dysphagia, for solid food at the beginning and total dysphagia afterwards, depending on the tumor evolution, but leading in the end to the alteration of the nutritional status [45]. This is often a sign of an advanced stage of this disease, but other symptoms are also present, such as weight loss, retrosternal pain, nausea, vomiting, dyspepsia, and anemia. Patients with pharyngoesophageal neoplasms often complain about paresthesia in the pharyngeal region, fetid halitosis, eructation, regurgitations, and foreign body sensation [45]. Metastases often develop in the liver, brain, lungs, and bones. According to HRQOL (health-related quality of life) questionnaires [46], the specific esophageal symptomatology persists or even deteriorates, leading to a poor quality of life in esophageal carcinoma survivors compared to the general population.

Squamous cell carcinomas in the hypopharynx (HP) and the cervical esophagus are two distinct diseases with different staging systems and treatment approaches. A pharyngoesophageal junction tumor involves both the hypopharynx and the cervical esophagus at the same time, but there have been few reports focused on pharyngoesophageal junction tumors. Although the hypopharynx and the cervical esophagus are anatomically adjacent, squamous cell carcinomas of the hypopharynx (HP) and cervical esophagus are distinct diseases with different staging systems and ways of treatment.

Cervical esophageal cancer is a very rare disease and is often locally advanced at the time of diagnosis, making local lesions difficult to control and survival rates low. The aggression of cervical esophageal carcinoma is high as it tends to grow in an abundant lymphatic drainage area and fails to produce early symptoms; it also easily and frequently extends towards the hypopharynx; these tumors are sometimes treated with schedules for locally advanced head and neck squamous cell carcinoma (LAHNSCC) which consist of 70 Gy in 35 fractions and 100 mg/m^2 cisplatin on days 1, 22, and 43 of radiotherapy (RT) (The National Comprehensive Cancer Network guidelines for head and neck cancers); dCRT is related to life-threatening adverse events in 5–10% of patients; thus, further research is needed to define the optimal treatment schedule with adequate survival and acceptable toxicity [47].

Local failure of a neoplasm is a significant predictor of survival of cancer patients. Uno et al. [48] found that after definitive chemoradiotherapy (dCRT), none of the patients with initial local failure as determined by endoscopic examination survived more than 20 months compared with 2–5-year survival rates of 60% and 40%, respectively, in patients with initial local control. Local recurrences can be treated with saving surgery, which has a high morbidity rate, but it is the only option for relatively long-term survival. If not, palliative care options must be considered. Because of delayed diagnosis, poor performance of the majority of patients, and the high malignancy potential associated with particular anatomic characteristics, local and distant metastases occur frequently, with a 12–30% increased synchronous or metachronous risk, the survival rates for these kinds of patients being very poor. Cervical esophageal carcinoma is a very rare disease and often locally advanced at the time of diagnosis, resulting in limited locoregional disease control and poor survival. Finally, we need to recognize that optimal clinical support is needed to maintain dietary intake and exercise to optimize patient outcomes and quality of life. Cervical esophageal cancer is uncharted territory for many practitioners. Treatment of cancer in this region is often challenging due to its location in the cervical region, and most tumors are locally advanced cancers that have invaded the surrounding vital structures. To improve the survival outcomes and decrease the morbidity and mortality rates, future research should focus on the early detection of these cancers and improve treatment design by investigating innovative radiation schedules and identifying the optimal backbone for systemic therapy.

Clinical nutrition is required in the case of such patients as their nutritional status is assessed upon admission using body mass index protocols. Clinical nutrition must be maintained throughout the hospitalization while clinical parameters for each patient are evaluated (required caloric intake, biochemistry). If the digestive tract is functional, enteral nutrition via nasogastric tube, jejunal or gastric stoma with standardized nutritional supplements should be started as soon as possible [45]. The best medical approach to this disease is determined by a variety of factors, including general status, systemic and local implications, type of neoplasm, medical resources, and the acceptance of illness by the patient and their approval for medical attention [49,50]. One of the most important modern concerns in the management of this type of neoplasms is multimodal therapy that includes different medical and surgical specialties, also including, and very importantly, a psychologist.

Hebra was the first to recognize that skin pigmentation can indicate presence of visceral cancer in 1868 [51]. Since then, more than 50 dermatologic conditions have been identified as potential cancer markers [52]. Malignant diseases may involve the skin directly or indirectly. Direct involvement denotes the presence of tumor cells in the skin as a result of direct tumor extension or metastasis. In turn, indirect involvement is caused by a variety of factors, such as inflammatory, proliferative, or metabolic factors related to the neoplasm, such as polypeptides, hormones, cytokines, antibodies, or growth factors that act as mediators and interfere with cell communication and, thus, activity. There are no neoplastic cells in the skin in this case, so this involvement is classified as a dermatologic paraneoplastic syndrome [10,53].

At first glance, paraneoplastic skin manifestations may appear benign, and it is not always easy to establish a link between a dermatologic finding and an internal malignancy, let alone define the frequency of this association in the general population [52,53].

4.1. Bazex Paraneoplastic Acrokeratosis or Bazex Syndrome—Pharynx, Esophagus

In 1965, Bazex et al. [23] described the first patient with this condition as follows: "paraneoplastic syndrome with hyperkeratosis of the extremities", because mainly it affects the nose, ears, hands, elbows, knees, and feet.

About 80% of cases are associated with upper aerodigestive tract tumors, such as of oral cavity, larynx, pharynx, trachea, esophagus, and lungs, and squamous cell carcinoma metastasis to cervical lymph nodes appears to be widespread in Bazex syndrome patients. In a retrospective study, the oropharynx and the larynx were involved in 48.6% of the cancers, followed by the lungs (17%) and the esophagus (10.6%) [10,15,54].

It appears as symmetrical erythematous–violaceous scaly patches on the dorsum of the helix, nose, and distal ends of the extremities, with a psoriasiform aspect [54]. Desquamations occur in the dorsal and palmoplantar regions as the disease progresses, and nails are affected by subungual hyperkeratosis, dystrophy, and onycholysis (Figures Figures 1–3). Other areas, such as the scalp, arms, knees, and legs, may be affected over time, with lesions spreading centripetally [24].

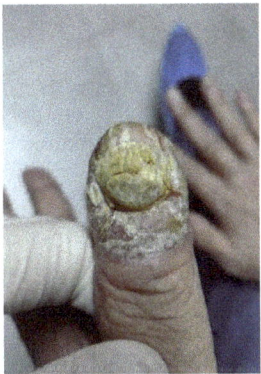

Figure 1. Bazex syndrome lesions.

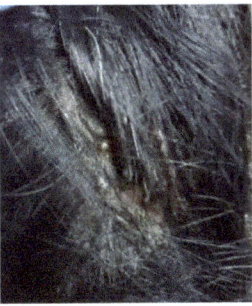

Figure 2. Bazex syndrome lesions.

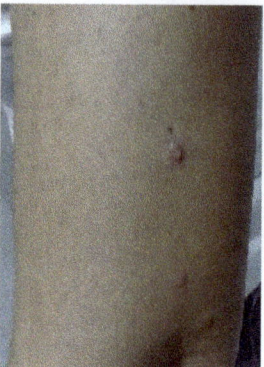

Figure 3. Bazex syndrome lesions.

Bologna et al. [14] reported the following findings in a retrospective study of the primary location of malignancies in 113 patients with Bazex syndrome: oropharynx and larynx, esophagus, lung, including one with an associated pyriform sinus carcinoma, and isolated cases of prostate, liver, stomach, vulva, bone marrow, and uterus.

4.2. Paraneoplastic Pemphigus—Hypopharynx, Esophagus

Paraneoplastic pemphigus is considered a rare autoimmune disorder usually associated with confirmed or occult malignancy [55]. Patients typically present with extensive and painful mucosal and cutaneous involvement, usually having an overall poor prognosis [25,26]. Patients present with a variety of lesions with different morphologies, ranging from flaccid vesicles to extensive eruptions, some of which may be intensely itchy [25,27] (Figure 4,Figure 5,Figure 6). Paraneoplastic pemphigus always shows early mucosal involvement in the form of vesicles or bullae leading to painful mucocutaneous erosions and severe stomatitis, which may morphologically resemble pemphigus vulgaris [25,28].

Histologically, paraneoplastic pemphigus can resemble lichenoid eruptions (such as lichen planus, erythema multiforme drug eruptions), and other immunobullous diseases (pemphigus vulgaris, linear IgA bullous dermatosis, pemphigus foliaceous, IgA pemphigus, herpetiform pemphigus, drug-induced pemphigus). Correlation with clinical findings and immunofluorescence is invaluable in arriving at the correct diagnosis because etiopathogenetic differentiation can lead to a favorable prognosis [29].

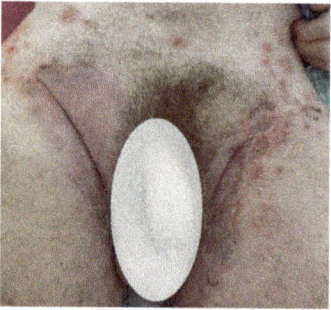

Figure 4. Pemphigus vegetans.

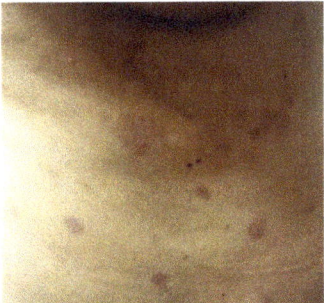

Figure 5. Pemphigus vulgaris.

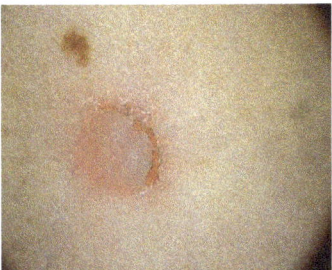

Figure 6. Pemphigus vulgaris—incipient phase.

Oral involvement with painful stomatitis is seen in almost all cases and can often be the first symptom, generally the least responsive to treatment. Oral lesions can be severe and diffuse, affecting the hypopharynx and the esophagus; they may also involve the conjunctival and anorectal mucosa. Skin manifestations range from erythema multiforme-like papules and plaques to pemphigus vulgaris-like vesicles and blisters and even lichen planus-like pruritic plaques [16]. In contrast to pemphigus vulgaris, acral and paronychial involvement is possible. Some patients develop respiratory complications such as bronchiolitis obliterans, which can lead to respiratory failure. Sepsis, hemorrhage, and respiratory failure are all associated with a high mortality rate in patients with paraneoplastic pemphigus [54].

4.3. Erythema Gyratum Repens—Esophagus

Erythema gyratum repens (EGR) is a paraneoplastic rash associated with a variety of malignancies and is considered one of the most prominent skin manifestations of solid tumors. EGR has a characteristic appearance consisting of undulating erythematous concentric bands that may be figural, circular, or annular [56,57].

Malignant neoplasms are found in 82% of patients with erythema gyratum repens [55,58,59]. Lung cancer is the most common (32%), followed by esophageal cancer (8%) and breast cancer (6%). Other malignancies such as colon, gastric, bladder, prostate, uterine, rectal, and pancreatic cancers, as well as multiple myeloma, have also been associated with erythema gyratum repens [30]. Approximately 80% of patients are diagnosed with erythema gyratum repens prior to the neoplasm, four to nine months prior to the diagnosis on average. Rarely, non-neoplastic diseases such as tuberculosis, pregnancy, calcinosis, esophageal dysmotility, sclerodactyly, Sjögren syndrome, and CREST syndrome may be associated with erythema gyratum repens [54,58].

4.4. Pityriasis Rotunda—Esophagus

The associated neoplasms include hepatocellular, gastric, and esophageal carcinoma, prostate cancer, chronic lymphocytic leukemia, and multiple myeloma [3]. Pityriasis commonly refers to flaking (or scaling) of the skin [55,59]. Although the conditions beginning with the name pityriasis have a different etiology, they do represent important dermatologic diseases, such as pityriasis versicolor or pityriasis folliculorum [59].

This disease is distinguished by multiple macules, which are circular, with hypo- or hyperpigmentation, usually found on the torso.

4.5. Palmoplantar Keratoderma—Esophagus

It is a disease characterized by changes in keratinization that may be inherited or acquired (Figure 7,Figure 8). Several associations with malignancy have been described [55]. The prototype of the inherited disease is Howel–Evans syndrome, in which the risk of developing oral or esophageal carcinoma in increased 36-fold [55]. Skin lesions usually begin in childhood, although neoplastic involvement occurs at an average age of 61 years [10]. The pathogenesis of the syndrome has been linked to chromosome 17q24, a site where keratin is formed [12].

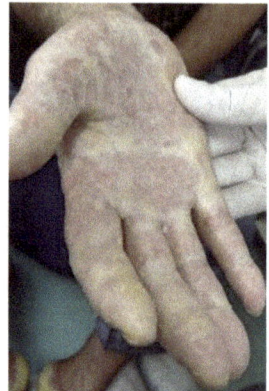

Figure 7. Palmar keratoderma.

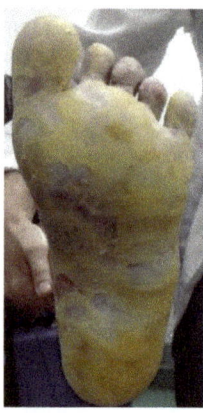

Figure 8. Plantar keratoderma.

4.6. Paraneoplastic Dermatomyositis–Pharynx

Dermatomyositis is a rare idiopathic inflammatory myopathy that presents clinically with proximal muscle weakness and characteristic cutaneous manifestations [22].

Skin lesions can be classified as pathognomonic, characteristic, and compatible with dermatomyositis [31], but periorbital heliotropic rash and erythematous maculopapular lesions covering bony prominences are the more specific or pathognomonic manifestations of dermatomyositis [31,32]. The heliotropic rash appears as a red-to-purplish confluent macular erythema that affects the eyelids, upper cheeks, forehead, and temples symmetrically and is frequently associated with eyelid and periorbital tissue edemas [56].

In Southeast Asia, the incidence of nasopharyngeal carcinoma in men with or without dermatomyositis is increasing [18]. Another retrospective study described 12 patients with internal malignancy among 64 patients with polymyositis and 28 patients with dermatomyositis. Four of these 12 patients had malignancies of the gastrointestinal tract (two 74- and 75-year-old male patients had gastric carcinoma, another 51-year-old female had pharyngeal carcinoma, and one female had pancreatic carcinoma) [19]. Erosions of the oral cavity, pharynx, conjunctiva, gastrointestinal mucosa, and even anogenital area are examples of mucosal involvement [20,21].

4.7. Leser–Trelat Syndrome (LTS)—Esophagus

Ulysse Trelat (1884) and Edmund Leser (1901) [33] were the first surgeons to propose a link between internal malignancies and multiple seborrheic keratoses. There is no evidence of dermatitis or erythroderma prior to the appearance of seborrheic keratoses on the skin, and pruritus is a leading symptom in approximately half of the cases [34].

This syndrome is a relatively rare clinical condition found to be associated with internal malignancies and characterized by the sudden and eruptive appearance of multiple seborrheic keratoses in association with underlying malignant disease [56] (Figure 9).

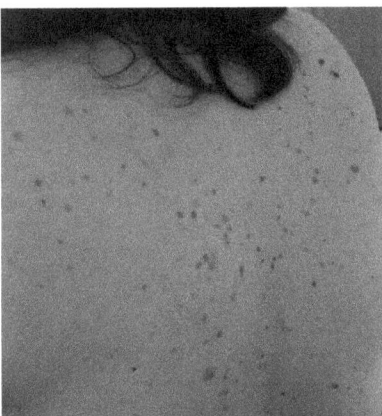

Figure 9. Leser–Trelat syndrome.

Most patients with LTS have adenocarcinomas, most commonly of the stomach [35,55], colon, or rectum [36–42] or, less commonly, carcinomas of the esophagus [22], duodenum [43], pancreas [44], gallbladder [4], or hepatocellular carcinoma [60–62].

Finally, 80% of the patients with paraneoplastic dermatoses found at our clinic, filtering for the pharyngoesophageal malignancies, were the ones with esophageal neoplasms, out of which seven were female and two were male, making esophageal cancer more common within paraneoplastic dermatoses within pharyngoesophageal malignancies.

5. Conclusions

Numerous systemic diseases can be diagnosed through the skin, including changes suggestive of internal malignancies. Cutaneous paraneoplastic syndromes are important clinical markers that may precede, co-occur with, or follow the diagnosis of a specific neoplasm. Plenty of dermatoses have been correlated with underlying neoplastic processes, many of which correlate with specific neoplasms, thus providing an important diagnostic aid. Skin manifestations suggestive of a malignancy are extremely useful in making a definitive early diagnosis. The knowledge of paraneoplastic syndromes is essential for first-line clinicians to improve the prognosis and the quality of life of patients. The data presented may contribute to the development of continuing postgraduate education programs for physicians of various specialties.

Author Contributions: Conceptualization, A.F. and I.F.; methodology, F.B.; software, E.S.; validation, L.B.B., O.M.D. and E.S.; formal analysis, A.I.P.; investigation, F.B.; resources, A.L.T.; data curation, A.I.P.; writing—original draft preparation, A.F.; writing—review and editing, A.F.; visualization, I.F.; supervision, A.L.T.; project administration, D.C.E.; funding acquisition, I.F. All authors have read and agreed to the published version of the manuscript.

Funding: This research was funded by the "Dunărea de Jos" University of Galati, VAT 27232142, and The APC was paid by the "Dunărea de Jos" University of Galati, VAT 27232142.

Institutional Review Board Statement: The study was conducted in accordance with the Declaration of Helsinki and approved by the Ethics Committee of the "Dunărea de Jos" University of Galati (477/CEU/01.09.2022).

Informed Consent Statement: Informed consent was obtained from all the subjects involved in the study. Written informed consent was obtained from the patients to publish this paper.

Data Availability Statement: Not applicable.

Conflicts of Interest: The authors declare no conflict of interest.

References

1. Saeed, A.; Hameem, Z.; Modi, D.; Park, R.; Saeed, A. Cutaneous Paraneoplastic Syndrome Associated with Anal Squamous Cel Carcinoma: A Rare Presentation of an Uncommon Cancer. *Curr. Oncol.* **2020**, *27*, 433–435. [CrossRef] [PubMed]
2. Ramos-e-Silva, M.; Carvalho, J.C.; Carneiro, S.C. Cutaneous Paraneoplasia. *Clin. Dermatol.* **2011**, *29*, 541–547. [CrossRef] [PubMed]
3. Pipkin, C.A.; Lio, P.A. Cutaneous Manifestations of Internal Malignancies: An Overview. *Dermatol. Clin.* **2008**, *26*, 1–15, vii. [CrossRef] [PubMed]
4. Kocygit, P.; Akay, B.N.; Anadolu, A.E.; Erdem, R.Y. Post-Renal Transplantation Leser-Trelat Sign Associated with Carcinoma of the Gallbladder: A Rare Association. *Scand. J. Gastroenterol.* **2007**, *42*, 779–781. [CrossRef] [PubMed]
5. Global Burden of Disease Cancer Collaboration; Fitzmaurice, C.; Allen, C.; Barber, R.M.; Barregard, L.; Bhutta, Z.A.; Brenner, H.; Dicker, D.J.; Chimed-Orchir, O.; Dandona, R.; et al. Global, Regional, and National Cancer Incidence, Mortality, Years of Life Lost, Years Lived with Disability, and Disability-Adjusted Life-Years for 32 Cancer Groups, 1990 to 2015: A Systematic Analysis for the Global Burden of Disease Study. *JAMA Oncol.* **2017**, *3*, 524–548. [CrossRef]
6. Bray, F.; Ferlay, J.; Soerjomataram, I.; Siegel, R.L.; Torre, L.A.; Jemal, A. Global Cancer Statistics 2018: GLOBOCAN Estimates of Incidence and Mortality Worldwide for 36 Cancers in 185 Countries. *CA Cancer J. Clin.* **2018**, *68*, 394–424. [CrossRef]
7. Global Burden of Disease Cancer Collaboration; Fitzmaurice, C.; Abate, D.; Abbasi, N.; Abbastabar, H.; Abd-Allah, F.; Abdel-Rahman, O.; Abdelalim, A.; Abdoli, A.; Abdollahpour, I.; et al. Global, Regional, and National Cancer Incidence, Mortality, Years of Life Lost, Years Lived with Disability, and Disability-Adjusted Life-Years for 29 Cancer Groups, 1990 to 2017: A Systematic Analysis for the Global Burden of Disease Study: A Systematic Analysis for the Global Burden of Disease Study. *JAMA Oncol.* **2019**, *5*, 1749–1768. [CrossRef]
8. Kamangar, F.; Nasrollahzadeh, D.; Safiri, S.; Sepanlou, S.G.; Fitzmaurice, C.; Ikuta, K.S.; Bisignano, C.; Islami, F.; Roshandel, G.; Lim, S.S.; et al. The Global, Regional, and National Burden of Oesophageal Cancer and Its Attributable Risk Factors in 195 Countries and Territories, 1990–2017: A Systematic Analysis for the Global Burden of Disease Study 2017. *Lancet Gastroenterol. Hepatol.* **2020**, *5*, 582–597. [CrossRef]
9. Lazăr, D.C.; Avram, M.F.; Faur, A.C.; Goldiș, A.; Romoșan, I.; Tăban, S.; Cornianu, M. The Impact of Artificial Intelligence in the Endoscopic Assessment of Premalignant and Malignant Esophageal Lesions: Present and Future. *Medicina* **2020**, *56*, 364. [CrossRef]
10. Thiers, B.H.; Sahn, R.E.; Callen, J.P. Cutaneous Manifestations of Internal Malignancy. *CA Cancer J. Clin.* **2009**, *59*, 73–98. [CrossRef]
11. Dourmishev, L.A.; Draganov, P.V. Paraneoplastic Dermatological Manifestation of Gastrointestinal Malignancies. *World J. Gastroenterol.* **2009**, *15*, 4372–4379. [CrossRef] [PubMed]
12. Ehst, B.D.; Minzer-Conzetti, K.; Swerdlin, A.; Devere, T.S. Cutaneous Manifestations of Internal Malignancy. *Curr. Probl. Surg.* **2010**, *47*, 384–445. [CrossRef] [PubMed]
13. McLean, D.I. Cutaneous Manifestations of Internal Malignant Disease. *Can. Fam. Physician* **1987**, *33*, 2357–2365. [PubMed]
14. Bolognia, J.L.; Brewer, Y.P.; Cooper, D.L. Bazex Syndrome (Acrokeratosis Paraneoplastica). An Analytic Review. *Medicine* **1991**, *70*, 269–280. [CrossRef]
15. Lee, A. Skin Manifestations of Systemic Disease. *Aust. Fam. Physician* **2009**, *38*, 498–505.

16. Edgin, W.A.; Pratt, T.C.; Grimwood, R.E. Pemphigus Vulgaris and Paraneoplastic Pemphigus. *Oral Maxillofac. Surg. Clin. N. Am.* **2008**, *20*, 577–584. [CrossRef]
17. Boyce, S.; Harper, J. Paraneoplastic Dermatoses. *Dermatol. Clin.* **2002**, *20*, 523–532. [CrossRef]
18. Leow, Y.H.; Goh, C.L. Malignancy in Adult Dermatomyositis. *Int. J. Dermatol.* **1997**, *36*, 904–907. [CrossRef]
19. Wakata, N.; Kurihara, T.; Saito, E.; Kinoshita, M. Polymyositis and Dermatomyositis Associated with Malignancy: A 30-Year Retrospective Study: Polymyositis and Dermatomyositis with Malignancy. *Int. J. Dermatol.* **2002**, *41*, 729–734. [CrossRef]
20. Joly, P.; Richard, C.; Gilbert, D.; Courville, P.; Chosidow, O.; Roujeau, J.C.; Beylot-Barry, M.; D'incan, M.; Martel, P.; Lauret, P.; et al. Sensitivity and Specificity of Clinical, Histologic, and Immunologic Features in the Diagnosis of Paraneoplastic Pemphigus. *J. Am. Acad. Dermatol.* **2000**, *43*, 619–626. [CrossRef]
21. Anhalt, G.J. Paraneoplastic Pemphigus. *J. Investig. Dermatol. Symp. Proc.* **2004**, *9*, 29–33. [CrossRef] [PubMed]
22. Tutakne, M.A.; Das, K.D.; Upadhyaya, V.K.; Ramachandra, S.; Narayanaswamy, A.S.; Sarkar, S.K. Leser Trelat Sign Associated with Carcinoma of Gastro-Oesophageal Junction. *Indian J. Cancer* **1983**, *20*, 32–34. [PubMed]
23. Bazex, A.; Salvador, R.; Dupre, A.; Christol, B. Syndrome Paraneoplasique a Type d'hyperkeratose Des Extremites. Guerson Apres Le Traitement de l'epithelioma Larynge. *Bull. Soc. Fr. Dermatol. Syphiligr* **1965**, *72*, 182.
24. Ljubenovic, M.S.; Ljubenovic, D.B.; Binic, I.I.; Jankovic, A.S.; Jovanovic, D.L. Acrokeratosis Paraneoplastica (Bazex Syndrome). *Indian J. Dermatol. Venereol. Leprol.* **2009**, *75*, 329. [CrossRef] [PubMed]
25. Kartan, S.; Shi, V.Y.; Clark, A.K.; Chan, L.S. Paraneoplastic Pemphigus and Autoimmune Blistering Diseases Associated with Neoplasm: Characteristics, Diagnosis, Associated Neoplasms, Proposed Pathogenesis, Treatment. *Am. J. Clin. Dermatol.* **2017**, *18*, 105–126. [CrossRef] [PubMed]
26. Helm, T.N.; Camisa, C.; Venezuela, R.; Allen, C.M. Paraneoplastic Pemphigus. A Distinct Autoimmune Vesiculobullous Disorder Associated with Neoplasia. *Oral Surg. Oral Med. Oral Pathol.* **1993**, *75*, 209–213. [CrossRef]
27. Kimyai-Asadi, A.; Jih, M.H. Paraneoplastic Pemphigus. *Int. J. Dermatol.* **2001**, *40*, 367–372. [CrossRef]
28. Choi, Y.; Nam, K.-H.; Lee, J.-B.; Lee, J.Y.; Ihm, C.-W.; Lee, S.E.; Oh, S.H.; Hashimoto, T.; Kim, S.-C. Retrospective Analysis of 12 Korean Patients with Paraneoplastic Pemphigus. *J. Dermatol.* **2012**, *39*, 973–981. [CrossRef]
29. Tatu, A.L.; Nwabudike, L.C. Bullous Reactions Associated with COX-2 Inhibitors. *Am. J. Ther.* **2017**, *24*, e477–e480. [CrossRef]
30. De La Torre-Lugo, E.M.; Sánchez, J.L. Erythema Gyratum Repens. *J. Am. Acad. Dermatol.* **2011**, *64*, e89–e90. [CrossRef]
31. Dourmishev, L.A.; Dourmishev, A.L.; Schwartz, R.A. Dermatomyositis: Cutaneous Manifestations of Its Variants. *Int. J. Dermatol.* **2002**, *41*, 625–630. [CrossRef] [PubMed]
32. Santmyire-Rosenberger, B.; Dugan, E.M. Skin Involvement in Dermatomyositis. *Curr. Opin. Rheumatol.* **2003**, *15*, 714–722. [CrossRef] [PubMed]
33. Leser, E. Ueber Ein Die Krebskrankheit Bein Menschen Haufig Begleitendes, Noch Wenig Gekanntes Symtom. *Munch. Med. Wochenschr.* **1901**, *51*, 2035–2036.
34. Swartz, R.A.; Hemold, M.E.; Janniger, C.K.; Gascon, P. Sign of Leser-Trelat with a Metastatic Mucinous Adenorcarcinoma. *Cutis* **1991**, *47*, 258–260.
35. Kameya, S.; Noda, A.; Isobe, E.; Watanabe, T. The Sign of Leser-Trélat Associated with Carcinoma of the Stomach. *Am. J. Gastroenterol.* **1988**, *83*, 664–666. [PubMed]
36. Cohn, M.S.; Classen, R.F. The Sign of Leser-Trélat Associated with Adenocarcinoma of the Rectum. *Cutis* **1993**, *51*, 255–257.
37. Dourmishev, L. Multimple Seborrheic Keratoses Associated with Rectal Adenocarcinoma. *CEEDVA* **2004**, *6*, 27–30.
38. Liddell, K.; White, J.E.; Caldwell, I.W. Seborrheic Keratoses and Carcinoma of the Large Bowel. Three Cases Exhibiting the Sign of Leser-Trelat. *Br. J. Dermatol.* **1975**, *92*, 449–452. [CrossRef]
39. Hodak, E.; Halevy, S.; Igbner, A.; Engerstein, S.; Sandbank, M. Leser-Trelat Sign in Adenocarcinoma of the Signoid Colon-a Rare Clinical Picture. *Z. Hautkrankh.* **1987**, *62*, 875–876.
40. Heng, M.C.Y.; Soo-Hoo, K.; Levine, S.; Petresek, D. Linear Seborrheic Keratoses Associated with Underlying Malignancy. *J. Am. Acad. Dermatol.* **1988**, *18*, 1316–1321. [CrossRef]
41. Brauer, J.; Happle, R.; Gieler, U.; Effendy, I. The Sign of Leser-Trelat: Fact or Myth? *J. Eur. Acad. Dermatol. Venereol.* **1992**, *1*, 77–80. [CrossRef]
42. Ginarte, M.; Sánchez-Aguilar, D.; Toribio, J. Sign of Leser-Trélat Associated with Adenocarcinoma of the Rectum. *Eur. J. Dermatol.* **2001**, *11*, 251–253. [PubMed]
43. Klimopoulos, S.; Kounoudes, C.; Pantelidaki, C.; Skrepetou, K.; Papoudos, M.; Katsoulis, H. The Leser-Trelat Sign in Association with Carcinoma of the Ampulla of Vater. *Am. J. Gastroenterol.* **2001**, *96*, 1623–1626. [CrossRef] [PubMed]
44. Ohashi, N.; Hidaka, N. Pancreatic Carcinoma Associated with the Leser-Trélat Sign. *Int. J. Pancreatol.* **1997**, *22*, 155–160. [CrossRef]
45. Hoeben, A.; Polak, J.; Van De Voorde, L.; Hoebers, F.; Grabsch, H.I.; de Vos-Geelen, J. Cervical Esophageal Cancer: A Gap in Cancer Knowledge. *Ann. Oncol.* **2016**, *27*, 1664–1674. [CrossRef]
46. SEER. Surveillance, Epidemiology, and End Results Program. Available online: https://seer.cancer.gov (accessed on 19 August 2022).
47. National Oesophago-Gastric Cancer Audit. 2010 Annual Report. Available online: https://www.nogca.org.uk/reports/2010-annual-report/ (accessed on 19 August 2022).
48. Bedell, A.; Taft, T.H.; Keefer, L.; Pandolfino, J. Development of the Northwestern Esophageal Quality of Life Scale: A Hybrid Measure for Use across Esophageal Conditions. *Am. J. Gastroenterol.* **2016**, *111*, 493–499. [CrossRef]

49. Li, X.; Ai, D.; Chen, Y.; Liu, Q.; Deng, J.; Zhu, H.; Wang, Y.; Wan, Y.; Xie, Y.; Chen, Y.; et al. Cancer of Pharyngoesophageal Junction: A Different Subtype from Hypopharyngeal and Cervical Esophageal Cancer? *Front. Oncol.* **2021**, *11*, 710245. [CrossRef]
50. Didona, D.; Fania, L.; Didona, B.; Eming, R.; Hertl, M.; Di Zenzo, G. Paraneoplastic Dermatoses: A Brief General Review and an Extensive Analysis of Paraneoplastic Pemphigus and Paraneoplastic Dermatomyositis. *Int. J. Mol. Sci.* **2020**, *21*, 2178. [CrossRef]
51. Sneddon, I.B. Cutaneous Manifestations of Visceral Malignancy. *Postgrad. Med. J.* **1970**, *46*, 678–685. [CrossRef]
52. Poole, S.; Fenske, N.A. Cutaneous Markers of Internal Malignancy. I. Malignant Involvement of the Skin and the Genodermatoses. *J. Am. Acad. Dermatol.* **1993**, *28*, 1–13. [CrossRef]
53. Ortega-Loayza, A.G.; Ramos, W.; Gutierrez, E.L.; de Paz, P.C.; Bobbio, L.; Galarza, C. Cutanous Manifestations of internal Malignancies in a Tertiary Health Care Hospital of a Developing Country. *An. Bras. Dermatol.* **2010**, *85*, 736–742. [CrossRef] [PubMed]
54. Da Silva, J.A.; Mesquita, K.D.C.; Igreja, A.C.D.S.M.; Lucas, I.C.R.N.; Freitas, A.F.; de Oliveira, S.M.; Costa, I.M.C.; Campbell, I.T. Paraneoplastic Cutaneous Manifestations: Concepts and Updates. *An. Bras. Dermatol.* **2013**, *88*, 9–22. [CrossRef]
55. Tajima, J.; Mitsuoka, S.; Ohtsuka, E.; Nakamura, Y.; Nakayama, T.; Satoh, Y.; Schima, M.; Nakata, K.; Kusumoto, Y.; Koji, T. A Case of Hepatocellular Carcinoma with the Sign of Leser-Trelat: A Possible Role of a Cutenous Marker for Internal Malignancy. *JPN J. Med.* **1991**, *30*, 53–55. [CrossRef] [PubMed]
56. Stone, S.P.; Buescher, L.S. Life-Threatening Paraneoplastic Cutaneous Syndromes. *Clin. Dermatol.* **2005**, *23*, 301–306. [CrossRef] [PubMed]
57. Serrão, V.; Martins, A.; Ponte, P.; Baptista, J.; Apetato, M.; Feio, A.B. Erythema Gyratum Repens as the Initial Manifestation of Lung Cancer. *Eur. J. Dermatol.* **2008**, *18*, 197–198. [CrossRef]
58. Tatu, A.L.; Cristea, V.C. Pityriasis Folliculorum of the Back Thoracic Area: Pityrosporum, Keratin Plugs, or Demodex Involved? *J. Cutan. Med. Surg.* **2017**, *21*, 441. [CrossRef]
59. Yeh, J.S.; Munn, S.E.; Plunkett, T.A.; Harper, P.G.; Hopster, D.J.; du Vivier, A.W. Coexistence of Acanthosis Nigricans and the Sign of Leser-Trélat in a Patient with Gastric Adenocarcinoma: A Case Report and Literature Review. *J. Am. Acad. Dermatol.* **2000**, *42* (Pt 2), 357–362. [CrossRef]
60. González, C.S.; Vivero, C.M.; López Castro, J. Paraneoplastic syndromes review: The great forgotten ones. *Crit. Rev. Oncol./Hematol.* **2022**, *174*, 103676. [CrossRef] [PubMed]
61. Uno, T.; Isobe, K.; Kawakami, H.; Ueno, N.; Shimada, H.; Matsubara, H.; Okazumi, S.; Nabeya, Y.; Shiratori, T.; Kawata, T.; et al. Concurrent Chemoradiation for Patients with Squamous Cell Carcinoma of the Cervical Esophagus. *Dis. Esophagus* **2007**, *20*, 12–18. [CrossRef]
62. Bertesteanu, S.V.G.; Popescu, C.R.; Grigore, R.; Popescu, B. Pharyngo-Espophageal Junction Neoplasia—Therapeutic Management. *Rev. Chir.* **2012**, *107*, 33–38.

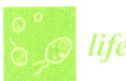

Case Report

Treatment of Severe Atopic Dermatitis with Dupilumab in Three Patients with Renal Diseases

Caterina Foti [1], Paolo Romita [1], Francesca Ambrogio [1,*], Carlo Manno [2], Raffaele Filotico [1], Nicoletta Cassano [3,4], Gino Antonio Vena [3,4], Aurora De Marco [1], Gerardo Cazzato [5,*] and Biagina Gisella Mennuni [1]

1. Section of Dermatology, Department of Biomedical Sciences and Human Oncology (DIMO), University of Bari "Aldo Moro", 70124 Bari, Italy
2. Section of Nefrology, Department of Emergency and Organ Transplantation (DETO), University of Bari "Aldo Moro", 70124 Bari, Italy
3. Dermatology and Venereology Private Practice, 76121 Barletta, Italy
4. Dermatology and Venerology Private Practice, 70100 Bari, Italy
5. Section of Pathology, Department of Emergency and Organ Transplantation (DETO), University of Bari "Aldo Moro", 70124 Bari, Italy
* Correspondence: dottambrogiofrancesca@gmail.com (F.A.); gerardo.cazzato@uniba.it (G.C.); Tel.: +39-3405203641 (G.C.)

Abstract: Background: Atopic dermatitis (AD) is a chronic relapsing inflammatory skin disease that can affect patients' quality of life. Dupilumab is the first biologic agent approved for the treatment of patients with inadequately controlled moderate-to-severe AD and its mechanism of action is based on the inhibition of the interleukin (IL)-4 and IL-13 signaling. There are only a few data on the safety of dupilumab in AD patients with comorbidities, including kidney disorders. Materials and Methods: Descriptive retrospective series of three patients with chronic kidney diseases (Alport syndrome, IgA nephropathy, and hypertensive nephrosclerosis, respectively) receiving dupilumab for their concomitant severe AD. Results: Treatment with a standard dosage of dupilumab caused a relevant improvement of AD in all patients without any adverse events or worsening of renal function. In a patient with severe renal failure, the drug was effective and well tolerated without the need for any dose adjustments, also after the initiation of peritoneal dialytic treatment. Conclusion: Our case series suggests the use of dupilumab as an effective and safe treatment for AD patients suffering from renal diseases, although additional studies are required to confirm such preliminary findings.

Keywords: atopic dermatitis; dupilumab; Alport syndrome; IgA nephropathy

1. Introduction

Atopic dermatitis (AD) is a chronic relapsing inflammatory skin disease that can have a significant impact on the quality of life of affected patients and their families. Dupilumab is a human monoclonal antibody that inhibits interleukin (IL)-4 and IL-13 signaling by binding the shared alpha-subunit of the IL-4 receptor, thus reducing the Th2 response [1]. Dupilumab is the first biologic agent that has been approved for the treatment of patients with inadequately controlled moderate-to-severe AD. There are only scant data on the safety of dupilumab and other systemic therapies in AD patients with comorbid conditions, including kidney disorders, as well as elderly patients, also because such patients are usually excluded from randomized clinical trials [2].

We describe three male adult patients with severe AD and kidney disease who were safely and successfully treated with a standard dosage of dupilumab (600 mg induction dose followed by 300 mg every 2 weeks thereafter).

2. Report of Cases

The first patient reported a long personal history of allergic rhinitis, asthma and severe AD, secondary arterial hypertension, and chronic kidney disease due to Alport

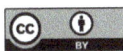

syndrome, a rare hereditary disease caused by mutations in the type IV collagen genes COL4A3, COL4A4, and COL4A5, affecting the renal glomerular basement membrane [3]. A reduction in the Eczema and Severity Index (EASI) of at least 90% from baseline (EASI 90) was reached after 16 weeks of treatment with dupilumab. One year after treatment initiation, an almost complete clearance of AD lesions and a slight improvement of renal function were noticed (Table 1). These effects persisted after two years of continuous treatment.

Table 1. Characteristics of three male patients with severe AD and chronic kidney disease and their laboratory parameters at baseline (T0) and after one year of treatment with dupilumab (T1).

	Patient 1		Patient 2		Patient 3	
Age at Baseline (yrs)	36		44		77	
Renal disease	Alport syndrome		IgA nephropathy		Hypertensive nephrosclerosis	
Concomitant treatment	Ramipril		Ramipril		Nifedipine	
Previous treatments for AD ^	Emollients, topical corticosteroids, phototherapy		Emollients, topical corticosteroids		Emollients, topical corticosteroids	
	T0	T1	T0	T1	T0	T1
EASI score	31	1	27	0	37.5	6
P-NRS	7	2	7	0	10	4
IGA score	4	1	4	0	4	1
DLQI score	20	1	15	0	25	2
Serum IgE (IU/mL)	50.1	40	145	58.7	103	55
Eosinophils (%)	5.1	4.5	2.1	2	13.3	10.7
Serum creatinine (mg/dL)	2.15	1.87	0.90	1.05	4.85	4.94
eGFR (mL/min/1.73 m^2)	38	43	97	86	12	12
Proteinuria (g/24 h)	2.40	2.50	1.61	1.39	1.2	1.1

^ Phototherapy was refused by patient 2 because of difficulties with work schedule and by patient 3 because of problems related to travel time and distance. AD, atopic dermatitis; DLQI, Dermatology Life Quality Index; EASI, Eczema Area and Severity Index; eGFR, estimated glomerular filtration rate; IGA, Investigator's Global Assessment; P-NRS, pruritus numerical rating scale. Normal range of laboratory parameters: eosinophils 0.3–6.2%; serum IgE < 100 IU/mL; eGFR > 90 mL/min/1.73 m^2; serum creatinine < 1.20 mg/dL; proteinuria < 0.20 g/24 h.

The second patient, affected by IgA nephropathy, reported a 10-year history of pollen allergy and a 4-year history of severe AD. AD manifestations rapidly improved with dupilumab leading to the achievement of EASI 90 in two months. After one year, a consistent reduction in AD scores was registered, while serum creatinine and glomerular filtration rate did not show remarkable changes; a slight reduction in proteinuria was observed (Table 1). Such results were maintained after 34 months of continuous therapy with dupilumab.

The third patient was an elderly subject with severe AD, chronic kidney disease probably due to hypertensive nephrosclerosis, and chronic obstructive pulmonary disease. After one year of therapy with dupilumab, AD scores dramatically improved and renal function remained stable (Table 1). Clinical results after 16 weeks of therapy are shown in Figure 1. However, due to the severity of the renal disease, peritoneal dialysis was initiated one year after dupilumab initiation, without the need for any dosage adjustments. During a 12-month follow-up period following the start of peritoneal dialysis, dupilumab treatment continued to be effective in controlling AD and did not induce any untoward effects or further deterioration of renal function.

All patients applied emollients and used short courses of topical corticosteroids on an as-needed basis, especially in the initial treatment phases.

Table 1 summarizes the main characteristics of patients and results after one year of treatment with dupilumab.

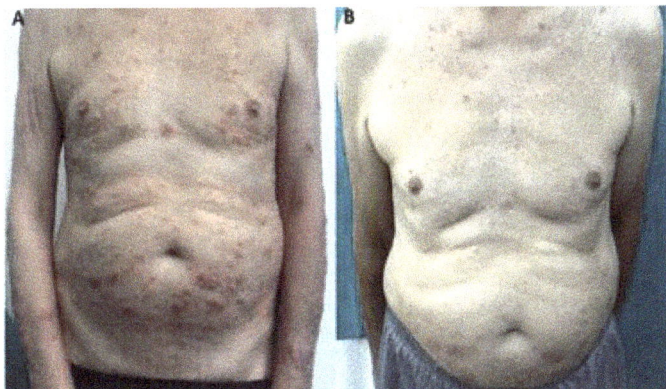

Figure 1. Patient 3 at T0 (**A**) and after 16 weeks of therapy with dupilumab (**B**).

3. Discussion

Dupilumab proved to be safe and effective in these three patients with severe AD and concomitant kidney disease, without any adverse events or worsening of renal function during treatment. Moreover, in the third patient affected by severe renal failure, the renal function remained stable during treatment with dupilumab, and no dose adjustments were required, even after the initiation of peritoneal dialytic treatment.

Only a few publications described the use of dupilumab for AD in patients with severe systemic comorbidities, including renal diseases [2,4]. However, the effects of dupilumab treatment on renal function or detailed safety data have been specified in a limited number of reports, mainly regarding isolated cases.

Renal disease is an obvious contraindication to cyclosporine, one of the most common therapeutic options for severe AD. Moreover, patients with chronic kidney disease, especially those with end-stage renal failure or on renal replacement treatment, frequently complain of chronic pruritus [5]. Therefore, concurrent renal disorder may influence itch intensity in patients suffering from concurrent AD or other pruritic dermatoses. Interestingly, Zhai et al. reported the response of various pruritic conditions to dupilumab, documenting the improvement of symptoms in five patients with uremic pruritus, one of whom in hemodialytic therapy [6].

Kha et al. described a renal transplant man with uremic pruritus, acute flare of AD and superimposed prurigo nodularis coinciding with recent transplant failure who was treated with dupilumab for 8 months [7]. Treatment was efficacious and well tolerated, and changes in the concurrent immunosuppressive therapy were not necessary. Similarly, another report demonstrated that dupilumab was safe and effective for severe and recalcitrant AD in an immunosuppressed renal transplant patient with an unspecified genetic renal syndrome [8].

Varma et al. presented the case of a 22-month-old child with a history of hydronephrosis and other pathological conditions, whose AD dramatically improved after receiving three doses of dupilumab [9]. A recent publication outlined the positive outcomes obtained with dupilumab in two children with AD and nephrotic syndrome [10].

Anecdotal and contrasting findings exist regarding the safety of dupilumab in patients with IgA nephropathy. IgA nephropathy is the most common primary glomerulonephritis in the world and is characterized by the deposition of IgA1-containing immune complexes in the glomerular mesangium responsible for glomerular injury. Pathogenesis of IgA nephropathy is only partially known and appears to be complex. Excessive activity of T lymphocytes, especially the Th2, Tfh, Th17, and Th22 subpopulations, is likely to have a relevant pathogenic role [11]. Moreover, it has been speculated that IgE might be involved in the pathogenesis of IgA nephropathy and serum IgE level might be associated with renal progression [12].

In our patient with IgA nephropathy, a slight reduction in proteinuria was detected during treatment with dupilumab. IgE levels were only slightly above the normal range at baseline and marginally decreased after one year of dupilumab treatment (Table 1). Tanczosova et al. reported similar positive results in a patient with IgA nephropathy whose severe AD worsened during prednisone tapering [13]. In their patient, after treatment with dupilumab for 9 months in association with a minimum dose of prednisone, such authors observed the achievement of EASI 90, an improvement of renal laboratory parameters, and a substantial decrease of serum IgE levels (from the baseline value of 12,500 IU/mL up to 3490 IU/mL). Tanczosova et al. hypothesized that reasons for the improved renal function after dupilumab therapy could be the inhibition of systemic inflammation and the reduction of IgE concentrations [13].

In another report (14), a relevant decline in serum IgE levels and an unexpected rapid deterioration in renal function were described during treatment with dupilumab in a patient with severe AD and minimal renal dysfunction. After stopping dupilumab, a renal biopsy was performed, and primary IgA nephropathy was diagnosed. The authors of this report suspected the involvement of IL-4 neutralization in IgA nephropathy exacerbation through the possible activation of Th17 cells or Toll-like receptor signaling [14]. Therefore, the role of dupilumab in IgA nephropathy is still controversial and requires further investigations.

In conclusion, the present cases suggest that dupilumab can be an effective and safe option in AD patients suffering from renal diseases. However, more data are necessary to better define the safety profile in subjects with relevant comorbidities and special patient populations, including patients with chronic kidney disease and subjects treated with dialysis.

Author Contributions: Conceptualization, F.A. and C.F.; methodology, P.R.; software, G.C.; validation, F.A., R.F. and N.C.; formal analysis, F.A.; investigation, G.C.; resources, B.G.M.; data curation, G.A.V.; writing—original draft preparation, F.A. and C.M.; writing—review and editing, F.A. and C.F.; visualization, A.D.M.; supervision, R.F. and C.F. All authors have read and agreed to the published version of the manuscript.

Funding: This research received no external funding.

Institutional Review Board Statement: Not applicable.

Informed Consent Statement: Informed consent has been obtained from the patients to publish this paper.

Data Availability Statement: Not applicable.

Conflicts of Interest: The authors declare no conflict of interest.

References

1. Gooderham, M.J.; Hong, H.C.; Eshtiaghi, P.; Papp, K.A. Dupilumab: A review of its use in the treatment of atopic dermatitis. *J. Am. Acad. Dermatol.* **2018**, *78* (Suppl. 1), S28–S36. [CrossRef] [PubMed]
2. Drucker, A.M.; Lam, M.; Flohr, C.; Thyssen, J.; Kabashima, K.; Bissonnette, R.; Dlova, N.C.; Aoki, V.; Chen, M.; Yu, J.; et al. Systemic Therapy for Atopic Dermatitis in older adults and adults with comorbidities: A scoping review and international eczema council survey. *Dermatitis* **2022**, *33*, 200–220. [CrossRef] [PubMed]
3. Martínez-Pulleiro, R.; García-Murias, M.; Fidalgo-Díaz, M.; García-González, M.Á. Molecular basis, diagnostic challenges and therapeutic approaches of alport syndrome: A primer for clinicians. *Int. J. Mol. Sci.* **2021**, *22*, 11063. [CrossRef] [PubMed]
4. Patruno, C.; Napolitano, M.; Argenziano, G.; Peris, K.; Ortoncelli, M.; Girolomoni, G.; Offidani, A.; Ferrucci, S.M.; Amoruso, G.F.; Rossi, M.; et al. DADE-dupilumab for atopic dermatitis of the elderly study group. dupilumab therapy of atopic dermatitis of the elderly: A multicentre, real-life study. *J. Eur. Acad. Dermatol. Venereol.* **2021**, *35*, 958–964. [CrossRef] [PubMed]
5. Makar, M.; Smyth, B.; Brennan, F. chronic kidney disease-associated pruritus: A review. *Kidney Blood Press Res.* **2021**, *46*, 659–669. [CrossRef] [PubMed]
6. Zhai, L.L.; Savage, K.T.; Qiu, C.C.; Jin, A.; Valdes-Rodriguez, R.; Mollanazar, N.K. Chronic pruritus responding to dupilumab-a case series. *Medicines* **2019**, *6*, 72. [CrossRef] [PubMed]
7. Kha, C.; Raji, K.; Chisolm, S. treatment of atopic dermatitis with dupilumab in a renal transplant patient. *Dermatitis* **2020**, *31*, 17–18. [CrossRef] [PubMed]
8. Elamin, S.; Murphy, B. Dupilumab in the management of atopic dermatitis in an immunosuppressed renal transplant patient. *Clin. Exp. Dermatol.* **2022**, *47*, 1191–1193. [CrossRef] [PubMed]

9. Varma, A.; Tassavor, M.; Levitt, J. The utility of dupilumab for use in the pediatric population. *JAAD Case Rep.* **2019**, *5*, 943–944. [CrossRef] [PubMed]
10. Yang, Y.Q.; Chen, H.; Qiu, L.R.; Zhu, R.F. Case report: The application of dupilumab in atopic dermatitis children complicated with nephrotic syndrome. *Front. Med.* **2022**, *9*, 813313. [CrossRef] [PubMed]
11. Ruszkowski, J.; Lisowska, K.A.; Pindel, M.; Heleniak, Z.; Dębska-Ślizień, A.; Witkowski, J.M. T cells in IgA nephropathy: Role in pathogenesis, clinical significance and potential therapeutic target. *Clin. Exp. Nephrol.* **2019**, *23*, 291–303. [CrossRef] [PubMed]
12. Lee, J.H.; Lee, S.Y.; Kim, J.S.; Kim, D.R.; Jung, S.W.; Jeong, K.H.; Lee, T.W.; Lee, Y.H.; Kim, Y.G.; Moon, J.Y.; et al. Elevated serum immunoglobulin E level as a marker for progression of immunoglobulin A nephropathy. *Kidney Res. Clin. Pract.* **2016**, *35*, 147–151. [CrossRef] [PubMed]
13. Tanczosova, M.; Arenberger, P.; Rychlik, I.; Arenbergerova, M.; Gkalpakiotis, S. Improvement of atopic dermatitis and IgA nephropathy in a patient treated by dupilumab. *Dermatol. Ther.* **2021**, *34*, 14708. [CrossRef] [PubMed]
14. Yamamoto, M.; Kawase, Y.; Nakajima, E.; Matsuura, Y.; Akita, W.; Aoki, R.; Suzuki, Y.; Mitsui, H. Exacerbation of IgA nephropathy in a patient receiving dupilumab. *JAAD Case Rep.* **2022**, *21*, 150–153. [CrossRef] [PubMed]

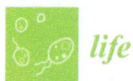

Review

Psoriasis Management Challenges Regarding Difficult-to-Treat Areas: Therapeutic Decision and Effectiveness

Alin Codrut Nicolescu [1], Marius-Anton Ionescu [2], Maria Magdalena Constantin [3], Ioan Ancuta [4,5,*], Sinziana Ionescu [6,7,†], Elena Niculet [8,9,*], Alin Laurentiu Tatu [10,11,†], Henner Zirpel [12] and Diamant Thaçi [13]

1. Medical Center "Roma" for Diagnosis and Treatment, 011773 Bucharest, Romania
2. Dermatology Department, University Hospital "Saint Louis", University of Paris, 75014 Paris, France
3. Department of Dermatology II, "Carol Davila" University of Medicine and Pharmacy, Colentina Clinical Hospital, 020125 Bucharest, Romania
4. Department of Rheumatology, "Carol Davila" University of Medicine and Pharmacy, "Dr. I. Cantacuzino" Clinical Hospital, 011437 Bucharest, Romania
5. Department of Dermatology III, "Carol Davila" University of Medicine and Pharmacy, 050474 Bucharest, Romania
6. General Surgery and Surgical Oncology Clinic I of the Bucharest Oncology Institute, "Carol Davila" University of Medicine and Pharmacy, 022328 Bucharest, Romania
7. "Prof Dr. Al Trestioreanu" Bucharest Oncology Institute, 022328 București, Romania
8. Department of Morphological and Functional Sciences, Faculty of Medicine and Pharmacy, "Dunarea de Jos" University of Medicine and Pharmacy, 800008 Galati, Romania
9. Pathology Department, "Sfantul Apostol Andrei" Emergency Clinical Hospital, 800578 Galati, Romania
10. Clinical Medical Department, Faculty of Medicine and Pharmacy, "Dunarea de Jos" University of Medicine and Pharmacy, 800008 Galati, Romania
11. Dermatology Department, "Sfanta Cuvioasa Parascheva" Hospital of Infectious Diseases, 800179 Galati, Romania
12. Research Institute and Comprehensive Center for Inflammation Medicine, University of Lübeck, 23538 Lübeck, Germany
13. Comprehensive Center for Inflammation Medicine, University of Lübeck, 23538 Lübeck, Germany
* Correspondence: iancuta@hotmail.com (I.A.); helena_badiu@yahoo.com (E.N.); Tel.: +40-728267435 (I.A.); +40-741398895 (E.N.)
† These authors had equal contributions to the first author.

Abstract: Psoriasis is not optimally controlled in spite of newly developed treatments, possibly due to the difficulty of objectively quantifying the disease's severity, considering the limitations of the clinical scores used in clinical practice. A major challenge addresses difficult-to-treat areas, especially in the absence of significant body surface involvement. It is controversial whether the severity evaluation of patients with several affected areas (having at least one difficult-to-treat area) should be done differently from current methods. Scores used for special areas (PSSI, NAPSI and ESIF) allow an accurate assessment of disease severity in difficult-to-treat areas, but the issue of whether to integrate these scores into PASI, BSA or DLQI remains. The review's purpose resides in providing an overview of the main current issues in determining psoriasis severity in patients with psoriasis in difficult-to-treat areas and suggesting possible solutions for the optimal integration of the area assessment in current scores: severity can be either established according to the highest calculated score (PASI or PSSI or NAPSI or ESIF) or by adding a correction factor in the calculation of PASI for special areas.

Keywords: psoriasis; psoriasis scores; difficult-to-treat areas

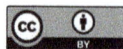

1. Introduction

Psoriasis, an autoimmune systemic skin disease, has joint involvement in 30% of cases (psoriatic arthritis—PsA) [1,2]. Psoriasis management brings many challenges, including an increased prevalence over the past years, chronicity, high grade of disability for some cases and associated comorbidities [3]. Psoriasis plaques are more common on the extensor surfaces but may be present in any area of the body, including the scalp, groins, and genital area. Nails are frequently affected and can be seen as isolated locations [1,2]. Genetic factors are various [1–3], and other factors that may trigger or exacerbate psoriasis can include: stress, body mass index (BMI), infection, drugs (beta-blockers, lithium, angiotensin-converting enzyme (ACE)-inhibitors, (synthetic) antimalarials, tetracyclines, non-steroidal anti-inflammatory drugs (NSAIDs)), withdrawal of systemic (or even potent local) corticosteroids, chronic alcohol consumption, smoking, friction, minimal trauma of the skin—even a slight irritation, radiotherapy, endocrine disorders, and many other [3–6].

Psoriasis is a persistent public health problem involving almost 125 million humans all around the globe [7], although 81% of the world's countries are lacking in psoriasis epidemiology [8]. The prevalence within adult populations estimates at between 0.91% in the United States of America (U.S.A.) and 8.5% in Norway, increasing in the world from 758/100,000 cases in 1990 to 812/100,000 cases in 2017. The highest incidence rates are in the European region, where an increase in incidence from 143.7 cases per 100,000 in 1990 to 147.2 in 2017 was reported [4,9,10]. This supports the statement that there is great variation in the prevalence rates among the world's regions, with variations from 0.73% (to even 2.9%) in Europe or 0.7 (even 2.6%) in the United States, to under 0.5% in Asia (China, Sri Lanka), Latin America, India, or Africa (Tanzania, Egypt) [11].

In Romania, psoriasis affects approximately 400,000 people, as evidenced by the first epidemiological study published recently in 2021 [12]. The prevalence of psoriasis vulgaris within this study was 4.99% [12] (although there are other sources reporting percentages as high as 5.18) [13]; this study is currently continuing in order to assess factors contributing to the increase in psoriasis prevalence over time [12].

Psoriasis displays diversity in presentation and treatment results, varying with disease extent in time, affected areas and affected body surface percentage. Perception of psoriasis severity differs at baseline from long-term disease course. Disease severity guides treatment decisions, choice of medication and the intensity of the treatment response, as well as eligibility criteria for participation in phase II or III clinical trials. In daily clinical practice, physicians evaluate psoriasis severity by combining subjective and objective parameters involving the skin involvement extension, signs and symptoms, and also the specific location of lesions and the impact on every patient's quality of life [14,15].

There is great variability in quantifying the severity of the disease worldwide, and we aimed to evaluate the current guidelines/recommendations and the severity scores in order to achieve better results as an integrated approach to the disease by combining the existing scores in current therapeutic guidelines, recommendations and protocols.

2. Materials and Methods

The current work is the outcome of conducting a thorough, comprehensive analysis of the current specialty literature, generating a narrative review type of article by using updated materials starting from the year 2000 and beyond, with the exclusion of prior materials and data reported in languages other than English. Database/record searches were carried out using Pubmed, Web of Science, and Google Scholar, by utilizing such keywords as: "psoriasis", "psoriasis scores", "PASI", "BSA", "PGA", "IGA", "DLQI", "PSSI", "NAPSI", "ESIF" and "difficult-to-treat areas", individually or combined, generating the current work after selection of the most representative, relevant and work-related, pertinent articles. After searching three databases and zero registers, eliminating articles irrelevant to the current subject, based on 59 relevant results, the following review was compiled.

3. Current Challenges in Disease Severity and Treatment Goals

In the past decade, new treatments and treatment strategies have become available, especially for those that suffer from moderate-to-severe forms of the disease. Amidst these newly developed drugs, biologics ensure the selective immune-mediated pathway inhibition involving cytokines: tumor necrosis factor (TNF), interleukin 23 (IL-23), IL-17,

IL-36, etc. [16,17]. Besides all of these advancements, psoriasis is still not always optimally treated; the patient satisfaction rate with the existing therapies remains modest; meanwhile, the disease burden is at high levels, in spite of the effectiveness of new treatments [17,18].

An explanation for the suboptimal response to treatment and outcomes could be the difficulty in quantifying the disease severity and the limitations brought by the commonly used clinical scores. Quantifying disease severity has implications for treatment selection and assessing therapeutic efficacy. There already exist many severity classification systems, but without reaching a general agreement or allowing the explicit separation into the moderate and the severe disease types, although making this clear-cut dissociation could make a difference in making the therapeutic choice. Reaching a consensus on setting a clear definition for severity is of special importance in medical research, clinical practice, and also for insurance and healthcare authorities in order to evaluate the extensive range of therapies now available for psoriasis [19–22].

Psoriasis severity includes the subjective or objective assessment of the disease: physical aspects, symptoms, the disease impact and the long-term disease and treatment response history categorization. There are numerous methods for assessing the severity of the disease: Body Surface Area (BSA) involved, Psoriasis Area and Severity Index (PASI), Physician's Global Assessment (PGA), Investigator Global Assessment (IGA), Dermatology Life Quality Index (DLQI). There is great variability in quantifying the severity of the disease worldwide; the PASI score is frequently used in Europe, both for assessing the disease severity and for treatment response monitoring. PASI is less frequently used in daily clinical practice in the USA, for example, where dermatologists make use of the BSA and IGA in their evaluation for making a therapeutic decision [19].

3.1. Body Surface Area (BSA)

BSA is a severity assessment tool that implies the estimation of the extent of body surface involvement by measuring the total area of the body affected by psoriasis. The "palm method" takes into account that the palm of the patient is the equivalent of 1% of the body surface (total BSA = 100% equivalent to 100 palms). Psoriasis may be considered: mild if <3% BSA, moderate 3% to 10% BSA, and severe > 10% BSA [19].

When using the percentage of BSA as an indicator of psoriasis severity, it is important that the measurement be made as accurate as possible. There are many question marks regarding the accuracy of BSA: does 'the palm' imply the actual palm or the palm's entirety, with the fingers and thumb? The full stretched hand area, with the digits, is almost 0.8% for males and 0.7% for females. Assuming incorrectly that the palm area is 1% BSA might lead to an almost 50% misrepresentation of the measurement. According to the recommendations, the entire surface of the palm with five digits is roughly 1% [23].

3.2. Physician's Global Assessment (PGA)

The PGA is another tool used in order to assess the severity of psoriasis, which uses a scale with 7 items ranging from clear to severe. Global assessments are used in evaluating extensive disease forms and also for localized plaques. Two disease forms are considered—the static one, measuring the doctor's disease assessment at a single point in the patient's disease course, and a dynamic one evaluating the global amelioration starting from the baseline. Starting from the idea that it is difficult for physicians to remember the severity of psoriasis at the time of initial diagnosis or in subsequent monitoring, the static PGA has become the standard option for practice use [24].

3.3. The Psoriasis Area and Severity Index (PASI)

PASI represents an extensively utilized tool in psoriasis trials that assesses and sets into grade the lesions' severity and the treatment response. This score evaluates the scaling, redness, induration, and extent of plaques per body region.

The PASI is limited in accuracy establishing. The first limitation comes from the specific PASI formula and location of lesions for hard-to-treat psoriasis. Considering the case of a patient with 3 affected areas, with minimal trunk involvement and a moderate-severe involvement of the scalp and/or face—the severity of the score using PASI could be deficient and lead to an under-treatment of the patient.

The second limitation is the estimation of the percentage of BSA extension—in which case, there is much variation in those suffering from limited lesions, resulting in poor detection of changes in mild or moderate psoriasis. The third limitation refers to patients having variable manifestations of psoriasis with identical PASI scores; for example, one has widespread but mild severity psoriasis lesions, and another has localized, severe lesions. Plaque elevation, erythema and scaling are scored equally, treatments improving erythema or scaling will change the score even more than equally useful treatments that do not—the latter being the fourth limitation. Absolute PASI is recommended as being a more accurate measurement for daily practice (PASI < 1 (minimal), PASI < 3 (very mild), PASI < 5 (mild), PASI 5–10 (moderate) and PASI > 10 (severe)) [25].

3.4. The Investigator Global Assessment (IGA) Scale

The IGA scale is frequently used as the final point to reach in psoriasis treatments [23–25]. The IGA scale is a visual assessment tool that consists of a score ranging from 0 (clear) to 4 (severe). For a treatment to be considered successful, the affected area must receive a score of 0 or 1 and experience a two-point improvement from the base line. The IGA scale is a visible evaluation device that consists of a rating ranging from zero (clear) to four (severe). The skin rated 4 is bright red, markedly elevated, with a thick, non-tenacious scale. A successful therapy considers that the area involved needs to have a score of 0/1, with a 2-point improvement from baseline.

3.5. The Dermatology Life Quality Index (DLQI)

The DLQI is a questionnaire reported by patients which were developed because the patient's life quality is crucial in proving that skin lesion severity has an effect on the latter. The questions that make up the DLQI are scored on a four-point scale, as follows: 0, not at all/not relevant; 1, a little; 2, a lot; and 3, very much, giving a total DLQI score from 0 to even 30 [26–28].

The DLQI assesses principally physical limitations, and few questions address the skin diseases' psychological involvement, aiming at decreased conceptual validity, specifically in psoriatic disease. Clinical practice proves that DLQI is a superior assessment tool for severe acute skin diseases and less for those with mild impact or few physical signs but with important psychological impact (vitiligo, basal cell carcinoma, alopecia areata). Another concern related to DLQI is that "not relevant" responses could be interpreted as "not at all" answers; this may lead to bias which could undervalue the severity of the disease. Recent studies highlighted the fact that the patients who responded as "not relevant" had a higher degree of severity than those who responded as "not at all". The rate of "not relevant" answers was high in moderate-to-severe disease patients supporting the statement that those using "not relevant" to one or more questions are going to indicate higher severity of the disease. Because a DLQI score of ≥10 is used for defining severe psoriasis and may influence the decision to initiate biological treatment, this underestimation of disease severity for patients with one or more "not relevant" answers could limit their access to more advanced treatments [26–28].

Treatment goals are a way of guiding physicians toward providing the best possible outcomes for patients so that, in the end, they can optimize patient care. Multiple definitions of psoriasis severity exist, which include disease classification mixtures of assessor- and patient-reported measures. The rule of "tens" is well known, and it describes a "severe psoriasis" if the BSA involved is >10% and/or PASI > 10 and/or DLQI > 10. There is a high degree of variability concerning the clinical guidelines establishing the treatment goal and the success or failure of the treatment (Table 1). At the beginning of 2021, a consensus was reached regarding (1) the clear separation between the best possible goals and those that are realistic in setting the therapeutic aim in psoriasis (moderate to severe); (2) the regulation of treatment aims needs to be adjusted indifferent to the existing treatment on the market; (3) the definition of treatment non-performance/inadequacy when not achieving PASI75; (4) that absolute PASI is to be favored to PASI improvement from what is considered baseline; (5) that treatment aims could be influenced by disorder attributes, the diseased's needs and doctors' judgment, as well as adherence [29,30].

Table 1. Treatment goals and response and/or failure definitions, with treatment changes in those with moderate to severe psoriasis [29–31].

Guideline	Moderate to Severe Psoriasis Treatment Aim Definitions	Treatment Response and/or Failure Definitions, with Changes in Those Suffering from Moderate to Severe Psoriasis
European guideline of systemic therapy	Any psoriasis treatment should aim at eliminating all symptoms of skin inflammation. Necessary: minimum improvement and particular drug analysis times.	Throughout the phases of induction and maintenance: ○ PASI 75—achieved, with treatment maintenance ○ PASI 50 improvement—not achieved, treatment change regimen should be modified ○ PASI response is across 50 to 75%, therapy change(if DLQI>5), therapy maintenance (if DLQI $\leq$ 5).
French guideline of systemic therapy	Factors when establishing treatment goals for systemic therapy: ○ Disease severity ○ PsA/any comorbidity presence ○ Physical, social and psychological patient disease impact ○ The positive benefit-risk balance of ongoing systemic treatment ○ Oppinion and satisfaction level of patient	An adequate treatment response: PASI 75 (from the baseline), or PASI 50 with DLQI $\leq$ 5.
British guideline of systemic therapy	Treatment choice according to the patient and other factors: ○ Psoriasis features (therapeutic aim, disorder phenotype, activity pattern, impact and severity of disorder, PsA presence) ○ Other factors (age, weight, comorbidities—past/present, pregnancy, views/preferences on treatmentfrequency and administration way, adherence).	○ Assessment whether the minimal response have been met defined as: at least 50% decrease in baseline severity of disease (a response of PASI 50, otherwise percentage BSA) and improvement of physical, social or psychological performance (DLQI—4-point).
Spanish consensus of systemic therapy	The ideal outcome is to achieve: PASI 90 and a PGA $\leq$ 1, or as an alternative, a minimal, topical treatment controllable localized disease (PGA $\leq$ 2 and PASI < 5), DLQI $\leq$ 1, prolonged remissions without loss of efficacy, no worsening of comorbidities. Criteria for an appropriate response initially and in the long term (more than 6 months), 1 of: PASI 75, PASI < 5, PGA $\leq$ 1 and DLQI < 5. Criteria for the minimum efficacy required: PASI 50, PASI < 5.	Therapeutic failure during initiation of the treatment: ○ a score is equal to or greater than those constituting the criteria for moderate-to-severe psoriasis at the end of the induction phase ○ there is no adequate response according to the physician and the patient by the end of the induction phase, ○ a decrease in 50% from the baseline PASI score has not been achieved (or this degree of response has been lost) after the induction phase.

Abbreviations. PsA—psoriatic arthritis; PASI—Psoriasis Area and Severity Index; BSA—Body Surface Area; DLQI—dermatology life quality index; RCT—randomized controlled trial; PGA—Physician's Global Assessment.

We consider it important to continuously monitor the treatment effects and make necessary changes during maintenance therapy. Treatment aims can be set for all patients, but treatment changes/adaptations need to be adapted to each patient when the aim is not attained [31].

3.6. The Psoriasis Scalp Severity Index (PSSI)

The PSSI measures the psoriasis skin extension and the severity of the scalp erythema, desquamation and infiltration. The psoriasis-affected skin and the degree of severity for the PSSI are established by doctors, which ranges from 0 to 72, 0 meaning absence of psoriasis, with increasing scores revealing more severe disease [32–39]. The PSSI excludes the face and neck areas. The scalp is a prevalent difficult-to-treat area for psoriasis; the visibility of lesions and pruritus degree that are associated with scalp lesions may adversely affect the quality of life of the patient.

3.7. The Nail Psoriasis Severity Index (NAPSI)

The NAPSI is a nail psoriasis objective assessment instrument that is used to assess the severity of nail bed and matrix psoriasis by the area of involvement of the nail unit (each nail is divided into 4 quadrants and given a score for nail bed psoriasis and nail matrix psoriasis, depending on the presence of any of the features of nail psoriasis in that quadrant–leukonychia, pitting, red spots in the lunula, crumbling (0 for none, 4 if present in 4 quadrants of the nail) and respectively, onycholysis, splinter hemorrhages, subungual hyperkeratosis, "oil drop" (0 for none, 4 for 4 quadrants)). Each nail gets a matrix score and a nail bed score, the total of which represents the score for that nail (0–8); the sum of all the nails' scores is the total NAPSI score (0–80 or 0–160 if the toenails are included in the calculation) [32].

Nail damage occurs in only 1 to 5% of patients, with 1 in 2 patients with psoriasis being affected by nail psoriasis at any given time; an estimated lifetime incidence of nail damage ranges between 80 to 90%.

3.8. The Erythema, Scaling, Induration, and Fissuring (ESIF)

ESIF is assessed for palm, and sole psoriasis using a 4-point scale (from 0 = clear to 3 = severe) and is determined with the addition of scores for the 4 sole signs, with a total from 0 (absence of disease)–24 (most severe involvement) [37].

A cross-sectional study that included more than 4000 adults with psoriasis from the Danish Skin Cohort evaluated the involvement of hard-to-treat areas. The most frequently difficult-to-treat areas are the scalp (in 43.0% of patients), the face (29.9%), nails (24.5%), soles (15.6%), genitals (14.1%), and palms (13.7%). Sixty-four point 8 percent, 42.4% and 21.9% of patients had involvement of at least one, and respectively at least 2 and at least three difficult-to-treat areas. According to its severity (Table 2), the prevalence of psoriasis in the face, scalp, nails genitals was directly proportional to the severity of psoriasis; for example, 66.1% of patients with severe psoriasis have lesions on the scalp. Among patients with mild psoriasis, 80.4% had an involvement ≥ 1 difficult-to-treat area, and the frequency among those with severe forms increased to 89.0%. Sixty-eight point eight percent and 43.7% of patients suffering from severe psoriasis had at least 2 and, respectively, 3 difficult-to-treat areas. Courses of action based on results among those with difficult-to-treat areas suggest that they are the population with the highest disease burden [38].

Table 2. Psoriasis frequency in difficult-to-treat areas with psoriasis severity [38].

Difficult-to-Treat Areas	% of Patients with Mild Psoriasis	% of Patients with Moderate Psoriasis	% of Patients with Severe Psoriasis
scalp	48.1%	57.8%	66.1%
face	27.6%	41.8%	53.3%
palms	13.5%	22.9%	19.5%
nails	25.6%	31.1%	42.4%
genitals	12.5%	18.1%	27.2%
soles	16.7%	24.7%	22.1%

These difficult-to-treat areas have a limited degree of response to local treatment and could be classified as moderate or severe psoriasis, even when BSA ≤ 10 and the PASI ≤ 10. Data collected from the Corrona Psoriasis Registry revealed that 2/3 of psoriasis patients undergoing biological treatment have psoriatic arthritis and/or at least one form of psoriasis in an area difficult to treat (scalp, nail psoriasis, palmoplantar). Scores dedicated to these special areas (PSSI—Psoriasis Scalp Severity Index, NAPSI, ESIF) allow a precise calculation of disease severity, but they are not integrated into the more commonly used scores such as BSA, PGA, or PASI [39].

The biggest challenge in establishing the disease severity, therapeutic choice and efficiency monitoring are "difficult-to-treat" areas, especially in the absence of significant involvement of the body surface elsewhere. The location and morphological features of scalp, nail, palmoplantar and genital psoriasis can often lead to ineffective topical treatment and often requires systemic treatment [37,40–42].

Determining psoriasis severity for those suffering from difficult-to-treat areas of psoriasis can be a demanding task due to the fact that some severity definitions depend on the involved area ratio. Dedicated scores allow a more accurate calculation of disease severity in special areas, but the dilemma remains whether or not to assess the overall severity of the disease by integrating these special area scores into scores such as PASI, PGA, BSA and DLQI. It is debatable whether, in patients with several affected areas (a common situation in clinical practice, with at least one special area), the classification of the degree of severity should be made differently from current methods or not.

We have an example of a psoriasis patient having 2 involved skin areas: scalp and trunk (Table 3). The scalp has erythema, induration and exfoliation of over 70%. Trunk lesions extend up to 10% with a severity of 4. The PASI score for this patient is 8, indicating a moderate form of the disease; if in this patient's case, we would use the PSSI score, the value will add up to 60 points, indicating a severe form, according to European guidelines. Severity framing can significantly influence therapeutic options and the choice of effective treatment for both areas involved [43].

Table 3. Examples of patients' scores involve difficult-to-treat areas.

Main Area	Additional Areas	Severity Assessment
trunk BSA less than < 10% severity 4 for erythema, induration and scaling PASI = 3.6	scalp >70% severity 4 for erythema, induration and scaling	PASI = 8 → PSO moderate or PSSI = 48 → PSO severe
	nails matrix and nail bed completely affected 10 nails	PASI = 6 → PSO moderate or NAPSI = 80 → PSO severe
	palmo-plantar both hands or both soles severity 4 for erythema, induration, scaling, fissuring	PASI = 8 → PSO moderate or ESIF = 24 → PSO severe

Abbreviations: PASI—Psoriasis Area and Severity Index; BSA—Body Surface Area; PSSI—Psoriasis Scalp Severity Index; NAPSI—Nail Psoriasis Severity Index; ESIF—Erythema, Scaling, Induration, Fissuring.

In a series of 26 psoriasis patients having nail psoriasis [44], there was an important (moderate) positive NAPSI and DLQI correlation ($p = 0.001$). A meta-analysis published in 2019 showed that the frequency of palmoplantar psoriasis (PPP) of both palms and soles (59%) was almost 3 times higher than the frequency of any single PPP location, be it palms (21%)/soles (20%). More than 60% of the patients from the 15 studies included in this meta-analysis had PPP with at least one additional area involved [45,46].

The severity assessment in patients with several affected areas and at least one difficult-to-treat area can also raise issues from the point of view of insurance and health authorities: the existence of country-specific therapeutic protocols limits the use of systemic therapy (biologics, small molecules) for severe psoriasis only to be done according to the PASI/PGA/BSA/DLQI scores. To meet psoriasis patients' needs while respecting the requirements of the authorities involved, we propose to be taken into account the score that represents the highest degree of severity.

The possible solutions for such practical issues reside in making the classification by the degree of severity according to the highest calculated score, regardless of whether it is PASI or PSSI, NAPSI, or ESIF. If, for the 3 examples mentioned above (affecting at least 2 areas, one of which being difficult-to-treat), the severity assessment would be done according to the specific scores of the special areas, then the patients would fall into the category of severe psoriasis, with all of the implications deriving from this classification (choosing the right treatment according to the involvement of a difficult-to-treat area, setting the therapeutic goal, evaluating the success or failure of the therapy). The challenge of this new possible classification could be the subsequent monitoring of the effectiveness of the treatment.

Since PASI is considered one of the standards in patient trials (with treatment comparison, having good correlation with multiple objective outcome measures, being the most validated objective measurement of psoriasis severity, with a test-retest variability of less than 2%), another solution could be to add a correction factor in the calculation of PASI for special areas, as in the example of the first patient with 2 areas involved, scalp and trunk (Table 3). The introduction of a correction factor for that area of the body defined as hard-to-treat could change the importance of the scalp involvement in the calculation of PASI and, consequently, the patient's framing in the severity degrees, reflecting the reality of usual clinical practice.

4. The Challenges of Individualized Treatment and Evaluating the Treatment Success

The issue of psoriasis in "difficult-to-treat" areas—Psoriasis localized in special areas—is difficult to treat and is often associated with important physical disability and discomfort. "Difficult-to-treat" areas are used for describing psoriasis located on the scalp, palms and soles, and nail, being frequently connected to high emotional and functional impact [32–37]. Some authors also include as part of this classification the psoriasis of the face and inverse psoriasis [37].

The biggest challenge after establishing the severity of the disease is choosing the optimal therapy adapted to the patient's needs, especially in cases with multiple site involvement and in difficult-to-treat areas [47,48].

Recent advances in systemic treatments may lead to more benefits in patients for whom topical approaches pose challenges. Scarce-controlled trials had results onsystemic therapy efficacy and safety (traditional or biological) for psoriasis management in difficult-to-treat areas. In general, the available evidence is obtained from sub-analyses of trials which included patients suffering from psoriasis and/or PsA, also having an assessment of the involvement of the nails, scalp, palms or soles [48].

Another reason for poorer clinical outcomes could be related to the patient. Conventional systemic therapies need various concentrations for local treatment response, toxicity being an important problem. In addition, selecting the appropriate treatment is problematic due to the lack of clinical trial data in such locations. Only patients with a minimum of 10% BSA are allowed in the clinical trials for newer targeted biological agents, and that's why extended evidence regarding the efficacy of new treatments in patients with lower BSA involvement or disease involving difficult-to-treat areas is lacking. This approach impacts the access of patients with decreased disease severity to new therapies in some national health systems and other payers refusing reimbursements for those lacking a BSA involvement of at least 10% [48,49].

5. Treatment Goals and Treat-to-Target

In order to reduce the risk of severe comorbidities, doctors should aim at establishing the goals of treatment so that treatment optimization is achieved, along with the long-term quality of life. Treatment goals need to be accustomed to disease severity and possible improvement degree. However, personal treatment aims can vary significantly, surprisingly, between patients with similar disease severity patients. Treatment goals need a clear discussion with the patient at initiation so that to meet both patient and physician expectations. Once target goals are defined, an aimed treatment manner can be contrasted with standard care in order to find the optimal management of the disease (Table 4) [47].

The introduction of biotherapies was accompanied by an increase in the therapeutic target, the PASI 75 response being replaced today by PASI 90 and PASI 100 with the new therapeutic classes. These types of aims may need reconsideration in those with lesions localized in difficult-to-treat areas (scalp, face, soles, palms, nails, genitals), having negative emotional effects, with increased disease severity (as compared to the disease severity evaluated with objective measures (like BSA or PASI) [50,51].

Table 4. Treatment goals in psoriasis are defined by European guidelines.

	Severity Scores to Achieve	Quality of Life
Treatment goals (assessed after 10–16 weeks and then every 8 weeks treatment goals	PASI 90 or PASI ≤ 2 PGA clear or almost clear	DLQI < 2
minimum efficacy (lowest hurdle for treatment modification)	PASI 50	DLQI < 5 or DLQI improvement ≥ 5

Abbreviations: PASI—Psoriasis Area and Severity Index; PGA—Physician's Global Assessment; DLQI—Dermatology Life Quality Index [47].

"Treat-to-target" is a concept that describes the changes in treatment as being suitable until a designated aim has been attained. The aimed treatment strategy may also be tough to enforce in world scientific medical practices if the goal purpose is too ambitious and past the attain of the majority of sufferers. PASI 100 needs to be an ideal aim, as only a few present treatments are able to reach it in over 50% of sufferers. The UNCOVER-1 study (Study in Participants With Moderate to Severe Psoriasis) revealed that 35.3% of ixekizumab-treated patients had PASI 100 in the 12th week. Conversely, PASI 90 is viable in many psoriasis patients (70–80%) medicated with IL-17 and IL-23 inhibitors [52–54].

Other treatment aims' analyses could be useful in setting a link between various PASI results. Data from clinical studies on secukinumab showed that achieving a PASI 90 was linked to an improved life quality (DLQI 0/1) in the 12th week, as compared to PASI 75–89. When defining treatment goals, it is necessary to accept the fact that a decrease in PASI is not relevant for all patients. As a result indicator, instead, the modification of absolute PASI might be even more pertinent. According to the Spanish Psoriasis Group consensus, absolute PASI is considered to be useful for medical care by superiorly correlating with DLQI, as opposed to relative PASI amelioration. A reduction of the biological therapy dosage might be attainable in those having complete/near complete results (PGA 0 or 1; PASI 90; absolute PASI from <2 to 3). The criteria necessary in order to go back to biological therapy (in full dosage) include that the absolute PASI values be ≥ 5 or that there be an absence of a PASI 75 response [55,56].

The European consensus on the treatment aim for psoriasis reveals the necessity of minimal improvement degree and treatment-specific assessment time points, but not all countries mention these minimum evaluation criteria in their guidelines.

6. Treatment Success or Failure for Patients with Difficult-to-Treat Areas

There is treatment failure in accordance with the overall treatment guidelines/consensus records—what was relevant was the absence of improvement in PASI 50 during the induction and maintenance phases. These concepts/theories adopted decreased improvement levels if there was good quality of life, with ≥ 2 taking into account other factors such as patient preference and treatment adherence.

One of the questions that have risen in recent years has been related to the implications of setting higher treatment targets, driven by the very good results of newer biologics [56]. Unfortunately, new biologic therapies are still restrictedly used in a small number of patients (mainly in those suffering from severe psoriasis). For many patients, there is the risk that failure in achieving the goals will be defined as treatment failure and therefore lead to an unnecessary change in therapy. We consider that a clear distinction is needed between the therapeutic goal (for which the doctor and the patient aim) and the minimum response criterion (which regulates the change in treatment).

The minimum response criteria are defined as a PASI 50 response and a DLQI score of 5 units lower than the baseline, assessed every 6 months; failure of treatment means that there is a lack of PASI 50 improvement. At the same time, if there exists an amelioration in PASI 50 with a DLQI of not less than 5 units from the beginning, then this situation is also considered treatment failure (Figure 1). The long-term treatment goal is similar to the recommendations from the EuroGuiDerm Guideline on the systemic treatment of Psoriasis vulgaris: at least PASI 90 and DLQI < 2. We consider that this approach in setting the therapeutic target takes into consideration clinical situations with patients having difficult-to-treat areas or patients with multiple areas, including at least one difficult-to-treat area while maintaining an equally ambitious therapeutic target [57].

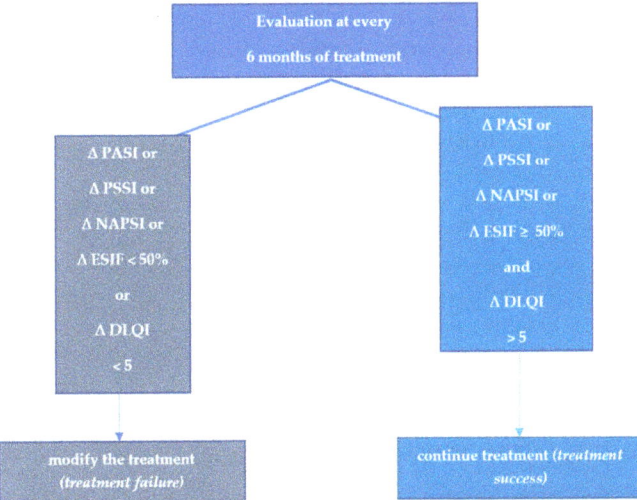

Figure 1. Minimum efficiency criteria for moderate-to-severe psoriasis; Δ = improvement of the score compared to baseline. Abbreviations: PASI—Psoriasis Area and Severity Index; BSA—Body Surface Area; PSSI—Psoriasis Scalp Severity Index; NAPSI—Nail Psoriasis Severity Index; ESIF—Erythema, Scaling, Induration, Fissuring.

7. Discussion

Psoriasis found on the face, scalp, intertriginous areas, hands, feet, nails and genitals are often diagnosed poorly and under-treated. In spite of the small surface area, which is commonly affected by psoriatic lesions in such areas, patients have increased physical impairment and emotional distress. Limitations in current disease severity scores do not fully assess the impact of disease on the quality of life of patients, and many are not receiving adequate care. In these cases, the therapeutic attitude to adapt is to adapt therapy (dose increase, therapeutic combination), change of treatment (switch) or continuation of treatment for the next 3 months with reevaluation [58]. Psoriasis severity classification is a major problem that needs to be addressed in order to guide the physician's decisions regarding treatment, always having in mind that the disease is heterogeneous in clinical expression and response to treatment, in its duration and involved areas (including the percentage of body area), being constantly variable [22].

Psoriasis is highly influenced by external factors; the list of triggering factors for flare-ups is extensive, starting with stress, mild localized skin trauma, different infections and drugs for different comorbidities, alcohol consumption, smoking, weather etc. A total of 73% of the patients have at least one comorbidity that can influence the disease evolution and response to treatment, especially for difficult-to-treat areas [58]. In the given example, the patient with 2 areas affected by psoriasis has been evaluated after 3 months of treatment with ΔPASI 90 for lesions on the trunk and ΔPASI < 50 for the scalp. The patient suffered a great level of stress during these 3 months, but according to aDLQI, there was a significant improvement.

There are many systems classifying psoriasis severity, but none have managed to reach a consensus, not having clear-cut demarcation between severity degrees (moderate and severe), the methodology disregarding the involvement of psoriasis in difficult-to-treat areas; the fact that current practices employ systems that are mainly used by physicians/dermatologists (such as PASI, PGA and/or BSI) and by patients (DLQI) alike is a step further in psoriasis severity assessment and treatment, the quality of life being of paramount importance [22]. Figure 2 reveals the raised issues, with point-by-point explanations and proposed solutions for the clinicians in their daily practice.

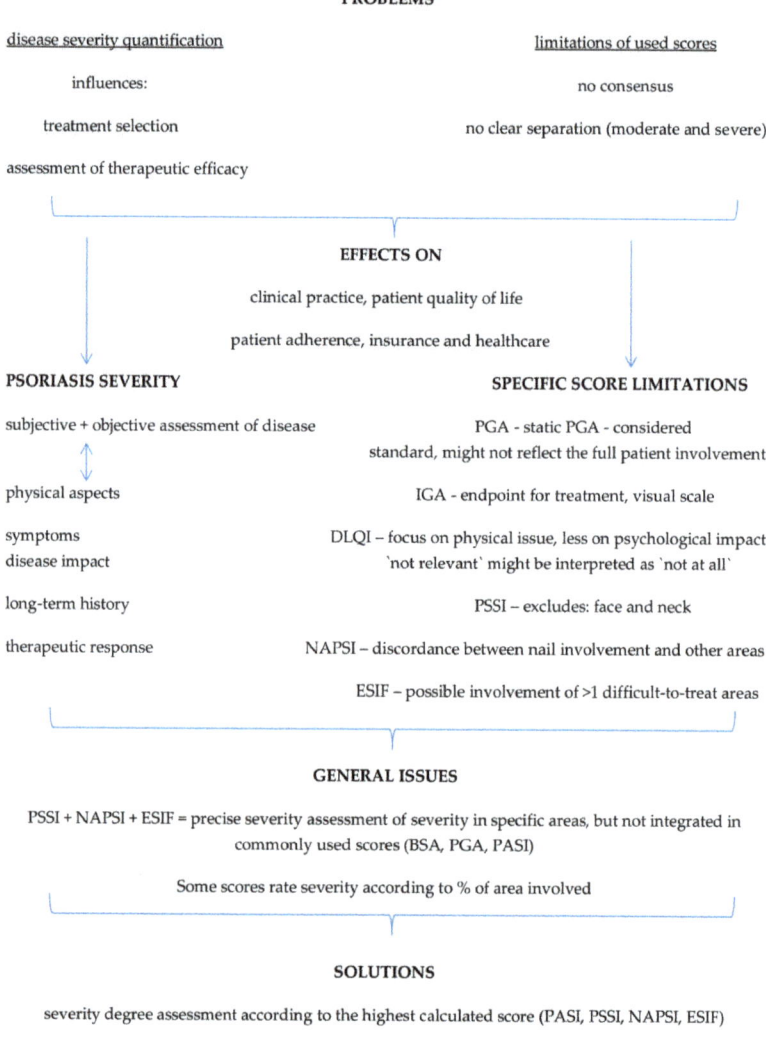

Figure 2. Issues and possible solutions in psoriasis severity effective calculation. Abbreviations: PASI—Psoriasis Area and Severity Index; BSA—Body Surface Area; PSSI—Psoriasis Scalp Severity Index; NAPSI—Nail Psoriasis Severity Index; ESIF—Erythema, Scaling, Induration, Fissuring.

For psoriasis involving difficult-to-treat areas, the challenge extends from establishing severity and choosing the optimal treatment to correctly evaluating the efficacy or failure of the therapy; this is a major problem that our paper addressed, having the advantage of bringing forth a practical, clinical issue which dermatologists face. There are several solutions to this issue; the first one is the evaluation of different scores for each area and the success or failure of the treatment to be evaluated by the area with the smallest improvement. The second solution is the inclusion of special areas in the treatment goal algorithm or to use of a completely different algorithm for psoriasis in difficult-to-treat areas by using the data obtained in different clinical studies or real-world experience. The current paper has made a summary of the literature at hand, examining the current knowledge on psoriasis and its score assessment, with the limitation of possibly having a broad area of research data (a wide range of psoriasis score reporting analysis), but with the advantage of identifying possible new research areas.

8. Conclusions

In clinical practice, psoriasis severity is usually categorized as "mild", "moderate", and "severe", using measurement tools that underestimate the actual disease severity in cases where skin lesions involve 'special areas such as the face, palms, soles, genitalia and scalp. It is necessary to consider the lesions' location and patients' quality of life in order to assess psoriasis severity more fully and accurately. The solutions considered for evaluating difficult-to-treat areas reside in establishing the severity according to the highest calculated score (PASI or PSSI, NAPSI, or ESIF) and/or in the addition of a correction factor when calculating PASI for special areas. The algorithms used to monitor and evaluate therapeutic efficacy should be upgraded with emphasis on the difficult-to-treat areas which greatly influence the overall severity degree.

The need to redefine disease severity with the inclusion of special areas is becoming increasingly obvious and should be done practically in order to prove its usefulness in clinics and research.

Author Contributions: All authors had substantial contributions to the conception or design of the work, in drafting the work or revising it critically for important intellectual content, in the final approval of the version to be published and have agreed to be accountable for all aspects of the work in ensuring that questions related to the accuracy or integrity of any part of the work are appropriately investigated and resolved. All authors have read and agreed to the published version of the manuscript.

Funding: The APC was paid by Carol Davila University of Medicine and Pharmacy, Bucharest.

Institutional Review Board Statement: Not applicable.

Informed Consent Statement: Not applicable.

Data Availability Statement: Not applicable.

Acknowledgments: The current paper was supported academically by the "Dunarea de Jos" University of Galati, Romania, through the Multidisciplinary Integrated Center of Dermatological Interface Research (MIC-DIR) [Centrul Integrat Multidisciplinar de Cercetare de Interfata Dermatologica—(CIM-CID)].

Conflicts of Interest: The authors declare no conflict of interest.

References

1. Global Burden of Disease Study 2010 (GBD 2010) Results by Cause 1990–2010. Available online: https://ghdx.healthdata.org/record/ihme-data/gbd-2010-results-cause-1990-2010 (accessed on 10 October 2022).
2. Reich, K.; Krüger, K.; Mössner, R.; Augustin, M. Epidemiology and clinical pattern of psoriatic arthritis in Germany: A prospective interdisciplinary epidemiological study of 1511 patients with plaque-type psoriasis. *Br. J. Dermatol.* **2009**, *160*, 1040–1047. [CrossRef] [PubMed]
3. Harden, J.L.; Krueger, J.G.; Bowcock, A.M. The immunogenetics of psoriasis: A comprehensive review. *J. Autoimmun.* **2015**, *64*, 66–73. [CrossRef] [PubMed]

4. Niculet, E.; Radaschin, D.S.; Nastase, F.; Draganescu, M.; Baroiu, L.; Miulescu, M.; Arbune, M.; Tatu, A.L. Influence of phytochemicals in induced psoriasis. *Exp. Ther. Med.* **2020**, *20*, 3421–3424. [CrossRef] [PubMed]
5. Kamiya, K.; Kishimoto, M.; Sugai, J.; Komine, M.; Ohtsuki, M. Risk factors for the development of psoriasis. *Int. J. Mol. Sci.* **2019**, *20*, 4347. [CrossRef] [PubMed]
6. Kim, G.K.; Del Rosso, J.Q. Drug-provoked psoriasis: Is it drug induced or drug aggravated?: Understanding pathophysiology and clinical relevance. *J. Clin. Aesthetic Dermatol.* **2010**, *3*, 32–38.
7. International Federation of Psoriasis Associations. World Psoriasis Day. 2015. Available online: https://ifpa-pso.com/our-actions/worldpsoriasis-day (accessed on 19 September 2022).
8. Parisi, R.; Iskandar, I.Y.K.; Kontopantelis, E.; Augustin, M.; Griffiths, C.E.M.; Ashcroft, D.M.; Global Psoriasis Atlas. National, regional, and worldwide epidemiology of psoriasis: Systematic analysis and modelling study. *BMJ* **2020**, *369*, 1590. [CrossRef] [PubMed]
9. Parisi, R.; Symmons, D.P.; Griffiths, C.E.M.; Ashcroft, D.M. Identification and management of psoriasis and associated comorbidity (IMPACT) project team. Global epidemiology of psoriasis: A systematic review of incidence and prevalence. *J. Investig. Dermatol.* **2013**, *133*, 377–385. [CrossRef]
10. AlQassimi, S.; AlBrashdi, S.; Galadari, H.; Hashim, M.J. Global burden of psoriasis—Comparison of regional and global epidemiology, 1990 to 2017. *Int. J. Dermatol.* **2020**, *59*, 566–571. [CrossRef]
11. Enamandram, M.; Kimball, A.B. Psoriasis epidemiology: The interplay of genes and the environment. *J. Investig. Dermatol.* **2013**, *133*, 287–289. [CrossRef]
12. Nicolescu, A.C.; Bucur, Ș.; Giurcăneanu, C.; Gheucă-Solovăstru, L.; Constantin, T.; Furtunescu, F.; Ancuța, I.; Constantin, M.M. Prevalence and characteristics of psoriasis in Romania—First study in overall population. *J. Pers. Med.* **2021**, *11*, 523. [CrossRef]
13. Boca, A.N.; Ilies, R.F.; Vesa, S.; Pop, R.; Tataru, A.D.; Buzoianu, A.D. The first nation-wide study revealing epidemiologic data and life quality aspects of psoriasis in Romania. *Exp. Ther. Med.* **2019**, *18*, 900–904. [CrossRef] [PubMed]
14. Krueger, G.G.; Feldman, S.R.; Camisa, C.; Duvic, M.; Elder, J.T.; Gottlieb, A.B.; Koo, J.; Krueger, J.G.; Lebwohl, M.; Lowe, N.; et al. Two considerations for patients with psoriasis and their clinicians. *J. Am. Acad. Dermatol.* **2000**, *43*, 281–285. [CrossRef] [PubMed]
15. Pariser, D.M.; Bagel, J.; Gelfand, J.M.; Korman, N.J.; Ritchlin, C.T.; Strober, B.E.; Van Voorhees, A.S.; Young, M.; Rittenberg, S.; Lebwohl, M.G.; et al. National psoriasis foundation. national psoriasis foundation clinical consensus on disease severity. *Arch. Dermatol.* **2007**, *143*, 239–242. [CrossRef] [PubMed]
16. Rider, P.; Carmi, Y.; Cohen, I. Biologics for targeting inflammatory cytokines, clinical uses, and limitations. *Int. J. Cell Biol.* **2016**, *2016*, 9259646. [CrossRef]
17. Raychaudhuri, S.P.; Raychaudhuri, S.K. Biologics: Target-specific treatment of systemic and cutaneous autoimmune diseases. *Indian J. Dermatol.* **2009**, *54*, 100–109. [CrossRef] [PubMed]
18. Feldman, S.R.; Goffe, B.; Rice, G.; Mitchell, M.; Kaur, M.; Robertson, D.; Sierka, D.; Bourret, J.A.; Evans, T.S.; Gottlieb, A. The challenge of managing psoriasis: Unmet medical needs and stakeholder perspectives. *Am. Health Drug Benefits* **2016**, *9*, 504–513.
19. Rhodes, J.; Clay, C.; Phillips, M. The surface area of the hand and the palm for estimating percentage of total body surface area: Results of a meta-analysis. *Br. J. Dermatol.* **2013**, *169*, 76–84. [CrossRef]
20. Weisman, S.; Pollack, C.R.; Gottschalk, R.W. Psoriasis disease severity measures: Comparing efficacy of treatments for severe psoriasis. *J. Dermatol. Treat.* **2003**, *14*, 158–165. [CrossRef]
21. Feldman, S.R.; Krueger, G.G. Psoriasis assessment tools in clinical trials. *Ann. Rheum. Dis.* **2005**, *64*, ii65–ii68. [CrossRef]
22. Salgado-Boquete, L.; Carrascosa, J.M.; Llamas-Velasco, M.; Ruiz-Villaverde, R.; de la Cueva, P.; Belinchón, I. A new classification of the severity of psoriasis: What's moderate psoriasis? *Life* **2021**, *11*, 627. [CrossRef] [PubMed]
23. Long, C.C.; Finlay, A.Y.; Averill, R.W. The rule of hand: 4 hand areas = 2 FTU = 1 g. *Arch. Dermatol.* **1992**, *128*, 1129–1130. [CrossRef] [PubMed]
24. Langley, R.G.; Ellis, C.N. Evaluating psoriasis with psoriasis area and severity index, psoriasis global assessment, and lattice system physician's global assessment. *J. Am. Acad. Dermatol.* **2004**, *51*, 563–569. [CrossRef]
25. Kirsten, N.; Rustenbach, S.; von Kiedrowski, R.; Sorbe, C.; Reich, K.; Augustin, M. Which PASI outcome is most relevant to the patients in real-world care? *Life* **2021**, *11*, 1151. [CrossRef]
26. Twiss, J.; Meads, D.M.; Preston, E.P.; Crawford, S.R.; McKenna, S.P. Can we rely on the dermatology life quality index as a measure of the impact of psoriasis or atopic dermatitis? *J. Investig. Dermatol.* **2012**, *132*, 76–84. [CrossRef] [PubMed]
27. Langebruch, A.; Radtke, M.A.; Gutknecht, M.; Augustin, M. Does the dermatology life quaslity index (DLQI) underestimate the disease-specific burden of psoriasis patients? *J. Eur. Acad. Dermatol. Venereol.* **2019**, *33*, 123–127. [CrossRef]
28. Rencz, F.; Poór, A.K.; Péntek, M.; Holló, P.; Kárpáti, S.; Gulácsi, L.; Szegedi, A.; Remenyik, É.; Hidvégi, B.; Herszényi, K.; et al. A detailed analysis of 'not relevant' responses on the DLQI in psoriasis: Potential biases in treatment decisions. *J. Eur. Acad. Dermatol. Venereol.* **2018**, *32*, 783–790. [CrossRef] [PubMed]
29. Belinchón Romero, I.; Dauden, E.; Ferrándiz Foraster, C.; González-Cantero, Á.; Carrascosa Carrillo, J.M. Therapeutic goals and treatment response evaluation in moderate to severe psoriasis: An expert's opinion document. *Ann. Med.* **2021**, *53*, 1727–1736. [CrossRef]
30. Smith, C.H.; Jabbar-Lopez, Z.K.; Yiu, Z.Z.; Bale, T.; Burden, A.D.; Coates, L.C.; Cruickshank, M.; Hadoke, T.; MacMahon, E.; Murphy, R.; et al. British association of dermatologists guidelines for biologic therapy for psoriasis 2017. *Br. J. Dermatol.* **2017**, *177*, 628–636. [CrossRef]

31. Mrowietz, U. Implementing treatment goals for successful long-term management of psoriasis. *JEADV* **2012**, *26* (Suppl. S2), 12–20. [CrossRef]
32. Wozel, G. Psoriasis treatment in difficult locations: Scalp, nails, and intertriginous areas. *Clin. Dermatol.* **2008**, *26*, 448–459. [CrossRef] [PubMed]
33. Van de Kerkhof, P.C.; Franssen, M.E. Psoriasis of the scalp. Diagnosis and management. *Am. J. Clin. Dermatol.* **2001**, *2*, 159–165. [CrossRef]
34. Farley, E.; Masrour, S.; McKey, J.; Menter, A. Palmoplantar psoriasis: A phenotypical and clinical review with introduction of a new quality-of-life assessment tool. *J. Am. Acad. Dermatol.* **2009**, *60*, 1024–1031. [CrossRef] [PubMed]
35. Reich, A.; Szepietowski, J.C. Health-related quality of life in patients with nail disorders. *Am. J. Clin. Dermatol.* **2011**, *12*, 313–320. [CrossRef] [PubMed]
36. Ryan, C.; Sadlier, M.; De Vol, E.; Patel, M.; Lloyd, A.A.; Day, A.; Lally, A.; Kirby, B.; Menter, A. Genital psoriasis is associated with significant impairment in quality of life and sexual functioning. *J. Am. Acad. Dermatol.* **2015**, *72*, 978–983. [CrossRef] [PubMed]
37. Sarma, N. Evidence and suggested therapeutic approach in psoriasis of difficult-to-treat areas: Palmoplantar psoriasis, nail psoriasis, scalp psoriasis, and Intertriginous psoriasis. *Indian J. Dermatol.* **2017**, *62*, 113–122. [CrossRef]
38. Egeberg, A.; See, K.; Garrelts, A.; Burge, R. Epidemiology of psoriasis in hard-to-treat body locations: Data from the Danish skin cohort. *BMC Dermatol.* **2020**, *20*, 3. [CrossRef] [PubMed]
39. Callis Duffin, K.; Mason, M.A.; Gordon, K.; Harrison, R.W.; Crabtree, M.M.; Guana, A.; Germino, R.; Lebwohl, M. Characterization of patients with psoriasis in challenging-to-treat body areas in the Corrona Psoriasis Registry. *Dermatology* **2021**, *237*, 46–55. [CrossRef]
40. Callis-Duffin, K.; Karki, C.; Mason, M.A.; Gordon, K.; Harrison, R.W.; Guana, A.; Gilloteau, I.; Herrra, V.; Lebwohl, M. Describing the clinical and patient reported outcomes of patients with scalp psoriasis enrolled in the Corrona Psoriasis Registry. *J. Am. Acad. Dermatol.* **2018**, *79*, AB105.
41. Callis-Duffin, K.; Karki, C.; Mason, M.A.; Gordon, K.; Harrison, R.W.; Guana, A.; Gilloteau, I.; Herrra, V.; Lebwohl, M. The burden of nail psoriasis: A real-world analysis from the Corrona Psoriasis Registry. *J. Am. Acad. Dermatol.* **2018**, *79*, AB283.
42. Duffin, K.C.; Herrera, V.; Mason, M.A.; Gordon, K.; Harrison, R.W.; Guana, A.; Gilloteau, I.; Karki, C.; Lebwohl, M. Impact of palmoplantar psoriasis on clinical and patient reported outcomes: Results from the Corrona Registry. *J. Am. Acad. Dermatol.* **2018**, *79*, AB159.
43. Mosca, M.; Hong, J.; Hadeler, E.; Brownstone, N.; Bhutani, T.; Liao, W. Scalp psoriasis: A literature review of effective therapies and updated recommendations for practical management. *Dermatol. Ther.* **2021**, *11*, 769–797. [CrossRef]
44. Arif, A.; Mahadi, I.D.R.; Yosi, A. Correlation between nail psoriasis severity index score with quality of life in nail psoriasis. *Bali Med. J.* **2021**, *10*, 256–260. [CrossRef]
45. Timotijević, Z.S.; Trajković, G.; Jankovic, J.; Relić, M.; Đorić, D.; Vukićević, D.; Relić, G.; Rašić, D.; Filipović, M.; Janković, S. How frequently does palmoplantar psoriasis affect the palms and/or soles? A systematic review and meta-analysis. *Adv. Dermatol. Allergol.* **2019**, *36*, 595–603. [CrossRef] [PubMed]
46. Kumar, B.; Saraswat, A.; Kaur, I. Palmoplantar lesions in psoriasis: A study of 3065 patients. *Acta Derm. Venereol.* **2002**, *82*, 192–195. [CrossRef]
47. Nast, A.; Smith, C.; Spuls, P.I.; Avila Valle, G.; Bata-Csörgö, Z.; Boonen, H.; De Jong, E.; Garcia-Doval, I.; Gisondi, P.; Kaur-Knudsen, D.; et al. EuroGuiDerm Guideline on the systemic treatment of Psoriasis vulgaris–Part 1: Treatment and monitoring recommendations. *JEADV* **2020**, *34*, 2461–2498. [CrossRef]
48. Mrowietz, U.; Steinz, K.; Gerdes, S. Psoriasis: To treat or to manage? *Exp. Dermatol.* **2014**, *23*, 705–709. [CrossRef]
49. Merola, J.F.; Abrar Qureshi, M.; Husni, E. Underdiagnosed and undertreated psoriasis: Nuances of treating psoriasis affecting the scalp, face, intertriginous areas, genitals, hands, feet, and nails. *Dermatol. Ther.* **2018**, *31*, e12589. [CrossRef] [PubMed]
50. Lakuta, P.; Marcinkiewicz, K.; Bergler-Czop, B.; Brzezinska-Wcislo, L.; Slomian, A. Associations between site of skin lesions and depression, social anxiety, body-related emotions and feelings of stigmatization in psoriasis patients. *Postepy Dermatol. Allergol.* **2018**, *35*, 60–66. [CrossRef] [PubMed]
51. Dopytalska, K.; Sobolewski, P.; Blaszczak, A.; Szymanska, E.; Walecka, I. Psoriasis in special localizations. *Reumatologia* **2018**, *56*, 392–398. [CrossRef]
52. Gordon, K.B.; Strober, B.; Lebwohl, M.; Augustin, M.; Blauvelt, A.; Poulin, Y.; Papp, K.A.; Sofen, H.; Puig, L.; Foley, P.; et al. Efficacy and safety of risankizumab in moderate-to-severe plaque psoriasis (UltIMMa-1 and UltIMMa-2): Results from two double-blind, randomised, placebo-controlled and ustekinumab-controlled phase 3 trials. *Lancet* **2018**, *392*, 651–661. [CrossRef] [PubMed]
53. Papp, K.; Thaçi, D.; Reich, K.; Riedl, E.; Langley, R.G.; Krueger, J.G.; Gottlieb, A.B.; Nakagawa, H.; Bowman, E.P.; Mehta, A.; et al. Tildrakizumab (MK3222), an anti-interleukin-23p19 monoclonal antibody, improves psoriasis in a phase IIb randomized placebo-controlled trial. *Br. J. Dermatol.* **2015**, *173*, 930–939. [CrossRef] [PubMed]
54. Blauvelt, A.; Papp, K.A.; Griffiths, C.E.; Randazzo, B.; Wasfi, Y.; Shen, Y.K.; Li, S.; Kimball, A.B. Efficacy and safety of guselkumab, an anti-interleukin-23 monoclonal antibody, compared with adalimumab for the continuous treatment of patients with moderate to severe psoriasis: Results from the phase III, double-blinded, placebo- and active comparator controlled VOYAGE 1 trial. *J. Am. Acad. Dermatol.* **2017**, *76*, 405–417. [PubMed]

55. Elewski, B.E.; Puig, L.; Mordin, M.; Gilloteau, I.; Sherif, B.; Fox, T.; Gnanasakthy, A.; Papavassilis, C.; Strober, B.E. Psoriasis patients with psoriasis Area and Severity Index (PASI) 90 response achieve greater health-related quality-of-life improvements than those with PASI 75-89 response: Results from two phase 3 studies of secukinumab. *J. Dermatol. Treat.* **2017**, *28*, 492–499. [CrossRef] [PubMed]
56. Carretero, G.; Puig, L.; Carrascosa, J.M.; Ferrándiz, L.; Ruiz-Villaverde, R.; de la Cueva, P.; Belinchon, I.; Vilarrasa, E.; Del Rio, R.; Spanish Group of Psoriasis; et al. Redefining the therapeutic objective in psoriatic patients' candidates for biological therapy. *J. Dermatol. Treat.* **2018**, *29*, 334–346. [CrossRef]
57. Lista Protocoalelor Terapeutice Aprobate Prin ORDINUL MS/CNAS NR 1462/347/2022—Valabila cu IUNIE 2022. Available online: https://cnas.ro/wp-content/uploads/2022/06/iunie.pdf (accessed on 10 October 2022).
58. Machado-Pinto, J.; Diniz Mdos, S.; Bavoso, N.C. Psoriasis: New comorbidities. *An. Bras. Dermatol.* **2016**, *91*, 8–16. [CrossRef] [PubMed]

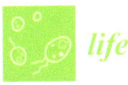

Case Report

Primary Cutaneous B-Cell Lymphoma Co-Existing with Mycosis Fungoides—A Case Report and Overview of the Literature

Doriana Sorina Chilom [1], Simona Sorina Farcaș [2,*] and Nicoleta Ioana Andreescu [2]

1. Department of Dermatology, University of Medicine and Pharmacy "Victor Babeș", Eftimie Murgu Sq. no.2, 300041 Timisoara, Romania
2. Department of Microscopic Morphology—Genetics, Center of Genomic Medicine, University of Medicine and Pharmacy "Victor Babes", Eftimie Murgu Sq. no.2, 300041 Timisoara, Romania
* Correspondence: farcas.simona@umft.ro

Abstract: The existence of two sequential lymphomas, one localized and one systemic, either both with B or T lymphocytes, or one with B cells and one with T cells, with the same patient, is a known possibility. The second lymphoma is often induced by immunodepression or by the initial treatment. However, the existence of two cutaneous lymphomas with different cell lines, without systemic involvement, represents an uncommon situation. In this report, we describe the case of a 37-year-old man with an initial diagnosis of PMZBCL that over 10 months also developed a MF patch/plaque on the left leg.

Keywords: B-cell lymphoma; Mycosis Fungoides; composite lymphomas; primary cutaneous lymphoma

1. Introduction

Primary cutaneous lymphomas (PCLs) are a group of T- and B-cell lymphomas that affect the cutaneous tissue without involving other organs at the time of diagnosis. PCLs are defined as non-Hodgkin lymphomas presenting in the skin with no evidence of extracutaneous disease at the time of diagnosis. The prevalence of PCL is of around 0.90/100,000 inhabitants in Europe and the USA [1]. Out of the total number of PCL, those with T-lymphocytes are the most common. In Western Europe, Primary cutaneous T-cell lymphomas (PCTCLs) represent about 75–80% of PCLs, while B-cell lymphomas (CBCLs) represent only 20–25% [2].

The most common type of PCTCLs is Mycosis Fungoides (MF), about 39% of PCTCL [2], and represents a proliferation of small to medium T-lymphocytes with hyper convoluted cerebriform nuclei. The risk factors for MF are male sex, advanced age and black race. MF develops from peripheral epidermotropic lymphocytes, which immunophenotype is positive for CD2, CD3, CD4 and CD5 and negative for CD8 and CD7 [3].

Primary marginal zone b-cell lymphoma (PMZBCL) is a rare disease, included in the group of extranodal marginal zone lymphoma of mucosa-associated lymphoid tissue (MALT). It is a low-grade malignant B-cell lymphoma that disseminates exceptionally and has a 5-year survival rate of 95% [4,5]. Immunohistochemically, the marginal zone cellular population is positive for CD20 and Bcl2, while the reactive germinal centers are positive for Bcl6, CD10 and negative for Bcl2 [6].

PCLs are extranodal non-Hodgkin lymphomas with broad clinical, histological, phenotypic, genetic, and prognostic spectrums. Therefore, it is necessary to collaborate in a large team of dermatologists, hematologists, pathologists, oncologists, radiotherapists and other specialists in order to obtain an accurate diagnosis and a targeted and personalized treatment. Even though CTCLs are a common lymphoproliferation in malignant skin pathology, the existence of CTCLs and CBCLs at the same time is a rare situation, with few cases being cited.

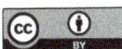

The coexistence of two lymphomas at a single anatomical site, is defined as composite lymphomas (CL). Immunohistochemical and genetic analyses have revealed that some types of lymphomas, classified as CL, represent the morphological manifestation of the same neoplastic clones. So, the presence of two lymphomas with different neoplastic cells, could represent a coexistence of them, without a proven association between the two lymphomas [7].

The aim of this study is to present a rare case of PMZBCL coexisting with MF plaque stage on a 37-year-old patient. The diagnosis of the two cutaneous lymphomas was based on the histopathological and immunohistochemical examination, and their primary character was established by excluding the involvement of other organs, except the skin.

2. Case Report

A 37-year-old man was evaluated at the University Dermatology Department of the Timisoara Municipal Emergency Hospital for a 5-year history of a non-itchy, papulo-erythematous plaque of 2–3.5 cm with a shiny surface on the antero-lateral part of the lower left leg, thus suggesting a granulomatous structure (Figure 1). The lesion appeared after mild, repeated traumas and began to grow in size in recent months. At the general clinical examination, the patient had a good general condition without palpable superficial adenopathy. Complete blood count and blood biochemistry (Serum creatinine, Alkaline phosphatase, GT Gamma, Blood glucose, TGO/AST, TGP/ALT, Serum urea) showed normal values, abdominal ultrasound and chest X-ray showed no pathological changes and the Mantoux test was negative. Following the first examination, the suspicion of cutaneous sarcoidosis with non-specific lesions was raised and treatment with topical corticoid of medium potency was initiated. There was no improvement after two weeks of topical treatment and so it was decided to perform a biopsy incision with histopathological examination.

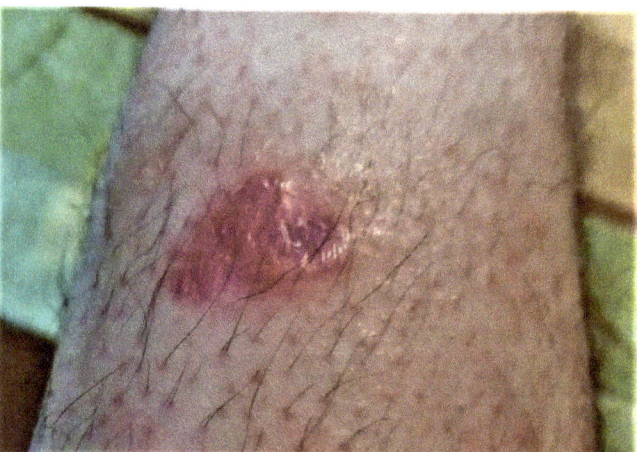

Figure 1. Primary marginal zone B-cell Lymphoma on the antero-lateral part of the lower left leg; purple–red plaque with shiny surface.

Histopathological (Figure 2) examination revealed ortokeratinized epidermis, hyalinization of the dermo-epidermal junction and flattening of the epidermal ridges. Papillary and deep dermis presented lymphoid proliferation with follicular and diffuse pattern that dissected the fascia of collagen fibers with periadnexial and perifollicular disposition. Lymphoid proliferation is composed of lymphoblasts, lymphocytes of centrocyte type-like with irregular nucleus and dense chromatin, quantitatively reduced cytoplasm, small lymphocytes, rare plasma cells, rare immunoblasts and very rare eosinophilic granulocytes. In different areas, the subcutaneous adipose tissue presented lymphoid infiltrates.

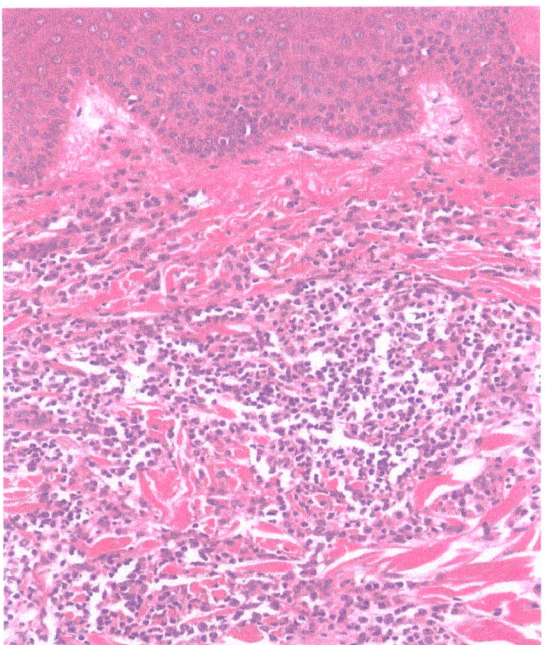

Figure 2. Primary marginal zone B-cell Lymphoma, Hematoxylin & Eosin stain, Ob ×20.

Immunohistochemistry (Table 1) revealed CD20-intense membrane immunoreaction in B-lymphocytes with nodular and focal interfollicular organization; Bcl2—intense cytoplasmic immunoreaction in B-lymphocytes in follicular and interfollicular areas, plasmocytes have clonal character (kappa/lambda ratio >10/1), positive for CD138, negative tumor proliferation for Bcl6 (positive in the remnants of reactive germination centers), negative for CD3 and the proliferation index measured by Ki67 was 10%. Based on these findings the diagnosis was B-cell lymphoma of the marginal area with immunophenotype CD20 positive (Figure 3a), Bcl2 positive (Figure 3b), and Ki67 = 10%.

To confirm the primitive cutaneous character of the proliferation, interdisciplinary consults and additional investigations were performed. The CT for abdomen-thorax-pelvis using contrast substance showed no thoraco-abdomino-pelvic secondary determinations and no adenopathy in the examined segments. Gastroscopy and colonoscopy presented a normal appearance; Osteo-medullary biopsy and aspirated medullary revealed medullary lymphocytes within normal limits and IgG and IgM for Borrelia were negative. Diagnosis of primary cutaneous lymphoma with B cells of the marginal area was established according to the data.

The patient received curative local radiotherapy using a Total dose = 40 gray/20 fractions (TD = 40Gy/20 fr). The treatment was well-tolerated.

After ten months from the initial diagnosis of primary cutaneous B-cell lymphoma of the marginal area, the patient returned to the dermatology clinic due to the appearance of a new plaque on the right inguinal fold (Figure 4). The plaque had an erythematous-squamous appearance, with slightly indurated well-defined edges and absent local itching or pain. The onset was reported about two months after minor trauma. The lesion has a tendency for superficial spread on the surface.

Table 1. Immunophenotypic features for the case presented.

Immunophenotypic Features of PMZBCL on the Antero-Lateral Antero-Lateral Part of the Lower Left Leg		Immunophenotypic Features of MF Plaque at the Right Inguinal Fold		Immunophenotypic Features of PMZBCL on the Lateral Part of the Left Forefoot	
Ki67	10%	Ki67	20%	Ki67	10–20%
CD20	positive	CD20	negative	CD20	positive
Bcl2	positive	Bcl2	negative	Bcl2	positive
CD3	negative	CD3	positive	CD3	positive
κ/λ	>10/1	CD4	positive	CD4	ND
CD5	negative	CD5	positive	CD5	negative
CD10	negative	CD7	negative	CD10	negative
CD23	negative	CD8	negative	CD23	negative
Bcl6	negative	Bcl6	negative	Bcl6	negative
CD138	positive	TCR βF1	negative	CD138	positive
		TCR γδ	negative	IgG	positive
		CD10	positive	IgA	negative
		CD56	negative	IgD	negative
		CD79	positive		
		Cyclin D1	positive		
		CD30	negative	IgM	negative

ND = not done, MF = Mycosis Fungoides, PMZBCL = Primary marginal zone B-cell Lymphoma, κ/λ = kappa/lambda ratio, TCR βF1 = T-cell receptor beta F1, TCR γδ = T-cell receptor gamma-delta.

A histopathological examination (Figure 5) was conducted that revealed superficial infiltration with small to medium-sized atypical lymphatic cells showing epidermotropism arranged in patches with "string of pearls" distribution along the junctional zone, under a regularly maturing ortokeratotic epidermis. There was no development of Pautrier microabscesses. Cells showed irregularly shaped, partially cerebriform hyperchromatic nuclei and sparse cytoplasm.

The immunohistochemical test (Table 1) revealed strong CD3 (Figure 6a), CD4 (Figure 6b) and CD5 expression with almost complete CD30 negativity and complete negativity for CD8, CD56, T-cell receptor betaF1, T-cell receptor gamma-delta and a complete antigen loss for CD7. In the CD20 stain, only extremely sparse small B-lymphocytes were found. The tumor cells were negative for Bcl2 and Bcl6. The lymphoid cells were positive for CD10, and just some of them were positive for CD79 and Cyclin D1. The proliferation activity index measured by Ki67 was 20%. The edges of the excision showed free tissue. The histopathological diagnosis was early MF.

After another 3 months from the diagnosis of MF in the patch/plaque stage, the patient developed another well-defined 5 × 3 cm oval erythematous plaque located on the lateral part of the left forefoot. No other general or local symptomatology was reported. The excision of the plaque was performed with the application of a graft of healthy skin tissue taken from the inguinal area.

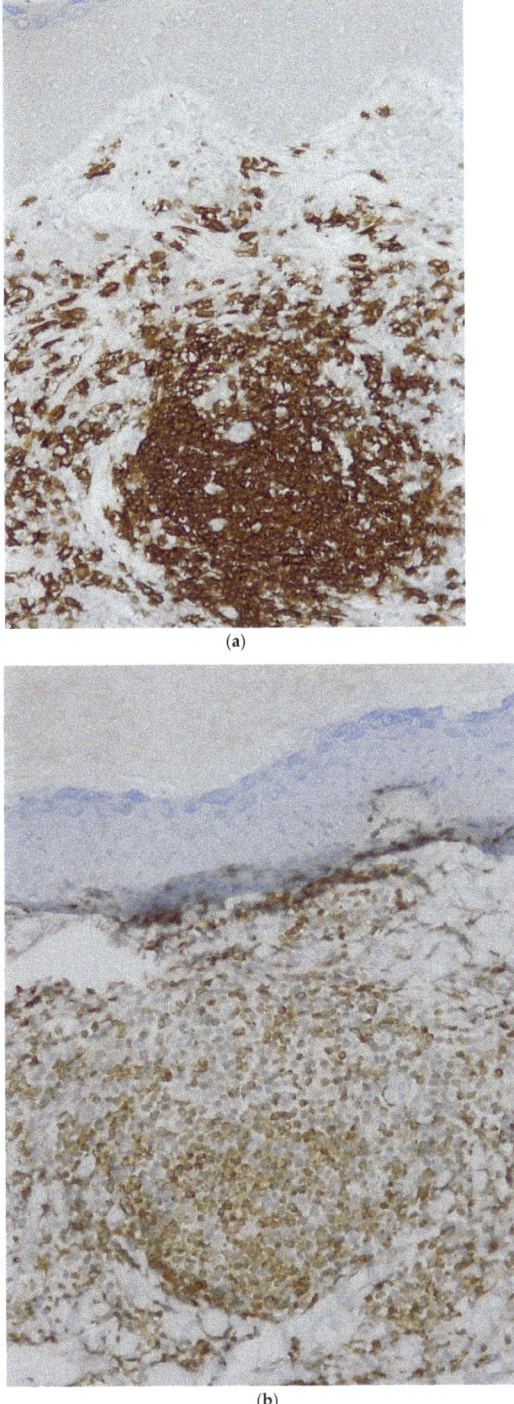

Figure 3. (**a**): Primary marginal zone B-cell Lymphoma, CD20 Ob ×20. (**b**): Primary marginal zone B-cell Lymphoma, Bcl-2, Ob ×20.

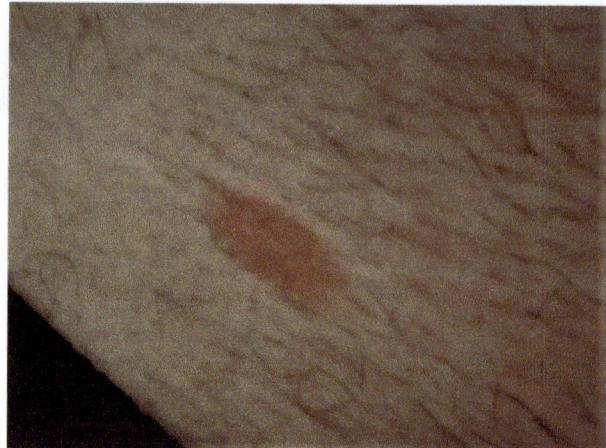

Figure 4. Mycosis Fungoides plaque at the right inguinal fold; oval erythematous and indurated plaque, with a fine scales surface.

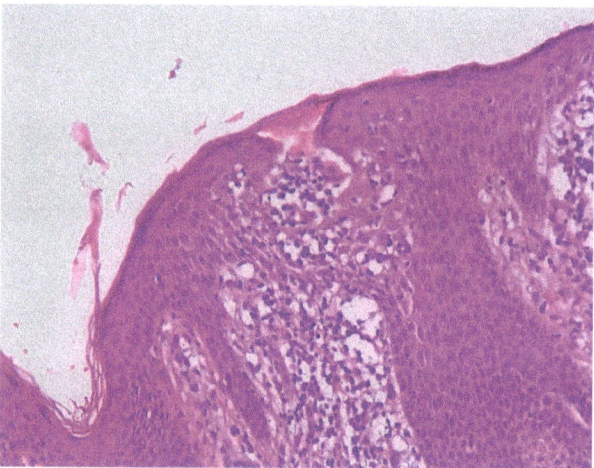

Figure 5. Mycosis Fungoides, Hematoxylin & Eosin stain, Ob ×20.

Immunohistochemical examination (Table 1): infiltrated cells are consistently positive for CD20, Bcl2 with simultaneous negativity for CD5, CD10, CD23 and Bcl6, high-proliferation physiological activity (ki-67) about 10% to 20%. In CD10 and Bcl6 staining the residual partially populated germ centers emerge, which are also physiologically negative for Bcl2. The germinal centers are based on partially compact and partially fragmented networks of follicular dendritic cells (CD23). Moderately abundant CD138-positive plasma cells without light chain restriction clearly detectable in light chain staining and a continuous positivity for IgG, with simultaneous negativity for IgA, IgD and IgM are present around the nodes. In IgD and IgM staining, mantle cells surrounding partially present residual germinal centers are revealed. The results indicate dermal-epidermal tissue (of the left foot) with infiltration by indolent non-Hodgkin lymphoma of the B-cell variety—especially around the marginal zone—compatible with a primary cutaneous marginal zone lymphoma.

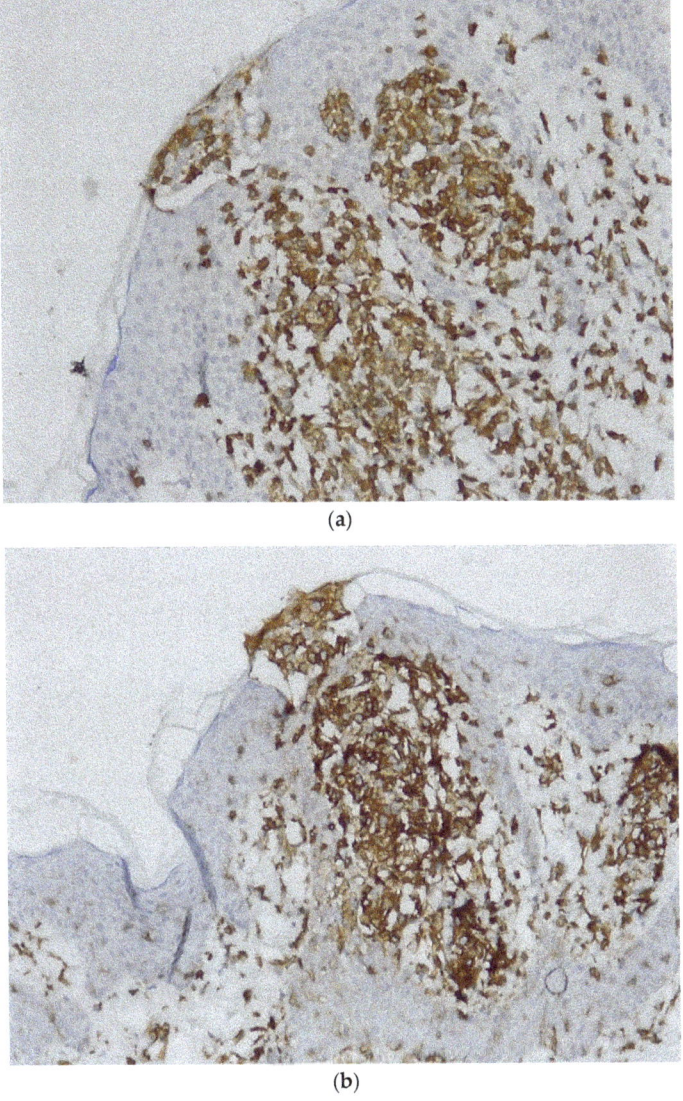

Figure 6. (**a**): Mycosis Fungoides, CD3, Ob ×20. (**b**): Mycosis Fungoides, CD4, Ob ×20.

3. Treatment

The patient performed radiotherapy for PMZBCL, located on the antero-lateral part of the lower left leg (DT = 40Gy/20fr on linear ACC with 6MV. Irradiation was well tolerated). The other two lesions, MF located at the right inguinal fold and the PMZBCL located on the lateral part of the left forefoot, were excised with negative safety margins. The skin healed without local relapse. The patient is still continuously monitored in dermatological, hematological and oncological services to ensure early diagnosis of relapsing lesions.

4. Discussion

Composite lymphomas (CL) are a combination of either two different B-cell lymphomas, two different T-cell lymphomas, or one B-cell lymphoma and one T-cell lymphoma that develop at a single tissue site simultaneously. The development of CL could be caused by chemotherapeutic agents, immunological defects or autoimmune diseases (Sjögren's syndrome, primary or acquired immunodeficiencies, and autoimmune lymphoproliferative syndrome) [8].

The incidence of CL is between 1% and 4.7%, and the most common associated lymphomas are two Non-Hodgkin B-cell Lymphomas, or a Non-Hodgkin B-cell lymphoma with a Hodgkin lymphoma. CL that associates T-cell lymphomas with B-cell lymphomas are rare, their location is frequently in the lymph nodes or lymphoid organs, and only rarely involve non-lymphoid organs [9].

Several mechanisms were proposed for explaining the occurrence of composite lymphomas with one being an immune deficiency secondary to an Epstein–Barr viral (EBV) infection [10]. There were several cases reported for which a EBV infection was documented, but there are also cases where the EBV infection was lacking, suggesting that other mechanisms can be involved in the development of CL [10–13]. For the case presented here, EBV infection was excluded by performing IgM and IgG serology for Epstein–Barr virus.

The appearance of a lymphoma or a new form of cancer in a patient treated for a pre-existing malignancy is a known possibility. The main cause is immunosuppression induced by the first malignancy or by its treatment. Herrmann & Sami reported a case of a 54-year-old man diagnosed with diffuse large B-cell lymphoma (DLBCL) on his right knee. A cutaneous T-cell lymphoma (CTCL MF-type) was diagnosed shortly after. The patient also had an ongoing symptomatic history of psoriasiform dermatitis starting 15 years prior, which the authors considered to represent the newly diagnosed MF. The patient received local radiation treatment for DLBCL and chemotherapy for CTCL. Shortly thereafter, he developed a tumor on the radiotherapy area that turned out to be CTLC type rather than a recurrent B-cell lymphoma [14]. In the case we are reporting, the patient received only radiotherapy, and the MF developed in a different area than the irradiated one.

A meta-analysis study which analyzed the risk for second malignancies in non-Hodgkin's lymphoma survivors concluded that patients with non-Hodgkin's lymphoma have a higher risk for a second malignancy than the general population even after controlling for treatment for non-Hodgkin's lymphoma (chemotherapeutic drugs, radiotherapy, combined-modality approaches including conventional-dose chemotherapy with radiotherapy or with total body irradiation) [15]. Multiple cases of association of non-Hodgkin lymphomas with other types of lymphomas have been reported over time [16,17], but the simultaneous presence of two cutaneous lymphomas is an unusual situation. However, the appearance of the second lymphoma occurs a few years after the first diagnosis [18]. Radiation therapy can also induce a second malignancy, but this risk is not clearly quantified, and it is assumed that it occurs after a long period of time [19].

In our case, the patient developed MF ten months after the first diagnosis of B-cell lymphoma (located on the antero-lateral part of the lower left leg). It is a small possibility that MF to be caused by the radiation therapy performed to treat PMZBCL, given the short period of occurrence of the second cutaneous lymphoma. In addition, the appearance of a cutaneous lymphoma due to local radiation therapy, occurs in the area where the radiation therapy was applied.

In regard to prognosis, most CL have an aggressive clinical course, and little data is available about treatment options and their outcomes [12]. A recent study reported a recovery rate of 60% when using a protocol including rituximab, cyclophosphamide, doxorubicin, vincristine, prednisone (R-CHOP) [20]. The patient presented here, followed the local curative radiotherapy for PMZBCL located on the antero-lateral part of the lower left leg, and the lesions of MF and the second PMZBCL, were excised within safety limits, without the need for another associated therapy.

5. Conclusions

This case report presents a case of PMZBCL followed 10 months later by the appearance of MF, and another 3 months later by a new lesion of PMZBCL, which is an unusual association. The CD20, Bcl2 with simultaneous negativity for CD5, CD10, CD23 and Bcl6 is the immunohistochemical profile for PMZBCL. The cutaneous lymphoid infiltration in small/medium T cell, diffuse positive for CD3, CD4 and CD5 with simultaneous almost complete negativity for CD30 and complete negativity for CD8, CD56, T-cell receptor betaF1, T-cell receptor gamma-delta and a complete antigen loss for CD7 revealed an MF diagnosis. Analyzing these data, we consider that these two cutaneous lymphomas coexist, with no direct connection between them. This requires a detailed genetic and molecular investigations to assess the oncogenic status and to exclude overlapping diagnoses.

Author Contributions: Conceptualization, D.S.C. and N.I.A.; writing—original draft preparation, D.S.C.; writing—review and editing, N.I.A. and S.S.F.; supervision, N.I.A. All authors have read and agreed to the published version of the manuscript.

Funding: This research received no external funding.

Institutional Review Board Statement: Not applicable.

Informed Consent Statement: Informed consent was obtained from all subjects involved in the study. Written informed consent has been obtained from the patient to publish this paper.

Acknowledgments: We would like to thank the medical personal from Bioclinica for their help with the histopathological examination.

Conflicts of Interest: The authors declare no conflict of interest.

References

1. Vermeer, M. Epidemiology of cutaneous lymphoma. *Br. J. Dermatol.* **2021**, *184*, 993–994. [CrossRef] [PubMed]
2. Willemze, R.; Cerroni, L.; Kempf, W.; Berti, E.; Facchetti, F.; Swerdlow, S.H.; Jaffe, E.S. The 2018 update of the WHO-EORTC classification for primary cutaneous lymphomas. *Blood* **2019**, *133*, 1703–1714. [CrossRef] [PubMed]
3. Yamashita, T.; Abbade, L.P.; Marques, M.E.; Marques, S.A. Mycosis fungoides and Sézary syndrome: Clinical, histopathological and immunohistochemical review and update. *An. Bras. Dermatol.* **2012**, *87*, 817–828; quiz 829–830. [CrossRef] [PubMed]
4. Hristov, A.C.; Tejasvi, T.; Wilcox, R.A. Cutaneous B-cell lymphomas: 2021 update on diagnosis, risk-stratification, and management. *Am. J. Hematol.* **2020**, *95*, 1209–1213. [CrossRef] [PubMed]
5. Hoefnagel, J.J.; Vermeer, M.H.; Jansen, P.M.; Heule, F.; van Voorst Vader, P.C.; Sanders, C.J.; Gerritsen, M.J.; Geerts, M.L.; Meijer, C.J.; Noordijk, E.M.; et al. Primary Cutaneous Marginal Zone B-Cell Lymphoma: Clinical and Therapeutic Features in 50 Cases. *Arch. Dermatol.* **2005**, *141*, 1139–1145. [CrossRef] [PubMed]
6. Ronchi, A.; Sica, A.; Vitiello, P.; Franco, R. Dermatological Considerations in the Diagnosis and Treatment of Marginal Zone Lymphomas. *Clin. Cosmet. Investig. Dermatol.* **2021**, *14*, 231–239. [CrossRef] [PubMed]
7. Chen, S.; Boyer, D.; Hristov, A.C. Primary Cutaneous Composite Lymphomas. *Arch. Pathol. Lab. Med.* **2018**, *142*, 1352–1357. [CrossRef] [PubMed]
8. Steinhoff, M.; Assaf, C.; Anagnostopoulos, I.; Geilen, C.C.; Stein, H.; Hummel, M. Three coexisting lymphomas in one patient: Genetically related or only a coincidence? *J. Clin. Pathol.* **2006**, *59*, 1312–1315. [CrossRef] [PubMed]
9. Szablewski, V.; Costes-Martineau, V.; René, C.; Croci-Torti, A.; Joujoux, J.-M. Composite cutaneous lymphoma of diffuse large B-cell lymphoma-leg type and subcutaneous panniculitis-like T-cell lymphoma. *J. Cutan. Pathol.* **2018**, *45*, 716–720. [CrossRef] [PubMed]
10. Gui, W.; Wang, J.; Ma, L.; Wang, Y.; Su, L. Clinicopathological analysis of composite lymphoma: A two-case report and literature review. *Open Med.* **2020**, *15*, 654–658. [CrossRef] [PubMed]
11. Suefuji, N.; Niino, D.; Arakawa, F.; Karube, K.; Kimura, Y.; Kiyasu, J.; Takeuchi, M.; Miyoshi, H.; Yoshida, M.; Ichikawa, A.; et al. Clinicopathological analysis of a composite lymphoma containing both T- and B-cell lymphomas. *Pathol. Int.* **2012**, *62*, 690–698. [CrossRef] [PubMed]
12. Wang, E.; Papavassiliou, P.; Wang, A.R.; Louissaint, A., Jr.; Wang, J.; Hutchinson, C.B.; Huang, Q.; Reddi, D.; Wei, Q.; Sebastian, S.; et al. Composite lymphoid neoplasm of B-cell and T-cell origins: A pathologic study of 14 cases. *Hum. Pathol.* **2014**, *45*, 768–784. [CrossRef] [PubMed]
13. Papalas, J.A.; Puri, P.K.; Sebastian, S.; Wang, E. Primary cutaneous, composite, Epstein-Barr virus-associated, diffuse large B-cell lymphoma and peripheral T-cell lymphoma. *Am. J. Dermatopathol.* **2011**, *33*, 719–725. [CrossRef]
14. Herrmann, J.L.; Sami, N. Large-Cell Transformation of Mycosis Fungoides Occurring at the Site of Previously Treated Cutaneous B-Cell Lymphoma. *Clin. Lymphoma Myeloma Leuk.* **2014**, *14*, e43–e46. [CrossRef]
15. Pirani, M.; Marcheselli, R.; Marcheselli, L.; Bari, A.; Federico, M.; Sacchi, S. Risk for second malignancies in non-Hodgkin's lymphoma survivors: A meta-analysis. *Ann. Oncol.* **2011**, *22*, 1845–1858. [CrossRef] [PubMed]
16. Chang, T.W.; Weaver, A.L.; Shanafelt, T.D.; Habermann, T.M.; Wriston, C.C.; Cerhan, J.R.; Call, T.G.; Brewer, J.D. Risk of cutaneous T-cell lymphoma in patients with chronic lymphocytic leukemia and other subtypes of non-Hodgkin lymphoma. *Int. J. Dermatol.* **2017**, *56*, 1125–1129. [CrossRef] [PubMed]

17. Miyagaki, T.; Sugaya, M.; Minatani, Y.; Fujita, H.; Hangaishi, A.; Kurokawa, M.; Takazawa, Y.; Tamaki, K. Mycosis Fungoides with Recurrent Hodgkin's Lymphoma and Diffuse Large B-cell Lymphoma. *Acta Derm. Venereol.* **2009**, *89*, 421–422. [CrossRef] [PubMed]
18. Barzilai, A.; Trau, H.; David, M.; Feinmesser, M.; Bergman, R.; Shpiro, D.; Schiby, G.; Rosenblatt, K.; Or, R.; Hodak, E. Mycosis fungoides associated with B-cell malignancies. *Br. J. Dermatol.* **2006**, *155*, 379–386. [CrossRef] [PubMed]
19. Braunstein, S.; Nakamura, J. Radiotherapy-Induced Malignancies: Review of Clinical Features, Pathobiology, and Evolving Approaches for Mitigating Risk. *Front. Oncol.* **2013**, *3*, 73. [CrossRef] [PubMed]
20. Esper, A.; Alhoulaiby, S.; Zuhri Yafi, R.; Alshehabi, Z. Composite lymphoma of T-cell rich, histiocyte-rich diffuse large B-cell lymphoma and nodular lymphocyte predominant Hodgkin lymphoma: A case report. *J. Med. Case Rep.* **2021**, *15*, 163. [CrossRef] [PubMed]

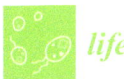

Systematic Review

Erosive Pustular Dermatosis: Delving into Etiopathogenesis and Management

Shashank Bhargava [1], Sara Yumeen [2], Esther Henebeng [2] and George Kroumpouzos [2,*]

1. Department of Dermatology, R.D. Gardi Medical College and C.R. Gardi Hospital, Ujjain 456006, India
2. Department of Dermatology, Warren Alpert Medical School, Brown University, Providence, RI 02903, USA
* Correspondence: gk@gkderm.com

Abstract: Erosive pustular dermatosis (EPD) is a chronic inflammatory skin disorder that usually affects mature individuals. It predominantly affects the scalp and can lead to scarring alopecia. Risk factors include actinic damage and androgenetic alopecia. A traumatic insult to the skin is considered a vital trigger of the condition. EPD is a diagnosis of exclusion; thus, several neoplastic, infectious, vesiculobullous, and inflammatory conditions should be ruled out. Biopsy and clinicopathologic correlation are required to differentiate between EPD and these entities. A dysregulated, chronic immune response is considered central to the etiopathogenesis of EPD. We performed an evidence-based systematic review of the management options. There were predominantly studies with level IV and V evidence and only two with level III. Despite the responsiveness of EPD to potent topical steroids, such as clobetasol propionate, recurrence occurs after treatment withdrawal. With the available data, tacrolimus 0.1%, curettage-assisted aminolevulinic acid-photodynamic therapy, and systemic retinoids can be considered second-line options for EPD with a role in maintenance regimens. However, controlled data and more powerful studies are needed to make solid recommendations.

Keywords: erosive pustular dermatosis; etiopathogenesis; differential diagnosis; management; treatment; therapy; corticosteroids

1. Introduction

The first case of erosive pustular dermatosis (EPD) was reported by Dr. Burton in 1977 [1]. Two years later, Pye et al. reported six elderly women "who developed chronic, extensive, pustular, crusted and occasionally eroded scalp lesions which produced scarring alopecia. Investigations were essentially negative, and skin biopsies showed only nonspecific atrophy and chronic inflammation changes. The condition did not respond to antibiotics but was suppressed by potent topical steroids" [2]. Since then, the etiopathogenesis of EPD has been poorly elucidated, and the management of the condition remains suboptimal. In this article, we focus on these aspects.

2. Epidemiology

The incidence is unknown, with fewer than 200 cases reported [3–5]. Paton and colleagues challenged that the condition is rare by reporting 11 cases in a small region over three years [6]. These authors concurred that the condition is not uncommon and indicated that underreporting may be due to misdiagnosis [7,8]. A female predominance is observed (female-to-male ratio of 2:1) [4,9], but a recent systematic review found that men are more frequently affected [5]. EPD has a mean age of onset of 60 to 70 years and has been reported from infancy to 95 years [6,10]. The median age of onset of 76 years was reported [5]. In a series of 50 patients, the average disease duration at diagnosis was 26 months (range, 3–144 months) [11]. Geographic or racial distribution has not been demonstrated [4]. EPD commonly develops in individuals with sun-damaged skin and androgenetic alopecia [7,12].

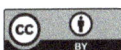

3. Clinical Presentation

The scalp is commonly involved, but the condition has also been reported on the face and legs [11,13]. The vertex is the most affected location, followed by the scalp's frontal, parietal, and temporal regions [12]. On examination, there are crusts and erosions (Figure 1A,B) and varying numbers of pustules on a background of atrophic skin [4]. The epidermis is easily detachable with forceps, and when removed, copious purulent exudate is exposed underneath (Figure 1B) [7,14]. Lesions are typically asymptomatic; however, pain, burning, or pruritus in the affected areas may develop [4]. These erosions typically develop over several months or years and, without improvement, can cause cicatricial alopecia (Figure 1C), skin atrophy, and telangiectasia [7].

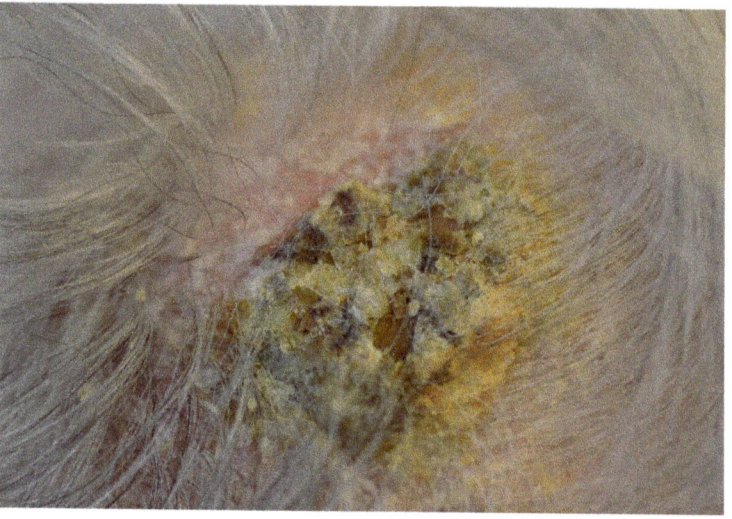

(A)

Figure 1. *Cont.*

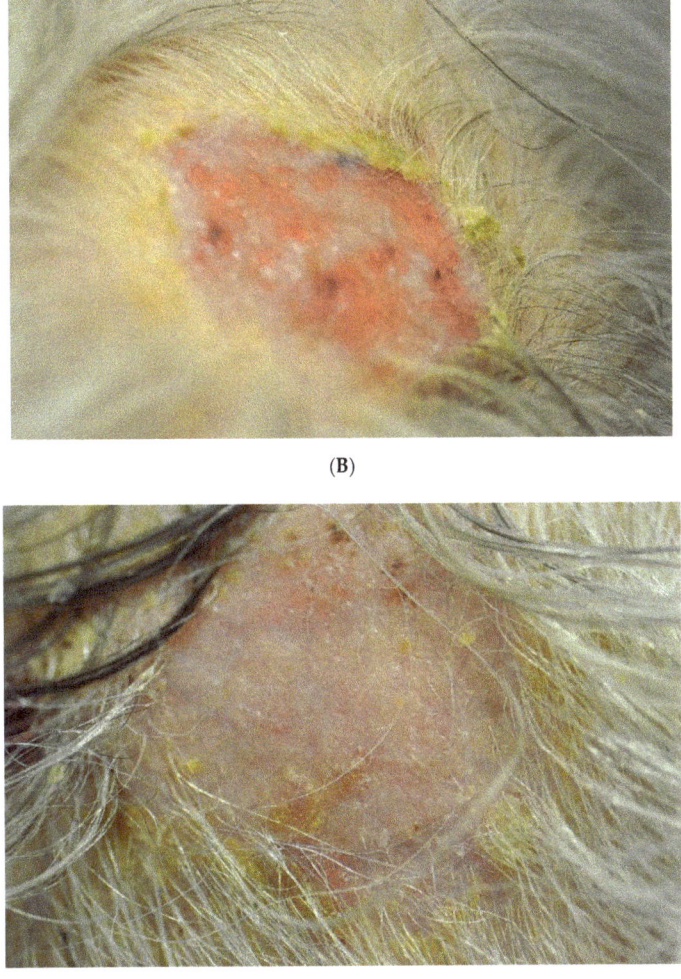

Figure 1. Female patient in her 80s with EPD of the scalp. (**A**), crusted plaques can show massive hyperkeratosis. (**B**), a large superficial erosion partially covered by purulent exudate; such exudate is noted when uplifting the crusts with forceps. (**C**), an area of scarring alopecia developed at the later stages of EPD.

4. Laboratory Investigations

There are no specific serologic findings. The erythrocyte sedimentation rate was elevated and seemed to correlate with disease activity in a small sample; however, the C-reactive protein was normal [14]. Cultures of the exudate are typically sterile or may grow normal skin flora [3]. However, patients can develop secondary superinfection with *Staphylococcus aureus*, *Pseudomonas*, or *Candida* species [14]. Appropriate bacteriologic and mycologic investigations are required when infection is suspected.

4.1. Histology

Two biopsies from an active area with intact hair follicles are required to rule out other scalp diseases. Specimens should be sent for histological analysis and immunofluorescent examination to rule out autoimmune blistering conditions [3]. The histopathologic findings vary depending on the lesion type and disease duration [15]. In the early stage (EPD lasting less than 1 year), the epidermis is hyperkeratotic (orthokeratosis and parakeratosis are both reported), and the papillary dermis shows a slightly mixed inflammatory infiltrate [12]. In the intermediate stage (EPD lasting 1–2 years), findings include squamous crusts, ortokeratosis, parakeratosis, psoriasiform epidermal hyperplasia, moderate mixed inflammatory infiltrate, extensive fibrosis, and reduced numbers of hairs and sebaceous glands. In the late stage (EPD lasting more than 2 years), the epidermis becomes more atrophic, the dermis becomes fibrotic, there are only "remainders" or a complete absence of hair follicles and sebaceous glands, and a slight mixed infiltrate [12].

Two types of pathologic changes have been identified: specific and nonspecific [11]. Infundibular spongiotic pustules are a characteristic finding; they are mostly observed in hair-bearing areas in patients with mild-to-moderate alopecia. Nonspecific changes have been noted in 78% of cases and include epidermal atrophy with pustulation and dermal scarring, epidermal thickening with subepidermal clefting, scarred dermis and perifollicular granulomas with remnants of hair shafts and multinucleated giant cells, and epidermal erosion with foci of pustulation and underlying granulation tissue [11]. Nonspecific histopathologic findings were the most common in patients with severe androgenetic alopecia or total baldness.

In the dermis, there is a mixed inflammatory infiltrate of neutrophils, lymphocytes, plasma cells, and foreign body giant cells [3,14]. Based on the finding of spongiotic vesiculopustules affecting the follicular infundibula, Tomasini and colleagues considered EPD of the scalp a neutrophilic superficial folliculitis [15]. Reschke et al. observed neutrophils mostly around ulcerations and suggested that the finding of plasma cells in the dermal infiltrate is the most characteristic feature of EPS [14]; however, the plasma cell predominance needs confirmation. Stains for microorganisms are negative [15].

4.2. Trichoscopy

Trichoscopy is of limited use in the diagnosis of EPD because its findings are related to hair cycle change, inflammation, and scarring alopecia, and most of them can be found in other scalp disorders. Such findings include hair shaft tortuosity, tapering hair, milky red areas, white patches, follicular keratotic plugging, and the absence of follicular openings. A unique tracheoscopy feature of EPD is the visualization of prominent telangiectasias, especially after detachment of the serous or pigmented crust. Additionally, other notable findings include enlarged dermal vessels or anagen bulbs on atrophic skin [3]. Severe atrophy allowing visualization of hair follicle bulbs through the epidermis and enlarged dermal vessels, erosions, and crusts, may elevate the index of suspicion and be useful in differentiating EPD of the scalp from other scarring alopecias [11].

5. Differential Diagnosis

Establishing an EPD diagnosis can be challenging because the condition has a clinical presentation that can mimic numerous other conditions [16]. EPD is a diagnosis of exclusion; thus, several neoplastic, infectious, vesiculobullous, and inflammatory conditions should be ruled out. Biopsy and clinicopathologic correlation are required to distinguish between EPD and these entities. Neoplastic conditions, such as field cancerization and nonmelanoma skin cancer (NMSC), including squamous cell carcinoma and basal cell carcinoma, should be considered when evaluating very hyperkeratotic or shiny papules in areas of actinic damage on the scalp [16]. As indicated by the group of Kroumpouzos, NMSC should be considered when crusted plaques become nodular and/or grow substantially within a relatively short period of time or erosions persist and/or become larger [17]. Cultures can exclude infections such as Gram-negative folliculitis, tinea capitis, and kerion celsi [12].

Vesiculobullous conditions such as subcorneal pustular dermatosis, pemphigus vegetans, and cicatricial pemphigoid should be considered and require appropriate laboratory investigation. Inflammatory conditions, such as eczema, pustular psoriasis, superficial pyoderma gangrenosum, and chronic vegetating pyoderma, should be considered. Pustular

PG, a rare variant of PG, is characterized by sterile, sometimes folliculocentric pustules on an erythematous base, most frequently involving the extremities and trunk, and occasionally the scalp, but these lesions do not develop into frank ulcerations and often heal without scarring. Other causes of cicatricial alopecia, such as discoid lupus erythematosus, lichen planopilaris, folliculitis decalvans, and folliculitis et perifolliculitis abscedens et suffodiens, may present similarly to EPD [16,18]. In addition, in cases showing erosions with geometric borders, factitial conditions such as dermatitis artefacta may be considered. Lastly, drug-induced EPD should be considered in patients receiving targeted therapies for cancer, such as gefitinib [19].

6. Etiopathogenesis

While the etiopathogenesis of EPD remains to be fully elucidated, clues may be obtained from the classic clinical course and histopathology of the condition. These observations suggest four key factors that may lead to the development of EPD: a predisposing environment on the scalp, including skin atrophy, actinic damage, and androgenetic alopecia; an initial inciting trauma or damage; resultant dysregulated, chronic immune response; culmination in fibrosis, atrophy, and scarring alopecia [6,12,20]. These key factors and possible mechanisms involved are discussed below.

6.1. Predisposing Factors

EPDS commonly occurs on the scalp in areas of actinic damage, skin atrophy, and androgenetic alopecia, all likely predisposing factors for the poor healing response seen in EPD [12]. Indeed, actinically damaged and atrophic skin is well known to have impaired healing [6]. Androgenetic alopecia further exposes the underlying skin to accumulation of more actinic damage and resultant atrophy. As wound healing involves re-epithelialization from the skin edge and adnexa, lack of hair follicles due to androgenetic alopecia may contribute to delays in healing [14,21]. These factors result in a milieu primed for developing the chronic inflammation and poor healing response observed in EPD.

6.2. Triggers

On a scalp with the predisposing factors outlined, EPD has commonly been reported to occur following several medical, surgical, or traumatic insults to the scalp, as outlined in Table 1 [14,22–37]. Mechanical trauma is an established precipitating factor, as a few cases have occurred in infants and children after prolonged labor, perinatal scalp injury, or cranial surgical procedures [38]. Removal of the trauma does not result in clearance, and the disease can recur with repeated trauma to the skin [12,22]. It has been postulated that these insults cause tissue damage and inflammation, resulting in a dysregulated inflammatory response. Systemic medications such as epidermal growth factor (EGFR) inhibitors, i.e., gefitinib and panitumumab, block the anagen-to-telogen phase transition and enhance ultraviolet light (UV)-induced apoptosis. These effects result in a loss of the hair follicle immune privilege and stimulation of inflammatory processes, apoptosis, and occlusion of follicular ducts, leading to their rupture [32]. A mechanism of contact dermatitis was postulated in a case of EPD triggered by a prosthetic hair piece [34]. The diagnosis of contact dermatitis was supported by the temporal association with the adhesive and a clinically consistent pruritic eruption following the adhesive pattern. However, in some cases, EPD may occur spontaneously without a known inciting factor. Infectious etiology is not thought to play a role in inflammation, as cultures often demonstrate only occasional colonization, the eradication of which did not improve the lesions [12,14].

Table 1. Suggested EPD triggers [14,22–33].

Locally Applied Medications
Diclofenac
5-Fluorouracil
Imiquimod
Ingenol mebutate
Latanoprost
Minoxidil
Sirolimus
Tretinoin
Systemic Medications
Afatinib
Gefinitinib
Nivolumab
Panitumumab
Surgery/Other Procedure
PDT (aminolevulinic acid-PDT, methyl aminolevulinate PDT)
Cryotherapy
X-ray radiation therapy
Electrodessication and curettage (ED & C)
Wide excision
Mohs micrographic surgery
Neurosurgery (corrective surgery for ossification of the posterior longitudinal ligament and craniotomy)
Cochlear implant
Hair transplant
Prosthetic hair piece
CO_2 laser resurfacing
Surgical closures (secondary intent, primary closure, skin graft, local flap)
Local Trauma
Perinatal (e.g., caput secundum)
Burns (sunburn, flame, scald, chemical)
Physical injury
Falls

CO_2, carbon dioxide; PDT, photodynamic therapy.

6.3. Mechanisms

6.3.1. Chronic Dysregulated Inflammatory Response

In EPDS, there is an accumulation of a mixed infiltrate, including neutrophils, lymphocytes, and plasma cells, leading to a chronic inflammatory state [14]. As mentioned above, EPD is considered by some researchers a neutrophil-mediated disorder, as neutrophils are observed in areas adjacent to ulceration [14], and there is neutrophilic spongiosis affecting the follicular infundibula with focal neutrophilic pustules [15]. As Tomasini and colleagues indicated, EPD of the scalp shows clinicopathologic similarities with other pathergic neutrophilic dermatoses, such as pyoderma gangrenosum [15]. Pathergy can explain the recurrence of EPD lesions after trauma. Several authors indicate that neutrophilic dermatoses have clinicopathological similarities with autoinflammatory diseases [39]. However, EPD lacks several features of monogenic autoinflammatory diseases, including a genetic defect and systemic manifestations, such as recurrent fever and arthropathy [40]. Like autoinflammatory dermatoses, neutrophilic dermatoses involve dysfunctional cellular signaling mediated by pathways including interleukin-1 (IL-1) [41]. Therefore, it would be worth trying in EPD treatment with medications such as anakinra, an IL-1 receptor antagonist.

Any type of local trauma, either alone or in combination with predisposing factors, such as skin atrophy caused by chronic sun damage or androgenetic alopecia, might have impaired skin wound healing mechanisms. As Ibrihim et al. state, "an aberrant wound healing response in the setting of actinically damaged skin seems to be a consistent theme in its presentation" [42]. The lack of hair bulge stem cells, estrogen deprivation, the poor restorative capacity of aged keratinocytes, and chronic inflammation may be implicated in delayed healing [6,43]. Delayed healing may lead to local immunologic dysregulation and abnormal neutrophil chemotaxis or chemoattractants and cytokine production against epidermal or follicular antigens [15]. Contrary to the self-limited inflammation associated with disrupted skin, patients with EPD of the scalp may experience persistent cellular influxes into a previously injured scalp–this results in the continuous formation of infundibular vesiculopustules, quickly turning into erosions and crusting followed by granulation tissue and scarring alopecia, even if the triggering factor occurred much earlier [27]. The response to topical and systemic steroids and dapsone further supports local neutrophilic dysregulation [2,4]. The pivotal role of exaggerated immune response in the etiopathogenesis of EPD is also supported by concomitant serum elevation of matrix metalloproteinase-3 in patients with EPD [44].

As the condition progresses, fibrosis develops, with the loss of follicles and sebaceous glands, with the eventual development of epidermal atrophy and complete loss of adnexal structures. These factors may further predispose the individual to the recurrence of this cycle, resulting in the chronic course of EPD.

6.3.2. Autoimmune Mechanisms

Autoimmune mechanisms may contribute to the dysregulated inflammatory response. EPD has been associated with autoimmune conditions such as rheumatoid arthritis, autoimmune hepatitis, Hashimoto thyroiditis, undifferentiated collagen vascular disease, Takyasu artiritis, and elevated ESR [11,14,20,45]. Positive antinuclear antibody testing was found in four of 11 patients in one study [6]. However, a direct pathogenetic link with autoimmunity has not been established [6,20,45].

6.3.3. Immunosenescence

As EPD is primarily a disease of mature individuals, immunosenescence, which is the decrease in the specificity and efficacy of the immune response that develops as individual ages, has also been implicated [12,20,46]. As the immune system ages, it loses tolerance to self-antigens, leading to increased "self-reactivity" [46]. As EPD may develop as an aberrant immune response to delayed wound healing, this increased self-reactivity may play a vital role in immune dysregulation. Chemotherapeutic drugs that lower the host's immune function have been associated with the development of EPD [47].

6.3.4. Ultraviolet Light

EPD characteristically occurs in areas of chronic sun damage, which supports the role of UV light in chronic inflammation that perpetuates EPD. Thuraisingam and Mirmirani suggested that chronic ultraviolet light exposure may lead to the modification of intracellular components [46]. These modified factors are kept hidden internally until cell damage (for example, in the form of trauma) occurs. In genetically susceptible individuals, these factors, once released into their environment, activate the innate and adaptive immune systems. The age-related over-activation of the innate immune system described above, combined with the inability to properly heal wounds, may contribute to the chronicity of EPD.

6.3.5. EPD of the Leg and Venous Insufficiency

Most of the EPD of leg cases have been associated with chronic venous insufficiency. In a study by Nicol et al., venous insufficiency was diagnosed in 33 of 36 EPD patients (91.7%) [48]. However, a direct etiopathogenetic link has not been established. Of interest, stasis dermatitis secondary to chronic venous insufficiency is a common condition, while EPD of the leg is rare even among these patients [46]. In one study, less than 0.5% of patients presenting to a leg ulcer clinic developed EPD of the leg [49]. EPD of the leg may also develop in the absence of stasis dermatitis [11,50]. Poor circulation in patients with venous stasis may impair the healing of EPD of the leg. However, as several authors indicate [11,46], these patients share an advanced age and a long history of sun exposure and previous trauma at the site of EPD development, which is most likely the primary contributing factor in the development of EPD of the leg.

7. EPD Linked to NMSC

Lovell et al. reported the first case of NMSC arising in EPDS [51]. Most recently, Negbenebor and colleagues reported six patients that developed NMSC in the setting of EPD [17]. The authors suggested that the chronic inflammation of EPD and UV light exposure may predispose patients to develop NMSC. EPD, actinic keratoses, and NMSC share a lymphoplasmacytic infiltrate. Carcinogenesis can be triggered by chronic inflammation that develops secondary to reactive oxygen species produced by UV exposure, oxidizers, or metabolic processes that damage cells and further induce inflammatory cascades [52,53]. Of note, Aigner and colleagues reported a case of sun-induced EPD, and sun exposure was thought to have induced the inflammation that caused EPD [54]. There is a well-established link between chronic and intermittent UV exposure with the development of NMSC. Lastly, Barilla et al. reported a case of SCC arising in chronic EPD, which further supports the relationship between chronic inflammation in the context of EPD and NMSC in some patients [55].

8. Management
8.1. Methods
8.1.1. Search Strategy

We conducted a search of the MEDLINE, EMBASE, and Google Scholar databases from inception to September 2022 for publications on the management of EPD. This evidence-based, systematic review of management options for EPD follows the Preferred Reporting Items for Systematic Reviews and Meta-analysis (PRISMA) guidelines. Search terms included 'erosive pustular dermatosis' AND ('therapy' OR 'management' OR 'treatment' OR 'phototherapy' OR 'photodynamic therapy' OR 'administration'). Furthermore, we checked the reference lists of included studies and review articles for further studies on therapy.

8.1.2. Study Selection

The study selection is detailed in Figure 2. An eligibility assessment was performed independently by two authors (S.B. and G.K.). Inclusion criteria were studies published in the English language and reporting therapy of EPD. Exclusion criteria were cell/animal studies, review/opinion articles, commentaries, consensus papers, editorials, studies not focusing on treatment (e.g., purely dermatopathology studies), reports without sufficient clinical data (e.g., missing name of corticosteroid or dosing of systemic medication) and reports with only 1 participant.

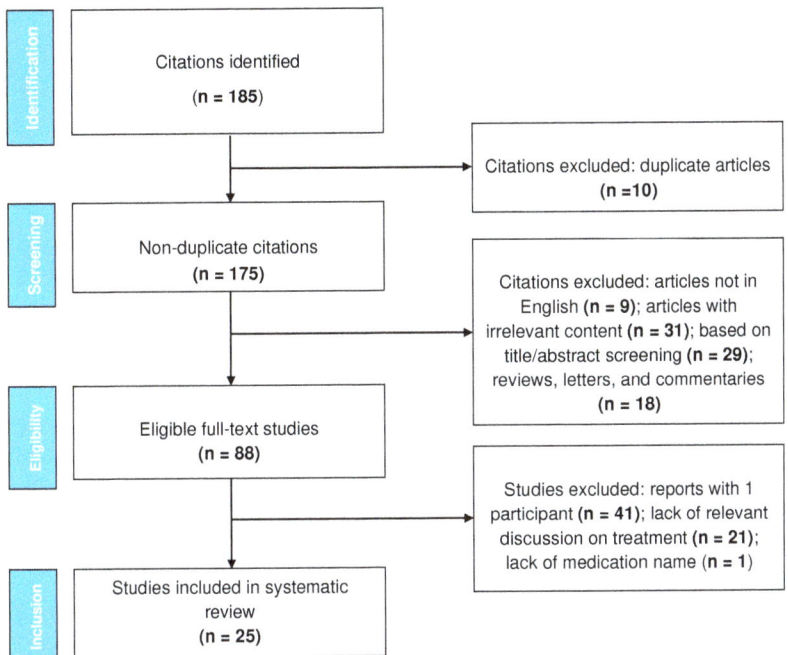

Figure 2. Flow diagram of literature search and study selection.

8.1.3. Extraction of Data

We extracted the following data: name of the first author, year of publication, study design, number of participants, male-to-female ratio, therapy, duration of treatment, duration of follow-up, primary outcomes, and secondary outcomes (adverse events).

8.2. Results

A total of 25 studies [2,6–8,12,15,16,25,49,56–70] with 162 participants (112 males, 50 females) met the selection criteria (Table 2).

Quality of Evidence Assessment

The quality of evidence of the studies included was ranked according to the established classification by Sullivan et al. [71] and is shown in Table 2. There were predominantly studies with level IV and V evidence and only two studies with level III [63,70]. The absence of a control group in most studies and the lack of randomization limit their quality. Another limitation is the small sample size (most studies on <20 subjects) that confers publication and sampling (selection) bias. The results were heterogeneous (interstudy variability, different study designs), and the methodological quality (e.g., lack of randomized controlled data, missing data) was low. Therefore, a meta-analysis was not feasible. Additionally, some studies included concomitant therapies, making it difficult to distinguish which agent was most responsible for improving the condition; this may affect the interpretation of results.

8.3. Topical Treatments

In a European study including 59 patients, most prescribed topical treatments were topical corticosteroids (TCS; 62.5%), in particular, clobetasol propionate 0.5%, followed by a combination of clobetasol with tacrolimus 0.1% (8.9%), and tacrolimus 0.1% monotherapy (5.4%) [72].

8.3.1. Corticosteroids

TCS is the most frequently used treatment for EPD. Ultrapotent (clobetasol, halobetasol) and potent/mid-potent (betamethasone, mometasone, triamcinolone, desoximetasone) TCS have been used, and infrequently, mild TCS (hydrocortisone, desonide) [2,15,38,64,68,73]. More than half of the patients achieved a partial response. Clobetasol was the most studied TCS (10 studies, Table 2). The duration of clobetasol treatment was 2 to 20 weeks. Most patients responded to clobetasol, but recurrence often occurred after cessation of treatment [15,25,73]. Tomasini et al. used clobetasol overnight for four weeks and tapered it to twice-weekly application for three months [15]. As shown in Table 2, skin atrophy was an adverse effect of clobetasol in four studies [12,16,58,61] (Figure 3) and of betamethasone in one study [46]. Betamethasone has been extensively used, but the results have been inferior compared to clobetasol [66]. It can be combined with topical antibiotics such as gentamycin and neomycin and oral nimesulide for better outcomes [2,64].

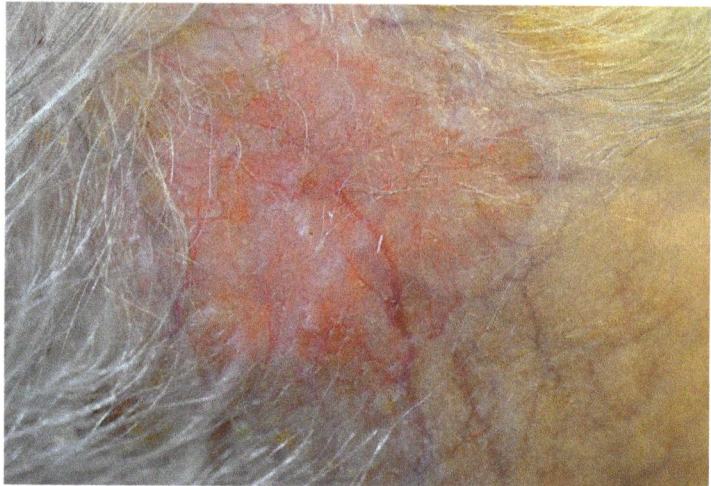

Figure 3. Female patient in her 70s with skin atrophy of the right frontal scalp that resulted from prolonged use of clobetasol propionate cream for EPD. The atrophic area is thin, erythematous, and shows prominent telangiectasias.

Table 2. Therapies used in erosive pustular dermatosis.

First Author, Year [Ref]	Type of Study	Level of Evidence	Patients (n), (M:F)	Affected Site	Therapy	Treatment Duration	Follow-Up	Primary Outcomes	Adverse Events
					Topical Treatments				
Bull et al., 1995 [56]	Case report	4	2 (0:2)	Leg	Clobetasol	NR	NR	CR with solo clobetasol; R* after Rx switched from clobetasol to methotrexate or minocycline	None
Patton et al., 2007 [6]	Case series	4	8 (3:5)	Scalp	Clobetasol	3–4 wks	NR	Immediate response	None
Rongioletti et al., 2016 [25]	Case report	5	2 (2:0)	Scalp	Clobetasol	8 wks	NR	CR (n = 2); R* after Rx withdrawal	None
Pileri A et al., 2017 [57]	Case series	4	5 (2:3)	Legs	Clobetasol	1–4 mos	20–72 mos	CR (n = 5); R* after Rx withdrawal	None
Starace et al., 2017 [12]	Case series	4	17 (12:5)	Scalp	Clobetasol	5 mos	NR	Inflammation improved (n = 14); R* 2–8 mos after Rx withdrawal in some pts but milder than the initial episode	Skin atrophy
Borgia et al., 2018 [58]	Case series	4	2 (1:1)	Scalp	Clobetasol	6 wks	NR	CR (n = 2)	Skin atrophy
Di Meo N et al., 2019 [59]	Case series	5	3 (2:1)	Scalp	Clobetasol	2–4 wks	NR	CR n = 2)	None
Piccolo et al., 2019 [16]	Case Series	4	8 (7:1)	Scalp	Clobetasol	2 wks	3 mos	CR (n = 7); R* (n = 1)	Atrophic scar after healing (n = 1)
Giuffrida et al., 2019 [60]	Case series	5	2 (2:0)	Scalp	Clobetasol	6 wks	NR	CR	None
Tomasini et al., 2019 [15]	Case series	4	30 (22:8)	Scalp	Clobetasol	4 mos (initial), 3 yrs (maintenance)	3 yrs	Marked improvement (n = 27); R* after Rx withdrawal at 4 mos	None

Table 2. Cont.

First Author, Year [Ref]	Type of Study	Level of Evidence	Patients (n), (M:F)	Affected Site	Therapy	Treatment Duration	Follow-Up	Primary Outcomes	Adverse Events
Lafitte et al., 2003 [61]	Case series	5	2 (2:0)	Scalp	Tacrolimus 0.1%	6 mos	12 mos	CR (n = 2)	Skin atrophy due to previous TCS Rx resolved after 6 (case 1) and 8 mos (case 2) of tacrolimus Rx
Starace et al., 2017 [12]	Case series	4	3 (2:1)	Scalp	Tacrolimus 0.1%	5 mos	NR	Inflammation improved (n = 3)	NR
Broussard et al., 2012 [62]	Case series	4	4 (2:2)	Scalp	Dapsone 5%	4-17 wks	7-24 mos	CR (n = 4); no R*	None
Photodynamic Therapy									
Yang et al., 2016 [7]	Case series	4	8 (5:3)	Scalp	Curettage (1 wk before ALA-PDT) + ALA-PDT (n = 8)	1 or 2 sessions	3-9 mos	CR with 1 session (n = 6) or 2 sessions (n = 2); R* after 5 mos in 1 pt required another session; CR lasted up to 9 mos	Well tolerated
Cunha et al., 2018 [8]	Case series	4	5 (5:0)	Scalp	Preprocedure curettage + (ALA-PDT) + postprocedure silicone gel bid	1 or 2 sessions	4-12 mos	CR with 1 session (n = 4) or 2 sessions (n = 1); R* after 9 mos in 1 pt required another session; CR lasted up to 12 mos	None
Misitzis et al., 2022 [63]	Comparative study	3	9 (6:3)	Scalp	*Protocol 1:* curettage (1 wk before ALA-PDT) + ALA-PDT	1 or 2 sessions	3-13 mos	CR with 1 session (n = 7) or 2 sessions (n = 2); R* after 5 mos in 1 pt required another session; mean length of remission was 6.4 mos (CR lasted up to 13 mos)	None

Table 2. *Cont.*

First Author, Year [Ref]	Type of Study	Level of Evidence	Patients (n), (M:F)	Affected Site	Therapy	Treatment Duration	Follow-Up	Primary Outcomes	Adverse Events
			8 (6:2)	Scalp	*Protocol 2:* preprocedure curettage + (ALA-PDT) + postprocedure silicone gel bid	1 session	4–12 mos	CR with 1 session (*n* = 8); 1 pt had R*, which was managed at 9th mo with another session; mean length of remission was 7.5 mos (CR lasted up to 12 mos); protocol 2 was superior to protocol 1 regarding easiness of Rx and postoperative healing (*p* = 0.005 for both)	None
Combination Treatments									
Pye et al., 1979 [2]	Case report	4	3 (0:2)	Scalp	Clobetasol, then hydrocortisone 1%, then betamethasone valerate 0.1%, neomycin 0.5% (*n* = 1); betamethasone valerate 0.1%, neomycin 0.5% (*n* = 1); clobetasol, neomycin 0.5%, nystatin (*n* = 1)	NR (case 1), 4 mos (case 2), 2 yrs (case 3)	NR, 2 yrs (case 3)	CR to clobetasol and betamethasone valerate, neomycin but flare with hydrocortisone (case 1); CR (cases 2, 3)	None

Table 2. Cont.

First Author, Year [Ref]	Type of Study	Level of Evidence	Patients (n), (M:F)	Affected Site	Therapy	Treatment Duration	Follow-Up	Primary Outcomes	Adverse Events
Caputo et al., 1993 [64]	Case report	5	3 (2:1)	Scalp	Betamethasone 0.05%, salicylic acid 2% lotion (n = 1); ketoconazole 2% biw, oral nimesulide (200 mg/d tapered) (n = 1); Betamethasone 0.05%, oral nimesulide (n = 1)	2 mos (cases 1,2), 1 mo (case 3)	NR	CR (case 1); PR (case 2); 50% improvement (case 3)	None
Ena et al., 1997 [65]	Case report	4	2 (1:1)	Scalp	Gentamycin-betamethasone, povidone-iodine, eosin 6% solution (with R*, dapsone 100 mg/d × 3 mos, then isotretinoin 40 mg/d × 3) (n = 1); isotretinoin 40 mg/d (n = 1)	7 mos (case 1), 2 mos (case 2)	NR	CR with R* after Rx withdrawal in the 1st case; SD (2nd case)	None
Brouard et al., 2002 [49]	Case report	4	3 (1:2)	Leg	Betamethasone 0.05%, tacrolimus (n = 1); betamethasone 0.05% (n = 1); betamethasone 0.05%, tacrolimus, prednisone 15 mg/d, then tacrolimus, split-thickness skin graft, then prednisone 20 mg/d, tacrolimus, colchicine 0.5 mg/d (n = 1)	3 mos	NR	CR (first 2 cases); PR (3rd case)	Skin atrophy (3rd patient)

Table 2. Cont.

First Author, Year [Ref]	Type of Study	Level of Evidence	Patients (n), (M:F)	Affected Site	Therapy	Treatment Duration	Follow-Up	Primary Outcomes	Adverse Events
Allevato et al., 2009 [66]	Case series	5	2 (1:1)	Scalp	Betamethasone 0.1%, prednisone 16 mg/d, zinc gluconate 50 mg tid, topical fusidic acid	2 mos	21 mos, 27 mos	CR (n = 2)	None
Dall'Olio et al., 2011 [67]	Case report	5	2 (0:2)	Leg (n = 1); scalp (n = 1)	Clobetasol, tacrolimus 0.1% (n = 1); betamethasone valerate 0.1%, oral dapsone 100 mg/d, tacrolimus 0.1% (n = 1)	12 mos	12 mos	CR (n = 2)	None
Mervak et al., 2017 [68]	Case series	5	2 (0:2)	Face	Tacrolimus 0.1%, prednisone 1 mg/kg/d, mupirocin, minocycline, then added dapsone 100 mg/d, isotretinoin 30 mg/d (n = 1); tacrolimus 0.1%, minocycline, dapsone 5%, triamcinolone acetonide 0.025% (n = 1)	3.5–4 yrs	3.5–4 yrs	PR with R* (n = 2); dapsone (2.5 yrs; maintenance dose 25–50 mg/d) and isotretinoin (3.5 yrs; maintenance dose 10–20 mg/d) provided further improvement in case 1	None
Sechi et al., 2019 [69]	Case series	4	4 (4:0)	Scalp	Betamethasone 0.05%, fusidic acid 2%, hyaluronic acid dressing bid	20–30 d	6 mos	CR (n = 4)	None

Table 2. Cont.

First Author, Year [Ref]	Type of Study	Level of Evidence	Patients (n), (M:F)	Affected Site	Therapy	Treatment Duration	Follow-Up	Primary Outcomes	Adverse Events
Siskou et al., 2021 [70]	Retrospective study	3	23 (22:1)	Scalp	TCS (n = 22); TCs + TCi (n = 7); TCS + Acitretin 25 mg/d (n = 9); TCi + acitretin 25 mg/d (n = 2)	NR		TCS: CR (n = 14), PR (n = 7), SD (n = 1); TCS + TCi: CR (n = 3), PR (n = 4); TCS + acitretin: CR (7), PR (2); TCi + acitretin: PR (n = 2); R* in 78.3% of pts after Rx cessation at a median of 8 wks; new R* in 22.2% of pts that received acitretin vs. 71.4% that received TCi as maintenance	None

Abbreviations: ALA-PDT, aminolevulinic acid photodynamic therapy; biw, twice weekly; CR, complete lesion resolution; d, day/days; mg/kg/d, milligram per kilogram per day; M:F, male to female ratio; mos, months; NR, not reported; PR, partial response; qhs, at night; R*, recurrence/deterioration; SD, stable disease; TCi, topical calcineurin inhibitor; TCS, topical corticosteroid(s); wks, weeks; yrs, years.

8.3.2. Calcineurin Inhibitors

Tacrolimus has the advantage of a better safety profile than TCS, a factor to consider, especially as EPD requires prolonged treatment and shows a high recurrence rate. It has been shown effective as early as one week of application, with complete clearance within two months [6,74,75]. Combining tacrolimus with TCS can help decrease the length of TCS therapy, which minimizes the adverse effects of TCS. It can also help prevent disease recurrence upon the TCS discontinuation [33,67]. Tacrolimus has been reported as the most effective medication for maintaining a disease-free state [76,77]. However, there is a lack of large series and controlled data, so its role as monotherapy requires further research.

8.3.3. Other Topical Treatments

Topical dapsone applied twice daily for 2–4.5 months was effective. No recurrence upon discontinuation was noted [62]. Topical gentamycin or neomycin have been combined to enhance the efficacy of topical steroids [2]. Calcipotriol cream has been effective in a case report but is limited by its slow action [78]. Recently, topical zinc oxide was effective in case reports and may be combined with other topical and/or systemic therapies for enhanced outcomes [79,80].

8.3.4. Wound Dressings/Allografts

The use of silicone dressing as monotherapy was effective in one case [81]. In addition, silicone dressing can be used after any minimally invasive modality, such as curettage-assisted photodynamic therapy (PDT), to enhance healing and decrease postprocedure inflammation [8]. Interestingly, case reports indicate that newer innovative dressings with umbilical remnant allograft and dehydrated human amnion/chorion membrane allograft can be successful in resistant cases of EPD [82,83].

8.3.5. Systemic Treatments

Systemic corticosteroids (SCSs) such as prednisone, methylprednisolone, or dexamethasone have been used most often in combination with TCS or tacrolimus after topical therapy failed [27,44,49,66] (Table 2). In a multi-center study, SCSs were taken by 7.1% of patients [72]. Prednisone doses such as 16–40 mg/day [12,66,84] or 0.5–1 mg/kg/d [15,68,85] were administered. Significant improvement or resolution was noted in most patients [15,84]. Gradual tapering was noted [12,15]. There are inadequate data regarding SCS used as monotherapy, with information about the dosing, length of therapy and follow-up, concomitant therapies, and response often missing. Prolonged SCS use is associated with adverse effects; therefore, proper tapering is recommended and can help prevent a flare that typically occurs with abrupt discontinuation [84,86,87].

Oral antibiotics such as dapsone or minocycline are ineffective or provide only partial response [48,54,88,89]; there are limited data on their use in combination therapies. In a retrospective study, acitretin was promising in patients experiencing recurrence after TCS treatment [70]. Several EPD cases have been treated with cyclosporine, isotretinoin, sulphasalazine combined with the excimer laser, or tofacitinib with a disease-free state over a follow-up period of a few months [90–94]. Oral zinc has been used as monotherapy [95] or as part of combination therapies [66,88,91]. A combination of oral dapsone, topical tacrolimus, and fractional 2940 nm laser successfully managed chronic, severe EPD [96].

8.3.6. Photodynamic Therapy

There are a few series showing the effectiveness of aminolevulinic acid-PDT (ALA-PDT) in the treatment of EPD [7,8,63]. The group reported the first 8 patients with EPD of the scalp were successfully treated with superficial curettage followed, 1 to 2 weeks later, by ALA-PDT [7]. One patient experienced a partial recurrence 5 months after therapy and was treated with another session of ALA-PDT. Clearance of lesions after curettage-assisted ALA-PDT can last up to 9 months, which indicates that this therapy, when used in a combination regimen, can allow more limited use of other therapies such as potent TCS.

The authors then attempted to revise the protocol by performing curettage immediately before ALA-PDT in 5 patients and enhancing the healing with the application of a silicone gel starting immediately after completion of ALA-PDT and continuing twice daily [8]. The revised protocol aimed at decreasing the number of visits and cost of treatment as well as minimizing postprocedure discomfort. Partial recurrence was noted in a patient at 9 months posttreatment and required another round of PDT. Clearance of lesions after the procedure lasted up to 12 months. A subsequent study by the group compared the protocols utilized in those series regarding efficacy, cost, and patient satisfaction: the first, 2-visit protocol and the second (revised), 1-visit protocol (all procedures in one visit with silicone gel application postprocedure) [63]. Both protocols were efficacious and provided similar lengths of remission. The second protocol was less costly. Patients treated using the second protocol were more satisfied because of the easiness of treatment completion in one visit and better postoperative healing.

However, methyl aminolevulinate PDT (MAL-PDT) has triggered EPD in 2 cases [27,97]. Kroumpouzos and colleagues recommend avoiding MAL-PDT because MAL is more lipophilic than ALA and, therefore, penetrates deeper into the skin and may cause excessive trauma [7]. In addition, the incubation period in MAL-PDT was 3 h [27,98] whereas, in the above ALA-PDT series was 1 h [7,8,63]–the more prolonged incubation of the MAL photosensitizer may also cause excessive tissue trauma that increases the risk of triggering PDT. A more prolonged incubation (2 h) of ALA may also explain why ALA-PDT triggered EPD in the case reported by Madray et al. [29]. The above observations show that ALA-PDT protocols using a short duration (1 h) of the photosensitizer may help minimize the risk of triggering EPD.

Another study showed that daylight PDT and conventional PDT have similar efficacy, which can be used in resource-limited settings for the best results in a single treatment [98]. PDT has been safely combined with fractional thulium 1927 nm laser with a complete response of EPD [99].

8.3.7. Therapeutic Challenges and the Search for Treatment Algorithm

The management of EPD remains a therapeutic challenge, especially because most therapies do not provide a long remission [70]. TCSs are a first-line treatment, especially as they help prevent the alopecia associated with ongoing EPD; however, EPD typically recurs upon discontinuation of TCS treatment [5,12]. In addition, TCS should be used for a short period of time because of an increased risk of adverse effects, such as steroid-induced atrophy that can lead to exposure of the skull and bacterial colonization associated with prolonged treatment [7,70]. Most topical EPD therapies have met with limited success partly because of difficulty penetrating the hyperkeratotic crust, especially in lesions exhibiting massive hyperkeratosis. Periodic in-office atraumatic removal of the hyperkeratotic crust with forceps or gentle curettage increases the penetration of topical medications; however, this increases the number of office visits and raises the cost of care.

Surgical treatments typically fail because EPD tends to recur after any procedure that induces trauma to the skin [100]. Dressings that have anti-inflammatory properties, such as silicone gel, may help minimize trauma and speed up the healing, helping prevent EPD recurrence after any minimally invasive procedure, such as curettage-assisted ALA-PDT. Some researchers have used silicone dressing as monotherapy [81]. These authors have witnessed the efficacy of a novel silicone gel dressing used after curettage-assisted ALA-PDT [8,63]. Interestingly, case reports indicate that newer innovative dressings with umbilical remnant allograft and dehydrated human amnion/chorion membrane allograft can be successful in resistant cases of EPD [82,83].

Siskou and colleagues advocated systemic retinoids as a superior maintenance treatment over calcineurin inhibitors [70], but the study's small sample size prevents definite conclusions. Curettage-assisted ALA-PDT that includes short incubation of the photosensitizer has a role as a primary therapeutic approach. Clearance of the lesions after curettage-assisted ALA-PDT can last up to 13 months [63]; therefore, this treatment should be considered in maintenance regimens as it allows more limited use of potent TCS. Considering the above, tacrolimus, curettage-assisted ALA-PDT, and systemic retinoids can be considered second-line options for EPD with a role in maintenance regimens.

While infrequently reported, topical dapsone and oral tofacitinib may be promising therapeutic options [62,94], but studies comparing them to TCS and the aforementioned second-line options are needed. There are inadequate, low-quality data to support the use of SCS as a second-line treatment option, and their suboptimal safety profile prohibits long-term use. There is some evidence supporting oral zinc in combination therapies [66,88,91], but further studies are needed.

9. Conclusions

EPD is a chronic inflammatory skin condition characterized by erosive crusts and superficial ulcerations. It predominantly affects the scalp and can lead to scarring alopecia. EPD is a diagnosis of exclusion; thus, several neoplastic, infectious, vesiculobullous, and inflammatory conditions should be ruled out. Biopsy and clinicopathologic correlation are required to differentiate between EPD and these entities. While the etiopathogenesis of the condition remains elusive, four key factors may contribute to the development of EPD: a predisposing environment on the scalp, including skin atrophy, actinic damage, and androgenetic alopecia; an initial inciting trauma or damage; resultant dysregulated, chronic immune response; culmination in fibrosis, atrophy, and scarring alopecia.

Management of EPD is challenging. Despite its responsiveness to TCS, such as clobetasol propionate, recurrence occurs after treatment withdrawal. Furthermore, prolonged use of TCS is associated with an increased risk of adverse effects such as steroid atrophy, necessitating the implementation of second-line therapies. With the available data, tacrolimus 0.1%, curettage-assisted ALA-PDT, and systemic retinoids can be considered second-line options for EPD with a role in maintenance regimens. However, as the level of evidence of the available therapy studies is low, it cannot guide the development of solid recommendations, and further studies are needed.

Author Contributions: S.B.: Formal analysis, Writing—original draft, review, and editing. S.Y.: Data curation, Writing—original draft, review, and editing. E.H.: Data curation, Writing—original draft. G.K.: Conceptualization, Data curation, Formal analysis, Writing—original draft, review, and editing. All authors have read and agreed to the published version of the manuscript.

Funding: This research received no external funding.

Institutional Review Board Statement: Not applicable.

Informed Consent Statement: Not applicable.

Conflicts of Interest: The authors declare no conflict of interest in the materials or subject matter dealt with in the manuscript.

References

1. Burton, J.L. Case for diagnosis. Pustular dermatosis of scalp. *Br. J. Dermatol.* **1977**, *97* (Suppl. 15), 67–69. [CrossRef] [PubMed]
2. Pye, R.J.; Peachey, R.D.G.; Burton, J.L. Erosive pustular dermatosis of the scalp. *Br. J. Dermatol.* **1979**, *100*, 559–566. [CrossRef] [PubMed]
3. Starace, M.; Alessandrini, A.; Baraldi, C.; Piraccini, B.M. Erosive pustular dermatosis of the scalp: Challenges and solutions. *Clin. Cosmet. Investig. Dermatol.* **2019**, *12*, 691–698. [CrossRef] [PubMed]
4. Semkova, K.; Tchernev, G.; Wollina, U. Erosive pustular dermatosis (chronic atrophic dermatosis of the scalp and extremities). *Clin. Cosmet. Investig. Dermatol.* **2013**, *6*, 177–182. [PubMed]
5. Junejo, M.H.; Kentley, J.; Rajpopat, M.; Tan, X.L.; Mohd Mustapa, M.F.; Harwood, C.A. Therapeutic options for erosive pustular dermatosis of the scalp: A systematic review. *Br. J. Dermatol.* **2021**, *184*, 25–33. [CrossRef]
6. Patton, D.; Lynch, P.J.; Fung, M.A.; Fazel, N. Chronic atrophic erosive dermatosis of the scalp and extremities: A recharacterization of erosive pustular dermatosis. *J. Am. Acad. Dermatol.* **2007**, *57*, 421–427. [CrossRef]
7. Yang, C.S.; Kuhn, H.; Cohen, L.M.; Kroumpouzos, G. Aminolevulinic acid photodynamic therapy in the treatment of erosive pustular dermatosis of the scalp: A case series. *JAMA Dermatol.* **2016**, *152*, 694–697. [CrossRef]

8. Cunha, P.R.; Tsoukas, M.M.; Kroumpouzos, G. Erosive pustular dermatosis of the scalp treated with aminolevulinic acid photodynamic therapy and postprocedure silicone gel. *Dermatol. Surg.* **2019**, *45*, 740–743. [CrossRef]
9. Yeh, R.; Polcz, M.; Wong, D. Erosive pustular dermatosis of the scalp. An Australian perspective: Insights to aid clinical practice. *Australas. J. Dermatol.* **2019**, *60*, e272–e278. [CrossRef]
10. Shimada, R.; Masu, T.; Hanamizu, H.; Aiba, S.; Okuyama, R. Infantile erosive pustular dermatosis of the scalp associated with Klippel-Feil syndrome. *Acta Derm. Venereol.* **2010**, *90*, 200–201. [CrossRef]
11. Michelerio, A.; Vassallo, C.; Fiandrino, G.; Tomasini, C.F. Erosive pustular dermatosis of the scalp: A clinicopathologic study of fifty cases. *Dermatopathology* **2021**, *8*, 450–462. [CrossRef] [PubMed]
12. Starace, M.; Loi, C.; Bruni, F.; Alessandrini, A.; Misciali, C.; Patrizi, A.; Piraccini, B.M. Erosive pustular dermatosis of the scalp: Clinical, trichoscopic, and histopathologic features of 20 cases. *J. Am. Acad. Dermatol.* **2017**, *76*, 1109–1114. [CrossRef] [PubMed]
13. Gallo, G.; Ribero, S.; Conti, L.; Baglioni, E.; Fierro, M.T.; Quaglino, P. Erosive pustular dermatosis: Not only scalp. *J. Eur. Acad. Dermatol. Venereol.* **2020**, *34*, e399–e402. [CrossRef]
14. Reschke, R.; Grunewald, S.; Paasch, U.; Averbeck, M.; Simon, J.C.; Wetzig, T. Erosive pustular dermatosis of the scalp: Clinicopathological correlation leading to a definition of diagnostic criteria. *Wounds* **2021**, *33*, 143–146. [CrossRef] [PubMed]
15. Tomasini, C.; Michelerio, A. Erosive pustular dermatosis of the scalp: A neutrophilic folliculitis within the spectrum of neutrophilic dermatoses. *J. Am. Acad. Dermatol.* **2019**, *81*, 527–533. [CrossRef]
16. Piccolo, V.; Russo, T.; Bianco, S.; Ronchi, A.; Alfano, R.; Argenziano, G. Erosive pustular dermatosis of the scalp: Why do we miss it? *Dermatology* **2019**, *235*, 390–395. [CrossRef]
17. Negbenebor, N.A.; Shayegan, L.H.; Cohen, L.M.; Kroumpouzos, G. Nonmelanoma skin cancer in the setting of erosive pustular dermatosis of the scalp: A case series and comment on management implications. *Dermatol. Ther.* **2022**, *35*, e15584. [CrossRef]
18. Lugović-Mihić, L.; Barisić, F.; Bulat, V.; Buljan, M.; Situm, M.; Bradić, L.; Mihić, J. Differential diagnosis of the scalp hair folliculitis. *Acta Clin. Croat.* **2011**, *50*, 395–402.
19. Toda, N.; Fujimoto, N.; Kato, T.; Fujii, N.; Nakanishi, G.; Nagao, T.; Tanaka, T. Erosive pustular dermatosis of the scalp-like eruption due to gefitinib: Case report and review of the literature of alopecia associated with EGFR inhibitors. *Dermatology* **2012**, *225*, 18–21. [CrossRef]
20. Van Exel, C.E.V.; English, J.C. Erosive pustular dermatosis of the scalp and nonscalp. *J. Am. Acad. Dermatol.* **2007**, *57*, S11–S14. [CrossRef]
21. Langton, A.K.; Herrick, S.E.; Headon, D.J. An extended epidermal response heals cutaneous wounds in the absence of a hair follicle stem cell contribution. *J. Investig. Dermatol.* **2008**, *128*, 1311–1318. [CrossRef] [PubMed]
22. Grattan, C.E.H.; Peachey, R.D.; Boon, A. Evidence for a role of local trauma in the pathogenesis of erosive pustular dermatosis of the scalp. *Clin. Exp. Dermatol.* **1988**, *13*, 7–10. [CrossRef] [PubMed]
23. Roche-Kubler, B.; Monnin, C.; Aubin, F.; Dupond, A.S. Erosive pustular dermatosis of the scalp and thigh associated with skin graft recipient and donor sites. *Eur. J. Dermatol.* **2015**, *25*, 269–271. [CrossRef] [PubMed]
24. Vaccaro, M.; Barbuzza, O.; Guarneri, B. Erosive pustular dermatosis of the scalp following treatment with topical imiquimod for actinic keratosis. *Arch. Dermatol.* **2009**, *145*, 1340–1341. [CrossRef]
25. Rongioletti, F.; Chinazzo, C.; Javor, S. Erosive pustular dermatosis of the scalp induced by ingenol mebutate. *J. Eur. Acad. Dermatol. Venereol.* **2016**, *30*, e110–e111. [CrossRef]
26. Vaccaro, M.; Barbuzza, O.; Borgia, F.; Cannavò, S.P. Erosive pustular dermatosis of the scalp following topical latanoprost for androgenetic alopecia. *Dermatol. Ther.* **2015**, *28*, 65–67. [CrossRef]
27. Guarneri, C.; Vaccaro, M. Erosive pustular dermatosis of the scalp following topical methylaminolaevulinate photodynamic therapy. *J. Am. Acad. Dermatol.* **2009**, *60*, 521–522. [CrossRef]
28. Suarez-Valle, A.; Diaz-Guimaraens, B.; Dominguez-Santas, M.; Fernandez-Nieto, D.; Saceda-Corralo, D. Afatinib-induced erosive pustular dermatosis of the scalp: Is there a synergistic effect between EGFR inhibitors and radiotherapy? *Dermatol. Ther.* **2020**, *33*, e14506. [CrossRef]
29. Madray, V.M.; Kent, S.M.; Davis, L.S. Aminolevulinic acid photodynamic therapy–induced erosive pustular dermatosis of the scalp. *Dermatol. Surg.* **2021**, *47*, 1140–1142. [CrossRef]
30. Khanna, U.; Semsarzadeh, N.; Glaser, K.; Fernandez, A.P. Erosive pustular dermatosis of the scalp associated with Sirolimus. *J. Eur. Acad. Dermatol. Venereol.* **2020**, *34*, e15–e16. [CrossRef]
31. Maglie, R.; Antiga, E. Nivolumab-induced erosive pustular dermatosis of the scalp. *Int. J. Dermatol.* **2020**, *59*, e399–e400. [CrossRef] [PubMed]
32. Nazzaro, G.; Giacalone, S.; Bortoluzzi, P.; Veraldi, S.; Marzano, A.V. Erosive pustular dermatosis of the scalp induced by gefitinib: Case and review of the literature. *Dermatol. Online J.* **2021**, *27*, 13030/qt8w87m82r. [CrossRef] [PubMed]
33. Marzano, A.V.; Ghislanzoni, M.; Zaghis, A.; Spinelli, D.; Crosti, C. Localized erosive pustular dermatosis of the scalp at the site of a cochlear implant: Successful treatment with topical tacrolimus. *Clin. Exp. Dermatol.* **2009**, *34*, e157–e159. [CrossRef] [PubMed]
34. Herbst, J.S.; Herbst, A.T. Erosive pustular dermatosis of the scalp after contact dermatitis from a prosthetic hair piece. *JAAD Case Rep.* **2017**, *3*, 121–123. [CrossRef]
35. Saridakis, S.; Giesey, R.L.; Ezaldein, H.H.; Scott, J.F. Erosive pustular dermatosis of the scalp following surgical procedures: A systematic review. *Dermatol. Online J.* **2020**, *26*, 13030/qt9d80k39g. [CrossRef]

36. Okuno, S.; Hashimoto, T.; Matsuo, S.; Satoh, T. Erosive pustular dermatosis of the scalp-like eruption from panitumumab. *Australas. J. Dermatol.* **2022**, *63*, 271–272. [CrossRef]
37. Karanfilian, K.M.; Wassef, C. Erosive pustular dermatosis of the scalp: Causes and treatments. *Int. J. Dermatol.* **2021**, *60*, 25–32. [CrossRef]
38. Siegel, D.H.; Holland, K.; Phillips, R.J.; Drolet, B.A.; Esterly, N.B.; Frieden, I.J. Erosive pustular dermatosis of the scalp after perinatal scalp injury. *Pediatr. Dermatol.* **2006**, *23*, 533–536. [CrossRef]
39. Marzano, A.V.; Borghi, A.; Wallach, D.; Cugno, M. A Comprehensive review of neutrophilic diseases. *Clin. Rev. Allergy Immunol.* **2018**, *54*, 114–130. [CrossRef]
40. Azizi, G.; Khadem Azarian, S.; Nazeri, S.; Mosayebian, A.; Ghiasy, S.; Sadri, G.; Mohebi, A.; Khan Nazer, N.H.; Afraei, S.; Mirshafiey, A. Monogenic auto-inflammatory syndromes: A review of the literature. *Iran. J. Allergy Asthma Immunol.* **2016**, *15*, 430–444.
41. Marzano, A.V.; Ortega-Loayza, A.G.; Heath, M.; Morse, D.; Genovese, G.; Cugno, M. Mechanisms of inflammation in neutrophil-mediated skin diseases. *Front. Immunol.* **2019**, *10*, 1059. [CrossRef] [PubMed]
42. Ibrihim, O.; Arndt, K.A.; Dover, J.S. Pathophysiology and treatment considerations for erosive pustular dermatosis. *JAMA Dermatol.* **2017**, *153*, 971–972. [CrossRef] [PubMed]
43. Archer, D.F. Postmenopausal skin and estrogen. *Gynecol. Endocrinol.* **2012**, *28* (Suppl. 2), 2–6. [CrossRef] [PubMed]
44. Aoshima, M.; Ito, T.; Tokura, Y. Erosive pustular dermatosis of the scalp arising concomitantly with elevation of serum matrix metalloproteinase-3 in a patient with rheumatoid arthritis. *J. Dermatol.* **2015**, *42*, 540–541. [CrossRef]
45. Yamamoto, T.; Furuse, Y. Erosive pustular dermatosis of the scalp in association with rheumatoid arthritis. *Int. J. Dermatol.* **1995**, *34*, 148. [CrossRef]
46. Thuraisingam, T.; Mirmirani, P. Erosive pustular dermatosis: A manifestation of immunosenescence A report of 8 cases. *Ski. Appendage Disord.* **2017**, *4*, 180–186. [CrossRef]
47. Black, J.M.; Hodari, K.T.; Rogers, N.; Farris, P.K.; Lewis, A.T.; Boh, E.E. Exudative, nonhealing scalp: A complication of systemic chemotherapy with capecitabine and bevacizumab. *Arch. Dermatol.* **2011**, *147*, 134–135. [CrossRef]
48. Nicol, P.; Perceau, G.; Barbe, C.; Bernard, P.; Members of GAD. Erosive pustular dermatosis of the leg: A prospective, multicentre, observational study of 36 cases. *Ann. Dermatol. Venereol.* **2017**, *144*, 582–588. [CrossRef]
49. Brouard, M.C.; Prins, C.; Chavaz, P.; Saurat, J.H.; Borradori, L. Erosive pustular dermatosis of the leg: Report of three cases. *Br. J. Dermatol.* **2002**, *147*, 765–769. [CrossRef]
50. Zhou, Z.; Zhang, Z.K.; Liu, T.H. Erosive pustular dermatosis of the leg mimicking lower limb cellulitis. *Clin. Exp. Dermatol.* **2015**, *40*, 865–867. [CrossRef]
51. Lovell, C.R.; Harman, R.R.; Bradfield, J.W. Cutaneous carcinoma arising in erosive pustular dermatosis of the scalp. *Br. J. Dermatol.* **1980**, *103*, 325–328. [CrossRef] [PubMed]
52. Neagu, M.; Constantin, C.; Caruntu, C.; Dumitru, C.; Surcel, M.; Zurac, S. Inflammation: A key process in skin tumorigenesis. *Oncol. Lett.* **2019**, *17*, 4068–4084. [CrossRef] [PubMed]
53. Ciążyńska, M.; Olejniczak-Staruch, I.; Sobolewska-Sztychny, D.; Narbutt, J.; Skibińska, M.; Lesiak, A. Ultraviolet radiation and chronic inflammation-molecules and mechanisms involved in skin carcinogenesis: A narrative review. *Life* **2021**, *11*, 326. [CrossRef] [PubMed]
54. Aigner, B.; Legat, F.J.; Schuster, C.; El Shabrawi-Caelen, L. Sun-induced pustular dermatosis of the scalp—A new variant of erosive pustular dermatosis of the scalp? *Acta Derm. Venereol.* **2014**, *94*, 457–458. [CrossRef] [PubMed]
55. Barilla, S.; Malviya, N.; Wang, H.; Sharon, V.R. Squamous cell carcinoma arising in chronic erosive pustular dermatosis. *Dermatol. Surg.* **2022**, *48*, 250–251. [CrossRef] [PubMed]
56. Bull, R.H.; Mortimer, P.S. Erosive pustular dermatosis of the leg. *Br. J. Dermatol.* **1995**, *132*, 279–282. [CrossRef]
57. Pileri, A.; Misciali, C.; Baraldi, C.; Sechi, A.; Faenza, M.; Fanti, P.A.; Stella, A.; Patrizi, A. Erosive pustular dermatosis of the leg: An uncommon entity? *G Ital. Dermatol. Venereol.* **2017**, *152*, 675–678. [CrossRef]
58. Borgia, F.; Giuffrida, R.; Caradonna, E.; Vaccaro, M.; Guarneri, F.; Cannavò, S.P. Early and late onset side effects of photodynamic therapy. *Biomedicines* **2018**, *6*, 12. [CrossRef]
59. di Meo, N.; Corneli, P.; Retrosi, C.; Conforti, C.; Fagotti, S.; Longone, M.; Vezzoni, R.; Bussani, R.; Zalaudek, I. Erosive pustular dermatosis of the scalp: Therapy is the diagnosis. *Dermatol. Ther.* **2019**, *32*, e13128. [CrossRef]
60. Giuffrida, R.; Borgia, F.; Cannavò, S.P. Two cases of erosive pustular dermatosis of the scalp occurring after topical 3.75% imiquimod for actinic keratoses. *Dermatol. Ther.* **2019**, *32*, e12770. [CrossRef]
61. Laffitte, E.; Kaya, G.; Piguet, V.; Saurat, J.H. Erosive pustular dermatosis of the scalp: Treatment with topical tacrolimus. *Arch. Dermatol.* **2003**, *139*, 712–714. [CrossRef] [PubMed]
62. Broussard, C.; Berger, T.G.; Rosenblum, M.; Murase, J.E. Erosive pustular dermatosis of the scalp: A review with a focus on dapsone therapy. *J. Am. Acad. Dermatol.* **2012**, *66*, 680–686. [CrossRef] [PubMed]
63. Misitzis, A.; Bhargava, S.; Cunha, P.R.; Kroumpouzos, G. Aminolevulinic acid-photodynamic therapy for erosive pustular dermatosis of the scalp: Comparison of two treatment protocols and participant satisfaction. *Skinmed* **2022**, *20*, 107–112. [PubMed]
64. Caputo, R.; Veraldi, S. Erosive pustular dermatosis of the scalp. *J. Am. Acad. Dermatol.* **1993**, *28*, 96–98. [CrossRef] [PubMed]
65. Ena, P.; Lissia, M.; Doneddu, G.M.E.; Campus, G.V. Erosive pustular dermatosis of the scalp in skin grafts: Report of three cases. *Dermatology* **1997**, *194*, 80–84. [CrossRef]

66. Allevato, M.; Clerc, C.; del Sel, J.M.; Donatti, L.; Cabrera, H.; Juárez, M. Erosive pustular dermatosis of the scalp. *Int. J. Dermatol.* **2009**, *48*, 1213–1216. [CrossRef]
67. Dall'Olio, E.; Rosina, P.; Girolomoni, G. Erosive pustular dermatosis of the leg: Long-term control with topical tacrolimus. *Australas. J. Dermatol.* **2011**, *52*, e15–e17. [CrossRef]
68. Mervak, J.E.; Gan, S.D.; Smith, E.H.; Wang, F. Facial erosive pustular dermatosis after cosmetic resurfacing. *JAMA Dermatol.* **2017**, *153*, 1021–1025. [CrossRef]
69. Sechi, A.; Piraccini, B.M.; Alessandrini, A.; Patrizi, A.; Tabanelli, M.; Sacchelli, L.; Misciali, C.; Savoia, F. Post-traumatic erosive dermatosis of the scalp: A hypergranulated variant. *Australas. J. Dermatol.* **2019**, *60*, e322–e326. [CrossRef]
70. Siskou, S.; Lallas, A.; Theodoropoulos, K.; Sgouros, D.; Trakatelli, M.; Patsatsi, A.; Trigoni, A.; Manoli, M.; Papageorgiou, C.; Liopyris, K.; et al. Diagnostic and management challenges of erosive pustular dermatosis of the scalp: A retrospective study in Greek population. *J. Eur. Acad. Dermatol. Venereol.* **2021**, *35*, e776–e779. [CrossRef]
71. Sullivan, D.; Chung, K.C.; Eaves, F.F., 3rd; Rohrich, R.J. The level of evidence pyramid: Indicating levels of evidence in Plastic and Reconstructive Surgery articles. *Plast. Reconstr. Surg.* **2021**, *148*, 68S–71S. [CrossRef] [PubMed]
72. Starace, M.; Iorizzo, M.; Trüeb, R.M.; Piccolo, V.; Argenziano, G.; Camacho, F.M.; Gallyamova, Y.; Rudnicka, L.; Umbert, I.; Lyakhovitsky, A.; et al. Erosive pustular dermatosis of the scalp: A multicentre study. *J. Eur. Acad. Dermatol. Venereol.* **2020**, *34*, 1348–1354. [CrossRef] [PubMed]
73. Din, R.S.; Tsiaras, W.G.; Mostaghimi, A. Two cases of severe erosive pustular dermatosis mimicking infection. *Wounds* **2018**, *30*, E84–E86. [PubMed]
74. Kim, K.R.; Lee, J.Y.; Kim, M.K.; Yoon, T.Y. Erosive pustular dermatosis of the scalp following herpes zoster: Successful treatment with topical tacrolimus. *Ann. Dermatol.* **2010**, *22*, 232–234. [CrossRef] [PubMed]
75. Erdmann, M.; Kiesewetter, F.; Schuler, G.; Schultz, E. Erosive pustular dermatosis of the leg in a patient with ankylosing spondylitis: Neutrophilic dysfunction as a common etiological factor? *Int. J. Dermatol.* **2009**, *48*, 513–515. [CrossRef] [PubMed]
76. Miller, A.L.; Esser, A.C.; Lookingbill, D.P. Extensive erosions and pustular lesions of the scalp–quiz case. *Arch. Dermatol.* **2008**, *144*, 795–800. [CrossRef]
77. Vano-Galvan, S.; Antonio, M.-C.; Pedro, J. Erosive pustular dermatosis of the scalp. *J. Pak. Med. Assoc.* **2012**, *62*, 501–502.
78. Boffa, M.J. Erosive pustular dermatosis of the scalp successfully treated with calcipotriol cream. *Br. J. Dermatol.* **2003**, *148*, 593–595. [CrossRef]
79. Di Altobrando, A.; Patrizi, A.; Vara, G.; Merli, Y.; Bianchi, T. Topical zinc oxide: An effective treatment option for erosive pustular dermatosis of the leg. *Br. J. Dermatol.* **2020**, *182*, 495–497. [CrossRef]
80. Di Altobrando, A.; Tabanelli, M. Topical zinc oxide: Breaking the vicious cycle of erosive pustular dermatosis of the scalp. *Int. J. Dermatol.* **2022**, *61*, e216–e217. [CrossRef]
81. Uva, L.; Aphale, A.N.; Kehdy, J.; Benedetto, A.V. Erosive pustular dermatosis successfully treated with a novel silicone gel. *Int. J. Dermatol.* **2016**, *55*, 89–91. [CrossRef] [PubMed]
82. Buttars, B.; Rashid, Z.; Al-Rubaie, V.; Brodell, R. Umbilical remnant allograft application in the treatment of erosive pustular dermatosis of the scalp. *JAAD Case Rep.* **2022**, *23*, 70–72. [CrossRef] [PubMed]
83. Kempton, D.M.; Maarouf, M.; Hendricks, A.J.; Shi, V.Y. Erosive pustular dermatosis of the scalp associated with lamellar ichthyosis successfully treated with dehydrated human amnion/chorion membrane allograft. *JAAD Case Rep.* **2018**, *4*, 1059–1061. [CrossRef] [PubMed]
84. Zahdi, M.R.; Seidel, G.B.; Soares, V.C.; Freitas, C.F.; Mulinari-Brenner, F.A. Erosive pustular dermatosis of the scalp successfully treated with oral prednisone and topical tacrolimus. *An. Bras. Dermatol.* **2013**, *88*, 796–798. [CrossRef]
85. Corradin, M.T.; Forcione, M.; Giulioni, E.; Fiorentino, R.; Ferrazzi, A.; Alaibac, M. Erosive pustular dermatoses of the scalp induced by imiquimod. *Case Rep. Dermatol. Med.* **2012**, *2012*, 828749.
86. Seckin, D.; Gurbuz, O.; Demirkesen, C. Erosive pustular dermatosis of the leg: An overlooked entity? *J. Cutan. Med. Surg.* **2009**, *13*, 160–163. [CrossRef]
87. Hiroyasu, S.; Tsuruta, D.; Yamane, T.; Shioi, A.; Toyoda, H.; Ishii, M.; Kobayashi, H. Atypical erosive pustular dermatosis of the scalp with eosinophilia and erythroderma. *J. Dermatol.* **2012**, *39*, 1089–1091. [CrossRef]
88. Feramisco, J.D.; Goerge, T.; Schulz, S.E.; Ma, H.L.; Metze, D.; Steinhoff, M. Disseminated erosive pustular dermatosis also involving the mucosa: Successful treatment with oral dapsone. *Acta Derm. Venereol.* **2012**, *92*, 91–92. [CrossRef]
89. Jacyk, W.K. Pustular ulcerative dermatosis of the scalp. *Br. J. Dermatol.* **1988**, *118*, 441–444. [CrossRef]
90. Di Lernia, V.; Ricci, C. Familial erosive pustular dermatosis of the scalp and legs successfully treated with ciclosporin. *Clin. Exp. Dermatol.* **2016**, *41*, 334–335. [CrossRef]
91. Petersen, B.O.; Bygum, A. Erosive pustular dermatosis of the scalp: A case treated successfully with isotretinoin. *Acta Derm. Venereol.* **2008**, *88*, 300–301. [PubMed]
92. Mastroianni, A.; Cota, C.; Ardigò, M.; Minutilli, E.; Berardesca, E. Erosive pustular dermatosis of the scalp: A case report and review of the literature. *Dermatology* **2005**, *211*, 273–276. [CrossRef] [PubMed]
93. Seckin, D.; Tekin, B.; Güneş, P.; Demirçay, Z. Erosive pustular dermatosis of the leg in a young girl successfully treated with sulfasalazine and 308 nm monochromatic excimer light. *Photodermatol. Photoimmunol. Photomed.* **2020**, *36*, 496–498. [CrossRef] [PubMed]

94. Leung, N.; Eldik, H.; Ramirez, M.R.; Sodha, P. Oral tofacitinib treatment of erosive pustular dermatosis of the scalp. *JAMA Dermatol.* **2019**, *155*, 752–754. [CrossRef]
95. Ikeda, M.; Arata, J.; Isaka, H. Erosive pustular dermatosis of the scalp successfully treated with oral zinc sulphate. *Br. J. Dermatol* **1982**, *106*, 742–743. [CrossRef]
96. Grubbs, H.E.; Robb, C.W. Successful use of a fractional 2940-nm laser in treating chronic, severe erosive pustular dermatosis of the scalp. *JAAD Case Rep.* **2019**, *5*, 188–190. [CrossRef]
97. López, V.; López, I.; Ramos, V.; Ricart, J.M. Erosive pustular dermatosis of the scalp after photodynamic therapy. *Dermatol. Online J.* **2012**, *18*, 13. [CrossRef]
98. Arteaga-Henriquez, M.; Gonzalez-Hernandez, S.; Garcia-Peris, E. Conventional versus daylight photodynamic therapy in the treatment of erosive pustular dermatosis of the scalp. *Dermatol. Ther.* **2020**, *33*, e13220. [CrossRef]
99. Brianti, P.; Paolino, G.; Mercuri, S. Fractional 1,927 nm Thulium laser plus photodynamic therapy for the treatment of erosive pustular dermatosis of the scalp. *Dermatol. Ther.* **2020**, *33*, e13246. [CrossRef]
100. Wilk, M.; Zelger, B.G.; Hauser, U.; Höpfl, R.; Zelger, B. Erosive pustular dermatoses of the scalp: Reappraisal of an underrecognized entity. *J. Dtsch. Dermatol. Ges.* **2018**, *16*, 15–19.

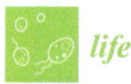 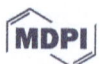

Review

Review: The Key Factors to Melanomagenesis

Cristina-Raluca (Jitian) Mihulecea [1,2,*] and Maria Rotaru [1,2,3]

1. Doctoral Studies, "Victor Babeș" University of Medicine and Pharmacy of Timișoara, 300041 Timișoara, Romania
2. Dermatology Clinic, Emergency Clinical County Hospital of Sibiu, 550245 Sibiu, Romania
3. Dermatology Department, Faculty of Medicine, "Lucian Blaga" University of Sibiu, 550169 Sibiu, Romania
* Correspondence: cristina.jitian@umft.ro

Abstract: Melanoma is the most dangerous form of skin cancer that develops from the malignant transformation of the melanocytes located in the basal layer of the epidermis (cutaneous melanoma). Melanocytes may also be found in the meninges, eyes, ears, gastrointestinal tract, genito-urinary system, or other mucosal surfaces (mucosal melanoma). Melanoma is caused by an uncontrolled proliferation of melanocytes, that at first may form a benign lesion (nevogenesis), but in time, it may transition to melanoma, determining what it is named, melanomagenesis. Some tumors may appear spontaneously (de novo melanoma) or on preexisting lesions (nevus-associated melanoma). The exact cause of melanoma may not be fully understood yet, but there are some factors that initiate and promote this malignant process. This study aims to provide a summary of the latest articles regarding the key factors that may lead to melanomagenesis. The secondary objectives are to reveal the relationship between nevi and melanoma, to understand the cause of "de novo" and "nevus-associated melanoma" and highlight the differences between these subtypes.

Keywords: nevi; melanoma; genetic tests; molecular tests; review

1. Introduction

Worldwide, melanoma is considered as one of the most aggressive forms of skin cancer, that affects individuals of any age. Melanoma develops from the malignant transformation of the melanocytes located in the basal layer of the epidermis (cutaneous melanoma) [1]. Melanocytes may also be found in the meninges, eyes, ears, gastrointestinal tract, genito-urinary system, or other mucosal surfaces (mucosal melanoma) [1]. Certain studies attest to a linear progression, from nevi, atypical nevi, to melanoma, that may occur under certain mutational factors, although the majority of melanomas may develop de novo (spontaneously) [2]. One of the most important factors known to activate melanomagenesis is exposure to ultraviolet light [3,4], which affects the tumoral DNA causing genetic mutations that could lead to nevi's progression to melanoma, through an abnormal proliferation of melanocytes [5]. Melanoma is known for its genomic instability and is one of the cancers with the most somatic mutations [6].

This study aims to provide a summary of the latest articles regarding the factors that lead to melanomagenesis, to get a better understanding of this cancer's biology. The secondary objectives are to reveal the relationship between nevi and melanoma, to understand the cause of "de novo" and "nevus-associated melanoma" and highlight the differences between these subtypes.

2. Materials and Methods

We analyzed over 90 of the most recent studies regarding the key factors responsible for the occurrence of melanoma, to provide a review of the possible causes of this neoplasia. We also assessed the relationship between nevi and melanoma by studying the latest articles on this topic, to understand the cause of "de novo" and "nevus-associated melanoma" and highlight the differences between these subtypes.

Citation: Mihulecea, C.-R.; Rotaru, M. Review: The Key Factors to Melanomagenesis. *Life* **2023**, *13*, 181. https://doi.org/10.3390/life13010181

Academic Editor: Alin Laurentiu Tatu

Received: 19 December 2022
Revised: 3 January 2023
Accepted: 5 January 2023
Published: 8 January 2023

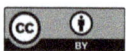

Copyright: © 2023 by the authors. Licensee MDPI, Basel, Switzerland. This article is an open access article distributed under the terms and conditions of the Creative Commons Attribution (CC BY) license (https://creativecommons.org/licenses/by/4.0/).

3. Results

Melanoma originates from melanocytes, neural crest-derived cells, that can be found in the skin, eye, and other tissues (ex. meninges, anogenital tract) [6]. The main function of melanocytes is to produce melanin and provide it to the keratinocytes, to absorb UV radiation and protect the keratinocyte's nucleus from the DNA damage induced by ultraviolet radiation. The data collected from the studied articles were separated into three categories, as follows: Section 3.1 the key factors to melanomagenesis; Section 3.2 from nevi to melanoma—a linear progression; Section 3.3 de novo vs. nevus-associated melanoma.

3.1. The Key Factors to Melanomagenesis

Melanoma can be classified based on: 1. the relationship between sun exposure and the location of the primary tumor (melanoma on skin with/without chronic sun damage (CSD)—CSD or non-CSD melanoma); acral melanoma—located on palm, soles, or nail bed; and mucosal melanoma); and 2. the tumoral growth pattern: superficial spreading melanoma (SSM), nodular melanoma (NM), lentigo maligna/melanoma (LM/LMM), and acral lentiginous melanoma (ALM) [7].

The exact cause of melanoma is not yet understood, but there are certain factors that may initiate and promote its development: ultraviolet (UV) radiation, indoor tanning [8–10], prolonged sun exposure/sunburn [11], burn scars [12–14], pesticides, genetic factors/heredity, geographical location, skin phototype, immunosuppression, hormonal changes, a high number of nevi, neuroendocrine factors, stress, depression [15], trauma, low socioeconomic status, non-melanoma skin cancers, autoimmune diseases, viral infections, biological/cytologic factors, smoking/alcohol, medicines, gender (melanoma has a higher incidence in men [16–20]), etc. [1,21–23]. The impact of a part of these factors will be explained in the following lines, see Table 1—the key factors to melanomagenesis.

3.1.1. UV Radiation

Exposure to UV radiation (UVR) is considered the main risk factor for melanomagenesis [1]. Both natural and artificial lighting systems are sources of UV radiation [1]. Melanocytes are known for their photoprotective function (they protect the nuclear DNA and reduce its damage) as a response to UV exposure through melanin synthesis [24]. The melanin pigment has a crucial role in the protection against the effects of UV radiation and other environmental factors [25]. While melanin protects against skin neoplasms, its presence is necessary for the oncogenic transformation of melanocytes, as melanogenesis may show mutagenic activities, which can lead to the initiation and progression of melanoma. The synthesis of this pigment is modulated by sun exposure and hormonal factors [25]. Melanin is then transferred to keratinocytes that cause tanning, due to UV exposure [24]. Some studies attest that melanoma is inversely related to skin pigmentation, having a lower incidence in individuals with dark skin tones and a higher incidence in individuals with fair skin tones [24].

Approximately 90% of melanomas are caused by ultraviolet radiation from sunlight, which induces DNA damage, leading to DNA mutations and contributing to melanomagenesis [24]. UV radiation can be classified into three categories: ultraviolet C (UVC; 200–290 nm), ultraviolet B (UVB; 290–320 nm), and ultraviolet A (UVA; 320–400 nm) [24]. UVB is the main cause of sunburns, it damages the epidermis, and has a central role in skin neoplasms. UVB waves are absorbed by the nuclear proteins and acids of the cutaneous cells [1]. The irreparable DNA damage promotes the onset of somatic mutations, with the transformation of normal cells into oncogenic cells [1]. UVA penetrates the skin deeper than UVB/UVC but is mainly responsible for its photoaging effect [24]. UV damages the skin cells and tissues and forms DNA mutations, altering the DNA integrity, which impairs many tumor-suppressing genes [24]. UV radiation may also suppress immunity: it inhibits antigen presentation, stimulates the release of immunosuppressive cytokines (ex. TNF-α), and determines the apoptosis of immune cells [24]. The immunity of the skin depends on the functioning of epidermal Langerhans cells (LCs)—the main antigen-presenting cells

(APCs) of the skin. UV also damages LCs, decreasing their numbers and inhibiting their antigen-presenting function [24].

All this considered, exposure to UV radiation either from sunlight or tanning beds contributes to cellular DNA damage, oxidative stress, immunosuppression, and skin inflammation, having a major role in melanomagenesis [26].

3.1.2. Genetic Factors

Melanoma is a neoplasm with complex pathogenesis, due to the genetic mutations within the molecular pathways that control cell proliferation, differentiation, and survival [7]. UV radiation is the most prevalent factor in determining somatic mutations that may cause the occurrence of melanoma [3]. Somatic mutations are produced by multiple mutational processes, which generate specific mutational signatures [4,26]. The most frequent mutational signatures found in melanoma were: signature 1B (associated with age and the spontaneous deamination of 5-methyl-cytosine), signature 7 (UV radiation-induced mutations), and signature 11 (associated with patients treated with the alkylating agent temozolomide) [3].

As for the genetic mutations, $BRAF^{V600E}$ is one of the most common mutations in melanoma (60% harbor this mutation) development [5]. This mutation activates the mitogen-activated protein kinase ($MAPK$) pathway and causes bursts of melanocytic proliferation followed by growth inhibition and senescence, an event known as oncogene-induced senescence, with senescence escape being thought of as a cause of melanomagenesis [5]. Epigenetic alterations and the loss of tumor suppressor $PTEN$ may also contribute to senescence escape [5]. The majority of BRAF mutations are represented by the substitution of valine at position 600 (V600) [7]. 75% of the BRAF variants are represented by the V600E mutation, 19% by the V600K mutation, and only 6% by V600D/V600R mutations [7].

Other mutations that contribute to melanomagenesis are: RAS (ex. TACC1, CTNNB1), and non-BRAF/non-RAS (ex. KIT, CDK4, MITF, CCND1, TERT, CDKN2A, WT1, EZH2, STK19, PIK3CA, RASA2, SNX31, FBXW7, PREX2, SF3B1, RB1, IDH1, MAPK2K1-2, DDX3X, RAC1, PPP6C, ARID2, NF1, TP53) [26–32]. TP53 and PTEN mutations are mostly found in advanced/invasive melanomas [33]. NRAS, HRAS, BRAF, and GNAQ, have also been identified in benign nevi, and their presence is associated with congenital nevi, Spitz, acquired, and blue nevi [34,35].

The characterization of melanoma molecular subtypes is very important for the right therapeutic decision. Melanoma can be classified into the following molecular subtypes [1,26,36]:

1. MAPK subtype: in melanoma patients, the MAPK (mitogen-activated protein kinase) pathway, is hyperactivated causing a cascade activation of NRAS, BRAF, MEK, and ERK (MAPK), intensifying the transcription of the genes involved in cell proliferation, growth, and mutation [1]. The BRAF kinase has a role in the regulation of the signaling pathway between MAPK and ERK (extracellular signal-regulated kinase), which controls cell division and differentiation [1]. The BRAF gene mutations cause uncontrolled cell division of the melanocytes and the development of melanoma [1]. BRAF mutations are often found in common or atypical nevi but are not enough to cause the occurrence of melanoma [1]. The most common mutation in BRAF is the conversion of thymidine to adenine (T→A), resulting in the substitution of valine with glutamate (V600E) [1]. The MAPK subtype with BRAF mutations (found in approximately 50% of melanomas, mostly in younger patients and in non-CSD melanoma) can be classified as follows:

(a) With the activation of the PI3K–AKT–mTOR pathway, increased AKT3 expression and/or the loss of PTEN. PI3K-AKT is involved in the modulation of cell survival, growth, and apoptosis. The increased activation of PI3K signaling is seen in melanomas triggered by the mutations, deletions, and promoter methylation of the coding genes of the PTEN inhibitor [1]. PTEN encodes a tumor suppressor protein that cannot fulfill its role if it is damaged, causing continuous cell proliferation (this gene is also involved in cell division by keeping cells from growing and dividing) [1,36]. mTOR is an activated protein found in 73% of human melanoma cell lines [1]. Therefore, this subtype can benefit from treatment with PI3K, AKT, and mTOR inhibitors [26]. A study by Leonardi et al. shows that the MAPK-pathway (mitogen-activated protein kinase) and PI3K-pathway (phosphoinositol-3-kinase) promote melanomagenesis through various genomic mutations on the components of these pathways [37].

(b) Alteration of the p16^{CDKN2A}–CDK4–RB pathway, with the inhibition of p16^{CDKN2A} and/or amplification of CDK4. CDKN2A (cyclin-dependent kinase inhibitor 2A) encodes two proteins—p16^{CDKN2A} and p14^{CDKN2A}. In normal conditions, p16^{CDKN2A} inhibits CDK4 (protein kinase cyclin-dependent kinase 4)/ CCND1 (cyclin D1) affecting the cell-cycle progression which depends on the retinoblastoma susceptibility protein (RB) [26]. In melanoma, p16^{CDKN2A} is inactivated and CCND1 amplified due to various epi/genetic mechanisms [26]. P16 acts as a CDK inhibitor, slowing the progression of the cell cycle [36]. On the other hand, p14^{CDKN2A} normally prevents the degradation of P53 and favors its control of cell-cycle progression [26]. In melanoma, P53 can be inactivated due to the mutations of p14^{CDKN2A} [26]. Taking all this into consideration, these patients may be treated with CDK4/6 inhibitors [26]. CDK4 is known for contributing to the regulation of the cell cycle, triggering metastasis, and interfering in the phosphorylation of RB [36].

(c) MITF gene amplification. MITF plays the most relevant role in melanoma, by controlling the differentiation and proliferation of the melanocytes [26]. A low/ absent expression of MITF leads to apoptosis, while overexpression determines cell differentiation and an anti-proliferative effect to some extent [26]. Patients could benefit from treatment with histone deacetylase (HDAC) inhibitors as they may interfere with the expression of MITF protein [26].

2. NRAS subtype: NRAS mutations (found in 15–20% of melanomas, but rare in nevi [1]; they have a more aggressive clinical course) are caused by prolonged sun exposure, mostly found in nodular melanomas and melanomas with a Breslow index of over 1 mm [1]. This mutation is important in the initiation and promotion of neoplasms, associated with possible activation of the PI3K-AKT pathway, therefore PI3K or MEK inhibitors treatment could be suitable in this case [26]. NRAS mutations result in a serial activation of serine/threonine kinases, stimulating cell cycle progression, transformation, and survival. This may be caused by the hyperactivation of either growth factor receptors like c-Met (tyrosine-protein kinase Met), EGFR (epidermal growth factor), c-KIT (tyrosine kinase receptor), or by the functional loss of the NF1 (neurofibromatosis type 1) gene [1].

3. cKIT subtype: cKIT (tyrosine kinase receptor) has an important role in cell differentiation/proliferation, melanocyte development, tumor formation, development, migration, and recurrence [26,36]. Its mutations could cause insufficient pigmentation and can activate multiple signaling pathways, especially the PI3K-AKT and MAPK pathways [1,36]. It is more frequently found in acral (10%), mucosal (15–20%), and CSD (5%) melanomas [1]. All this considered, the cKIT inhibitors could be utilized in the presence of certain activating mutations [26].

4. GNAQ/GNA11 subtype: GNAQ/GNA11 mutations are found in 80–90% of uveal melanomas [38]. These genes encode the alpha subunits of the heterotrimeric G proteins (Gq/G11) and their mutations activate various signaling pathways, acting as driver genes in the oncogenic process [38]. Patients may be treated with MEK inhibitors since these genes' activation leads to the activation of the MAPK pathway with MEK enzymes being one of its main effectors [26].

A family history of melanoma is associated with an increased risk due to shared genetic mutations and/or lifestyle habits (ex. outdoor hobbies, sun exposure, etc.) [39]. There are certain inherited genes (*CDKN2A, CDK4, MITF, TP53, XPC, XPD, XPA, TERT, POT1, ACD, TERF2IP, BRCA 1/2, BAP 1,* and *PTEN*) whose mutations may be causing hereditary melanoma [1]. For example, *CDKN2A* mutations (located on chromosome 9) are found in 3–20% of the families with a history of melanoma [1,39]. When this gene suffers mutations there is a loss of cancer suppression and it leads to uncontrolled cancer cell proliferation [39]. Patients with familial atypical multiple mole melanoma (FAMMM) syndrome have a high risk for melanoma development [40]. Patients with FAMMM syndrome have a 10.7%

risk of melanoma and a higher risk of melanoma also depends on the number of family members affected (approximately 100% risk if two or more relatives have atypical nevi and melanoma) [21].

Table 1. The key factors to melanomagenesis, [1,3–5,7,26,34,35,37,39], UV = ultraviolet, UVA = ultraviolet A, UVB = ultraviolet B, HIV = human immunodeficiency virus, AIDS = acquired immunodeficiency syndrome.

Melanoma: Trigger Factors				
UV Radiation	Genetic Mutations	Skin Phototypes	Immunosuppresion	Other Factors
Sunlight (UVA, UVB) Indoor tanning	BRAF^{V600E} Other mutations: PTEN, RAS, TP53, NRAS, HRAS, GNAQ, CDKN2A, CDK4	I/II—fair skin, blonde/red hair, a high number of freckles, blue/green eyes.	HIV/AIDS Immunosuppressive therapies	Inflammation Autoimmune diseases Metabolic syndrome Hormonal factors Aging Stress

Aside from genetic mutations, epigenetics is another important factor involved in melanomagenesis [36]. Epigenetics focuses on the change of the gene's functions that are meiotically and/or mitotically inherited [36]. Epigenetic factors modify the expression of microRNAs, and they target genes involved in cell differentiation, and growth/death, having a role in melanoma progression [36]. The main mechanisms of epigenetics identified in melanoma are: chromatin modifications (DNA methylation), histone alterations (they cause post-transcriptional modifications altering the chromatin state, useful for cancer progression), modifications of histones acetyl and methyl groups (they affect cancer progress, modulate the response to anticancer drugs and have a critical role in melanoma's signaling pathways), and the noncoding RNAs/microRNAs (involved in melanoma genesis, cell cycle regulation, tumoral growth, cell invasion/migration/apoptosis and drug resistance) [36]. All this considered, epigenetics mechanisms should be furtherly studied, as they could predict the outcome of certain melanoma therapies [36].

3.1.3. Skin Phototypes

There are six types of skin phototypes, with I as the lightest and VI being the darkest. Individuals with skin phototypes I/II have fair skin, blonde/red hair, a high number of freckles, and blue/green eyes, making these two phototypes the most sensitive to UV exposure [1]. These patients are more prone to develop melanoma, as they have a lower resistance to UVB rays [1].

3.1.4. Immunosuppression

Patients with immunosuppressive conditions, such as AIDS/HIV are predisposed to melanomagenesis as prolonged immunosuppression cannot protect the individual from the onset or progression of melanoma or other neoplasms [1]. The systemic immunosuppression caused by agents like cyclosporine in renal transplantation patients determines the inhibition of tumor suppressor factors like p53 and the activation of proto-oncogenes (HRAS, KRAS, or NRAS) [1]. This causes DNA damage and somatic mutations, inducing the onset and progression of melanoma [1]. If cutaneous melanoma occurs in patients with an intact immune system, it will develop mechanisms to evade the body's immune response, which includes the activation of immunosuppressive cytokines that will further modulate antigen-specific immune cells to initiate tumorigenesis [41,42].

3.1.5. Autoimmune Diseases/Inflammation

Chronic inflammation is recognized for its capacity to determine epidermal cell transformation and malignant progression, contributing to approximately 20% of all human cancers, including melanoma [43]. Under various factors (for example, trauma, and infections) inflammation determines the transformation of cancer-originating cells by producing reactive nitrogen intermediates (RNI) and reactive oxygen species (ROS) that cause DNA damage and genomic instability [43]. Some studies indicate that periostin (a contributing factor in tumorigenesis) and M2 macrophages may play a crucial role in melanoma progression through inflammation [44]. Many pro-inflammatory exogenic factors may promote neoplasm development through the nuclear factor-κB (NF-κB) and STAT3 signaling pathways [45]. Increased levels of miR-21 (an inhibitor of key tumor suppressors) are associated with inflammation, for example, in diabetes mellitus (type 1 and 2), atopic conditions, and chronic renal fibrosis [45]. Chronic inflammation may thus promote melanomagenesis, through a high level of miR-21. There are reports that neutrophilic cutaneous inflammation promotes angiotropism and metastatic spread of melanoma [46].

As for autoimmune diseases, some studies show that in type 1 diabetes mellitus, there is an increased response to inflammatory cytokines, demonstrating that this type of diabetes T1DM might be involved in melanoma development, through chronic inflammation [45]. In the literature, it is noted that psoriasis patients have a higher risk of developing certain cancers, due to the inflammation that these patients have [47]. Regarding psoriasis' therapy it seems that the biological treatments do not necessarily raise the risk for melanoma development and are considered safe [48,49]. One of the most common chronic inflammatory skin diseases is atopic dermatitis (AD) and there is a lot of controversy regarding the extent of skin cancer risk that these patients have [50]. These patients have a hyperactive immune system, which could prevent skin cancers [50]. Some studies, also report that patients with AD have fewer nevi, which implies that this pathology could prevent melanoma, as a higher count of nevi is considered a risk factor for developing it [50]. Marasigan et al. report that there is an inverse correlation between atopy and melanoma and that there is not enough evidence that supports an association between AD and melanoma progression or survival [50]. While some studies attest that there is a negative or inverse association between atopy and melanoma, other studies report that AD patients could have a high risk of developing it [50]. Since there is no strong scientific evidence, AD patients should use photoprotection, avoid excessive exposure to the sun, and monitor their nevi by self-examination and regular dermatologist appointments.

Considering the role of inflammation in tumor initiation, promotion/progression, angiogenesis, and metastasis, inflammatory pathways may become future targets for melanoma prevention [51–53].

3.1.6. Other Factors

Aside from the factors listed above, there are also other factors associated with melanoma development, such as the microenvironment, metabolic syndromes, hormonal factors, aging, etc.

The onset of melanoma could be associated, through direct/indirect interactions, with the *cancer microenvironment* formed by different types of cells (fibroblasts, macrophages, lymphocytes, keratinocytes, other immune system cells, adipocytes, and cells that form the cutaneous blood vessels) that interact with each other through signaling proteins and cytokines [54]. Studies examining the microenvironment of melanomas and macrophages associated with tumors have shown that they may be involved in all stages of melanomagenesis: in neoplasm initiation, they determine an inflammatory microenvironment and suppress the antitumoral activity of the immune system, they stimulate angiogenesis, enhance migration/invasion of the oncogenic cells, and are involved in the metastatic process [54]. Some studies suggest that keratinocytes and fibroblasts may contribute to melanomagenesis, as they inhibit certain mechanisms that prevent uncontrolled melanocytic proliferation [5]. Keratinocytes inhibit senescence-related genes, promote the uncontrolled proliferation of melanocytes, and affect the balance of the melanocyte-secreted factors that aid in the process of tumorigenesis [5].

Melanin biosynthesis and reactive oxygen species (ROS)—Melanogenesis is a process during which melanin is synthesized and distributed [55]. There are several factors that are known for modulating melanogenesis, such as UVR, MITF (microphthalmia-associated transcription factor), the ERK/MAPK pathway, immune regulation, or mitochondrial dynamics [55]. The main function of melanin is photoprotection by absorbing UVR, but it can also lead to high levels of intracellular ROS (reactive oxygen species) increasing melanoma susceptibility [55]. UVR is responsible for increasing ROS levels in the melanocytes and keratinocytes causing DNA damage and impairing the natural antioxidant defenses, eventually leading to melanomagenesis [55]. Melanin is known for its protective effect against reactive oxygen species and toxic radicals [56]. However, melanin biosynthesis has the potential to produce reactive oxygen species that determine DNA damage and the malignant transformation of the melanocytes [56]. Oxidative stress (OS) has been reported to be involved in all the phases of melanoma (from genesis to metastasis), it may alter gene expression by inhibiting key epigenetic enzymes' interaction with the DNA and it also determines chemoresistance [55,57]. This may lead to genomic instability and global hypomethylation [55]. ROS-induced abnormal DNA methylation pattern alterations can determine malignant transformation and cancer progression [55]. ROS may be generated by the increased metabolism of transformed cells, enzyme activity, UVR, melanin production, an immune reaction against tumors, an altered oxidant system, and exogenous factors (UVR, air pollution, ozone, infections, chemicals, cosmetics, drugs, toxins, or non-ionizing radiation) [55,57]. Additionally, the production of hydrogen peroxide and the consumption of reduced glutathione (GSH) during melanin biogenesis are responsible for a high level of ROS in melanoma [55]. Despite the skin's antioxidant defense mechanisms, excessive ROS production cannot be fully neutralized [57]. A controlled level of ROS is beneficial for the skin's homeostasis and the epidermal keratinocyte's proliferation, but excessive levels of ROS may lead to DNA damage, aberrant gene expression, cell death/mutations, injury of the local tissues, cancer progression, and metastasis [55,57].

Persister melanoma cells are considered dormant cells in a mass of cancer cells that can tolerate a high level of drugs [58]. A study by Karki et al. attests that persister cells could be induced by chemotherapy [58]. These cells experience metabolic alteration to improve the survival of tumoral cells, sustain cell proliferation, avoid the action of drugs, and fulfill energy requirements [58]. Travnickova et al. report that melanoma persister cells originate from the primary tumor and that they contribute to cancer recurrence and drug resistance [59]. Melanoma is thought to be a chemotherapy-resistant cancer, and this resistance could be attributed to persister cells [58,59]. The further study of persister cells could help develop novel cancer therapeutic strategies.

Metabolic syndrome and melanoma—A patient with metabolic syndrome (formed of at least three of the following: hypertension, impaired glucose tolerance, abdominal obesity, high triglycerides levels, and low HDL levels) may have a higher risk of developing melanoma [45]. Adipocytes activate AKT and mTORC1 in melanoma cells and stimulate their proliferation, migration, and invasion (they promote melanoma aggressiveness through high fatty acids oxidation) [45].

Hormonal factors—There is epidemiological evidence that associates acne, prostate cancer, and melanoma with the androgenic hormones as a possible link [45]. Apparently, patients with positive androgen receptors have a worse survival as opposed to melanoma patients with negative androgen receptors, as they also promote melanoma metastases through MITF signaling [45]. Metastatic melanoma cell lines have also been shown to have an increased level of growth hormone receptor (GHR) [45]. Melanoma metastases occur rapidly and are caused by a complex of factors, out of which genetic mutations are some of the most important factors [60]. The growth hormone influences different oncogenic signaling pathways, especially JAK2-STAT3 [45]. Vitamin D deficiency has also been associated with a poor prognosis in melanoma. A high level of vitamin D is associated with a low tumoral thickness and protects against relapses and death caused by melanoma [45,61]. Some studies suggest that neuroendocrine factors may play a role in melanoma development, influencing the tumoral cells' proliferation and metastasis capability [62]. For example, catecholamines stimulate proliferation, motility, and invasion of melanoma cells, while glutamate may activate angiogenesis [62].

Aging—it seems that the incidence of melanoma may increase with age and that melanoma in young individuals may be attributed to a complex of genetic factors, multiple nevi, as opposed to the older individuals where exogenic factors play the most important role [63–65]. A higher age often leads to a poor prognosis in stages I, II, or III, and is associated with high levels of miR-21, reaching the highest level at around 66 years of age (coinciding with the median age of melanoma incidence) [45].

Smoking/alcohol—Some studies have identified smoking as a predictor of poor outcomes in melanoma patients [45]. It seems that nicotine induces the expression of miR-21 and promotes melanoma cell proliferation and migration [45]. The same goes for pollution, a factor that increases miR-21 expression and activates the PI3K/AKT pathway, leading to melanomagenesis [45]. Cigarette smoking is known to determine premature skin aging, aggravate psoriasis, inhibit wound healing, and may also cause squamous cell carcinoma [22]. Alcohol may also be associated with an increased risk of invasive melanoma with white wine consumption having the highest risk of developing melanoma [66]. It seems that regarding this factor mostly UV-spared sites (trunk) were affected by melanoma [66].

Stress—chronic stress can be an important factor in cancer progression and melanoma spreading [67]. Moreover, catecholamines (stress hormones) may promote the aggression of melanoma cells through the interaction with specific receptors [67]. Some studies state that oxidative stress is a major force involved in all the phases of melanomagenesis, from initiation to the progression of melanoma, up until the onset of the metastases and chemoresistance, making it a target for therapy [55]. All this considered, there is a clear involvement of chronic stress in melanoma initiation and progression [68].

Therapies/medicines—immunomodulating medicines may increase cutaneous photosensitivity and suppress the immune system's responses, determining a higher melanoma risk [69]. Certain papers report that immunosuppressive agents like methotrexate (MTX) may increase skin cancer risk in patients with psoriasis [48]. As for melanoma suppression, it appears that resveratrol (a natural polyphenolic phytoalexin) has been demonstrated to inhibit melanoma cell viability, migration, and invasion, blocking melanoma progression [70].

Mucosal (oral) melanoma risk factors—Mucosal melanoma is a very rare and aggressive melanoma subtype that arises from the oncogenic transformation of the mucous membranes' melanocytes [71]. This type of melanoma is biologically, epidemiologically, and molecularly different from cutaneous melanoma [72]. The risk factors and causes of mucosal melanoma's development are not fully understood and there is little information regarding its molecular markers [71]. Mucous melanoma develops most frequently in the head and neck cavities (including the oral/nasal cavity and accessory sinuses), followed by the rectum/anus and the feminine genital tract [72]. Oral melanoma often presents clinically as heavily melanin-pigmented lesions but may also appear amelanotic [56]. The prevalence of this type of melanoma increases with age, affecting both females and males aged between 40 and 70 years [73]. It rarely affects the white population and is most often found in black, Japanese, and Indian individuals [73]. Unlike cutaneous melanoma, oral melanoma is not related to UVR exposure [73]. This type of melanoma may appear de novo, but approximately 30-37% of them occur on preexisting lesions possibly under the influence of various factors (denture irritations, cigarette smoking, infections) [56,73]. As of yet, oral melanoma is not associated with any confirmed oncogenic agents [56]. About 30% of oral melanomas develop on hyperpigmented melanin lesions which may lead to the conclusion that dysregulation of melanin biosynthesis, its products (reactive oxidative species (ROS), intermediates—semi/quinones, which are potentially mutagenic and may promote cytogenetic instability) or a loss of the melanosomal membrane's integrity, with the leakage of toxic melanin particles, could have a role in the carcinogenic transformation of melanocytes [56]. Regarding de novo oral mucosal melanoma, it is not understood if it is caused by an overproduction of melanin as an early/late event in melanomagenesis due to the acquisition of a malignant phenotype [56]. All this considered, melanin seems to be a risk factor for melanoma development [56]. As for the genetic mutations and oral melanoma's molecular pathways, the following are reported as risk factors for its development [56]: (a) the gain-of-function mutations in KIT protooncogene (dysregulated cKIT intracellular signaling pathways—PI3K, JAK/STAT, Ras-Raf-MAPK pathway which causes increased cell survival and proliferation) [56]; (b) MC1R polymorphism—determines damaged DNA repair mechanisms, promotion of toxic melanin particles synthesis, and increased survival and proliferation of the melanocytes [56]. Normally, MC1R (melanocortin receptor 1) regulates the proliferation and survival of melanocytes and promotes DNA repair in case of damages caused by oxidative stress [56]; and (c) the altered expression of cell adhesion molecules, which causes the downregulation of E-cadherin and the upregulation of N-cadherin that contribute to the increase of migration, proliferation, and invasivity of melanoma cells [56].

3.2. From Nevi to Melanoma—A Linear Progression?

There is a genetic overlap between nevi and melanoma, having a shared environmental influence of UV radiation, yet nevi remain localized, while melanoma can spread from its primary location to distant organs [74]. Some studies attest that there may be a linear progression from nevi to melanoma under certain mutational factors [2]. To confirm this theory, a study by Damsky et al. states that 33% of melanomas could be derived from nevi [75], while a study by Sondermann et al. suggests that 30-50% of melanomas and more than half of melanomas in young patients evolve from benign lesions, and neither clinicians nor artificial intelligence (AI) algorithms are yet able to predict a nevus' oncologic transformation [76]. Additionally, the Clark model of melanoma pathogenesis attests that there are certain steps that occur during a progression from normal melanocytes to melanoma cells [40]. These steps include the formation of common nevi, then atypical nevi, then melanoma in situ, and later, invasive melanoma. This linear progression is thought to be driven by the accumulation of genetic mutations and epigenetic changes [40]. A study by Eddy et al. [77] suggests that melanomagenesis is based on the following phases: 1. normal melanocytes acquire an initiating driver mutation that causes melanocyte hyperplasia and nevi development (breakthrough phase, with a low number of mutations); 2. in the expansion phase some of the nevi progress into atypical nevi and later into melanoma in situ, associated with a high number of mutations; and 3. after the accumulation of numerous mutations (ex. *CDKN2A, TP53, PTEN*) the primary melanoma goes into an invasive phase [77]. Melanomas that develop on non-sun-exposed anatomical sites are associated mostly with BRAF V600E mutations' which are considered one of the key factors to nevogenesis (formation of common nevi) [6]. The frequency of initiation of the BRAF V600E mutation is influenced by UV radiation, and the patient's genotype, while the number or morphological appearance of nevi may be influenced by the individual's phenotype (e.g., fair skin, low tanning ability) [6].

Whether nevi are melanoma precursors remains controversial [78]. Pathology-based studies have found that 20%-30% of melanomas contain nevus cells, suggesting a direct transformation of nevi into melanoma [78]. According to some studies, after acquiring different mutations, the melanocytes will proliferate to form nevi [6,78]. Common nevi develop in the first two decades of life, mainly on sun-exposed anatomical sites (acquired nevi), and may tend to regress after the sixth decade [6]. After the acquisition of certain mutations, another category of melanocytic lesion arises, one that is an intermediate form between common nevi and melanoma–atypical nevi. These lesions have clinical, dermoscopic, and histological similarities with early melanomas [2,24].

Recent studies have shown that common nevi have mainly one driver mutation—BRAF^{V600E}, whereas atypical nevi may have multiple mutations (ex. NRAS and BRAF^{nonV600E}) [6]. This contradicts the linear progression theory that common nevi may evolve into atypical nevi, as this type of lesions rarely have BRAF^{V600E} mutations, suggesting that some sporadic atypical nevi may follow a separate evolutionary trajectory [6]. Tschandl et al. report that the presence of BRAF/NRAS mutations does not predict the chance of malignant transformation of a nevus [79]. In this study, the frequency of BRAF mutation was similar in melanoma (63%) and nevi (65.2%) and the BRAF/NRAS transformed nevi did not have a higher chance of being associated with melanoma than a wild type of nevi [79]. This study states that BRAF/NRAS mutations within a nevus do not play a major role in the development of melanoma from nevi [79]. Other studies report that mutational signatures imply that UV radiation-mediated mutagenesis of superficial melanocytes of the nevus is the predominant pathogenic mechanism that drives the progression of nevi to melanoma [6].

A study by Ulanovskaya et al. states the cytosolic enzyme NNMT (nicotinamide N-methyltransferase) promotes migration, invasion, proliferation, and survival of cancer cells and that aggressive cancer lines possess a higher level of NNMT [80]. It is also stated that it supports tumorigenesis and may be used as a potential anticancer target [80]. According to an article by Ganzetti et al., it is reported that NNMT is overexpressed in melanoma, in comparison to nevi, but that there is an inverse relationship between the Breslow index, Clark level, mitoses, and ulceration (prognostic factors) [81]. This idea is also supported by a study made by Campagna et al. [82]. All this considered, the enzyme NNMT could be used as a prognostic biomarker for melanoma, and since it plays a role in tumorigenesis and cancer progression, if encountered in nevi, it could be involved in a linear progression from nevi to melanoma, as under oncogenic factors, nevi may eventually transform into melanoma.

3.3. De Novo vs. Nevus-Associated Melanoma

Melanoma may arise "de novo" (spontaneously) or on preexisting lesions (common or atypical nevi). This sustains the theory that under the circumstance of certain mutational factors, there can be a linear progression model, from common nevi, atypical nevi, to melanoma. Melanomas arising from nevi, common or atypical, normally develop intra-epidermally [6].

There are few known facts about the endogenic/exogenic factors that may cause melanoma to arise in normal skin or on a preexisting nevus [78]. Certain studies attest that only 20%–30% of melanomas are "nevus-associated" (NAM), with the majority of melanomas (70–80%) arising spontaneously (de novo—DNM) [78,83,84]. However, some authors report that this might not be the correct percentage of DNM as preexisting nevi may have been overgrown/destroyed by melanoma cells [85]. Studies show that de novo melanomas (DNM) are mostly associated with poorer outcomes and shorter survival compared to nevus-associated melanomas (NAM) [78]. DNM usually have a tumoral thickness greater than 1.0 mm, and are associated with the nodular melanoma subtype located mostly on extremities, a higher stage than stage I, older age onset, a low number of nevi, and tumor ulceration [78]. Some studies highlight that the lentigo maligna melanoma (LMM) subtype is very rarely associated with remnants of nevi [85,86].

It seems that, on histologic examination, nevus-associated melanomas present either as tumors growing on preexisting nevi or as a transformation of a common nevus into an atypical nevus and, later, fully developing into a melanoma [85]. In a study by Pandeya et al., NAM was associated with the superficial spreading melanoma subtype, with a younger age onset, blonde hair, fair skin, green/hazel eye color, no/fewer facial freckles, a high number of nevi, tumors located on the trunk, a tumoral thickness of under 0.5 mm, and BRAF^{V600E} mutation [40,87]. Apparently, patients with nevus-associated melanomas had many more moles on their skin as teenagers, but with less dermal elastosis as opposed to DNM [87]. These findings may suggest that NAM may arise through a different sequence of causal events, compared to those leading to other types of melanomas [87]. A study by Tas et al. suggests that even though DNM is associated with poor outcomes, the survival rates of DNM and NAM are similar, see Table 2—de novo melanoma vs. nevus-associated melanoma [88].

Table 2. De novo melanoma (DNM) vs. nevus-associated melanoma (NAM), [6,40,78,85–88]. BI = Breslow index.

Melanoma Characteristics	
De Novo Melanoma	Nevus-Associated Melanoma
Prevalence—70–80%	Prevalence—20–30%
Spontaneous development	Develops on preexisting lesions (nevi)
Associated with—poor outcome, BI > 1 mm, nodular melanoma, located mostly on extremities, older age onset, tumor ulceration, low number of nevi.	Associated with—better prognosis, superficial spreading melanoma, younger age onset, fair skin, a high number of nevi, BI < 0.5 mm, $BRAF^{V600E}$ mutation, tumors located on the trunk.

4. Discussion

Melanoma is a skin cancer with a very complex pathogenesis, caused by molecular and genetic mechanisms that are not yet fully understood and it is one of the cancers with the most somatic mutations according to a study by Alexandrov et al. [3,4,26]. Exposure to intense UV radiation, a high number of nevi, heredity, age, and light skin are some of the most important risk factors associated with increased melanoma incidence [43,55,57,89]. It is crucial to avoid all factors that could lead to melanomagenesis, if possible, and especially, to limit sun exposure and use photoprotection products.

According to a study by Conforti et al., although the epidemiological data from 1980–1990 suggest an increase in the incidence of melanoma across all ages, the studies from the last 10 years indicate a 5% reduction in the incidence of melanoma in young individuals (between 15–24 years) [90].

A family history of melanoma is associated with an increased risk due to shared genetic mutations and/or lifestyle habits. A healthy lifestyle may also have a positive influence on reducing the effect of some mutational factors [45]. In a study by Haenssle et al., patients with FAMMM syndrome or/and with multiple melanomas developed less frequently nevus-associated melanoma compared to patients with a high count of common nevi/ no previous melanoma [40]. It is thought that the onset of de novo melanoma in these patients is caused by genetic factors related to the FAMMM syndrome, as genetic analyses often reveal *CDKN2A* mutations associated with this syndrome [40].

Aside from genetic alterations, epigenetics is another factor that could determine the occurrence of melanoma [36]. The main epigenetic mechanisms involved in melanoma are: chromatin modifications, histone alterations (modifications of histones acetyl and methyl groups), and the noncoding RNAs/microRNAs (involved in melanoma genesis, tumoral growth, cell invasion/migration/ apoptosis, and drug resistance) [36]. We consider that epigenetics mechanisms should be furtherly studied, as they could predict the outcome of certain melanoma therapies.

Another important factor involved in melanomagenesis is persister cells. While some studies report that persister cells could be induced by chemotherapy [58], other studies attest that melanoma persister cells originate from the primary tumor and that they contribute to cancer recurrence and drug resistance [59]. These cells go through metabolic alteration to improve the survival of tumoral cells, sustain cell proliferation, avoid the action of drugs, and fulfill energy requirements [58].

The clinicopathological examinations for melanoma diagnosis should be integrated with molecular techniques, to increase the accuracy of melanoma detection and to have a better understanding of its pathogenesis [26]. The introduction of novel techniques for genetic and molecular analyses may lead to a better understanding of melanoma pathogenesis [7]. According to a study by Bastian et al. [91], melanomas may be categorized into multiple biological categories, which differ in types of origin cells, clinical/histologic presentation, the age of onset, the type of metastasis, the ethnic/gender distribution of patients, the role of UV radiation, mutational processes [91].

More research should be conducted to elucidate the clinical relevance of certain melanoma molecular mechanisms, to improve the clinical management, preventive strategies, and the prognosis of patients [7,88,92,93]. The exact cause of melanoma is not yet fully understood, but there are numerous factors that may initiate and promote its development: from ultraviolet (UV) radiation, genetic factors, geographical location, skin phototype, immunosuppression, viral infections [94], a high number of nevi, stress, biological/cytologic factors to gender. Despite the recent advances in the diagnosis and treatment of advanced melanoma, as stated in some studies, the best chance of survival is based on prevention/early detection [95–97].

5. Conclusions

Melanoma is an aggressive form of skin cancer that may occur spontaneously or through a linear progression from nevi under various key factors. Discovered in its early stages, it can be curable, with high survival rates, but with advanced/metastatic melanoma the patient's prognosis worsens. There is hope that in the next years, there will be a better understanding of melanoma's pathogenesis that will help discover it in its early stages and may aid in developing new effective treatments that could better the patient's prognosis.

Author Contributions: C.-R.M. was responsible for the manuscript design, conception, drafting, analysis, acquisition, and interpretation of the data; M.R. contributed to the manuscript's conception, drafting, analysis, interpretation of the data, and critical revision of the manuscript for important intellectual content. All authors contributed significantly to this publication and read and approved the final manuscript. All authors have read and agreed to the published version of the manuscript.

Funding: This research received no external funding.

Institutional Review Board Statement: The study was conducted in accordance with the Declaration of Helsinki and approved by the Ethics Committee of the Emergency Hospital of Sibiu County.

Informed Consent Statement: Not applicable.

Data Availability Statement: The datasets used and/or analyzed during the present study are available from the corresponding author upon reasonable request.

Conflicts of Interest: The authors declare no conflict of interest.

References

1. Strashilov, S.; Yordanov, A. Aetiology and Pathogenesis of Cutaneous Melanoma: Current Concepts and Advances. *Int. J. Mol. Sci.* **2021**, *22*, 6395. [CrossRef] [PubMed]
2. Mihulecea, C.R.J.; Frățilă, S.; Rotaru, M. Clinical-dermoscopic similarities between atypical nevi and early stage melanoma. *Exp. Ther. Med.* **2021**, *22*, 854. [CrossRef] [PubMed]
3. Alexandrov, L.B.; Nik-Zainal, S.; Wedge, D.C.; Aparicio, S.A.J.R.; Behjati, S.; Biankin, A.V.; Bignell, G.R.; Bolli, N.; Borg, A.; Børresen-Dale, A.-L.; et al. Signatures of mutational processes in human cancer. *Nature* **2013**, *500*, 415–421. [CrossRef]
4. Alexandrov, L.B.; Kim, J.; Haradhvala, N.J.; Huang, M.N.; Ng, A.W.T.; Wu, Y.; Boot, A.; Covington, K.R.; Gordenin, D.A.; Bergstrom, E.N.; et al. The repertoire of mutational signatures in human cancer. *Nature* **2020**, *578*, 94–101. [CrossRef] [PubMed]
5. Sadangi, S.; Milosavljevic, K.; Castro-Perez, E.; Lares, M.; Singh, M.; Altameemi, S.; Beebe, D.J.; Ayuso, J.M.; Setaluri, V. Role of the Skin Microenvironment in Melanomagenesis: Epidermal Keratinocytes and Dermal Fibroblasts Promote BRAF Oncogene-Induced Senescence Escape in Melanocytes. *Cancers* **2022**, *14*, 1233. [CrossRef]
6. Shain, A.H.; Bastian, B. From melanocytes to melanomas. *Nat. Rev. Cancer* **2016**, *16*, 345–358. [CrossRef]
7. Palmieri, G.; Colombino, M.; Casula, M.; Manca, A.; Mandalà, M.; Cossu, A.; Italian Melanoma Intergroup for the Italian Melanoma Intergroup (IMI). Molecular Pathways in Melanomagenesis: What We Learned from Next-Generation Sequencing Approaches. *Curr. Oncol. Rep.* **2018**, *20*, 86. [CrossRef] [PubMed]
8. Lazovich, D.; Vogel, R.I.; Weinstock, M.A.; Nelson, H.H.; Ahmed, R.L.; Berwick, M. Association Between Indoor Tanning and Melanoma in Younger Men and Women. *JAMA Dermatol.* **2016**, *152*, 268–275. [CrossRef] [PubMed]
9. Le Clair, M.Z.; Cockburn, M.G. Tanning bed use and melanoma: Establishing risk and improving prevention interventions. *Prev. Med. Rep.* **2016**, *3*, 139–144. [CrossRef]
10. Ghiasvand, R.; Rueegg, C.S.; Weiderpass, E.; Green, A.C.; Lund, E.; Veierød, M.B. Indoor Tanning and Melanoma Risk: Long-Term Evidence From a Prospective Population-Based Cohort Study. *Am. J. Epidemiology* **2017**, *185*, 147–156. [CrossRef]
11. Køster, B.; Meyer, M.; Andersson, T.; Engholm, G.; Dalum, P. Development in sunburn 2007–2015 and skin cancer projections 2007–2040 of campaign results in the Danish population. *Medicine* **2018**, *97*, e12738. [CrossRef] [PubMed]

12. Lee, H.B.; Han, S.E.; Chang, L.S.; Lee, S.H. Malignant melanoma on a thermal burn scar. *Arch. Craniofacial Surg.* **2019**, *20*, 58–61. [CrossRef] [PubMed]
13. Cantwell, P.; Brooks, A. Multiple melanoma in a burns scar. *BMJ Case Rep.* **2018**, *11*, e227295. [CrossRef] [PubMed]
14. Ostojic, N.; Stepic, N.; Rajovic, M.; Koncar, J.; Novakovic, M. Melanoma and squamous cell carcinoma developing on a burn scar. *Vojn. Pregl.* **2022**, *79*, 291–295. [CrossRef]
15. Ramírez-de Los Santos, M.L.; López-Navarro, A.; Ramírez-de Los Santos, S.; Guzmán-Flores, J.; Pereira-Suárez, A.; López-Pulido, E. Relation between personality dimensions and symptomatology of depression in skin cancer patients. *Biopsychosoc. Med.* **2021**, *15*, 18. [CrossRef]
16. Bellenghi, M.; Puglisi, R.; Pontecorvi, G.; De De Feo, A.; Carè, A.; Mattia, G. Sex and Gender Disparities in Melanoma. *Cancers* **2020**, *12*, 1819. [CrossRef]
17. Schwartz, M.R.; Luo, L.; Berwick, M. Sex Differences in Melanoma. *Curr. Epidemiology Rep.* **2019**, *6*, 112–118. [CrossRef]
18. Morgese, F.; Sampaolesi, C.; Torniai, M.; Conti, A.; Ranallo, N.; Giacchetti, A.; Serresi, S.; Onofri, A.; Burattini, M.; Ricotti, G.; et al. Gender Differences and Outcomes in Melanoma Patients. *Oncol. Ther.* **2020**, *8*, 103–114. [CrossRef]
19. Olsen, C.M.; Thompson, J.F.; Pandeya, N.; Whiteman, D.C. Evaluation of Sex-Specific Incidence of Melanoma. *JAMA Dermatol.* **2020**, *156*, 553–560. [CrossRef]
20. D'Ecclesiis, O.; Caini, S.; Martinoli, C.; Raimondi, S.; Gaiaschi, C.; Tosti, G.; Queirolo, P.; Veneri, C.; Saieva, C.; Gandini, S.; et al. Gender-Dependent Specificities in Cutaneous Melanoma Predisposition, Risk Factors, Somatic Mutations, Prognostic and Predictive Factors: A Systematic Review. *Int. J. Environ. Res. Public Health* **2021**, *18*, 7945. [CrossRef]
21. Heistein, J.B.; Acharya, U. Malignant Melanoma. In *StatPearls [Internet]*; StatPearls Publishing: Treasure Island, FL, USA, 2022. Available online: https://www.ncbi.nlm.nih.gov/books/NBK470409/ (accessed on 5 December 2022).
22. Sondermeijer, L.; Lamboo, L.G.; de Waal, A.C.; Galesloot, T.E.; Kiemeney, L.A.; van Rossum, M.; Aben, K.H. Cigarette Smoking and the Risk of Cutaneous Melanoma: A Case-Control Study. *Dermatology* **2020**, *236*, 228–236. [CrossRef]
23. Zhang, N.; Wang, L.; Zhu, G.; Sun, D.; He, H.; Luan, Q.; Liu, L.; Hao, F.; Li, C.; Gao, T. The association between trauma and melanoma in the Chinese population: A retrospective study. *J. Eur. Acad. Dermatol. Venereol.* **2014**, *28*, 597–603. [CrossRef]
24. Sun, X.; Zhang, N.; Yin, C.; Zhu, B.; Li, X. Ultraviolet Radiation and Melanomagenesis: From Mechanism to Immunotherapy. *Front. Oncol.* **2020**, *10*, 951. [CrossRef] [PubMed]
25. Slominski, R.M.; Sarna, T.; Płonka, P.M.; Raman, C.; Brożyna, A.A.; Slominski, A.T. Melanoma, Melanin, and Melanogenesis: The Yin and Yang Relationship. *Front. Oncol.* **2022**, *12*, 842496. [CrossRef]
26. Palmieri, G.; Ombra, M.; Colombino, M.; Casula, M.; Sini, M.; Manca, A.; Paliogiannis, P.; Eascierto, P.A.; Cossu, A. Multiple Molecular Pathways in Melanomagenesis: Characterization of Therapeutic Targets. *Front. Oncol.* **2015**, *5*, 183. [CrossRef]
27. Lugović-Mihić, L.; Ćesić, D.; Vuković, P.; Bilić, G.N.; Šitum, M.; Špoljar, S. Melanoma Development: Current Knowledge on Melanoma Pathogenesis. *Acta Dermatovenerol. Croat.* **2019**, *27*, 163–168. [PubMed]
28. Ha, L.; Merlino, G.; Sviderskaya, E.V. Melanomagenesis: Overcoming the barrier of melanocyte senescence. *Cell Cycle* **2008**, *7*, 1944–1948. [CrossRef]
29. Reddy, B.Y.; Miller, D.; Tsao, H. Somatic driver mutations in melanoma. *Cancer* **2017**, *123*, 2104–2117. [CrossRef]
30. Davis, E.J.; Johnson, D.B.; Sosman, J.A.; Chandra, S. Melanoma: What do all the mutations mean? *Cancer* **2018**, *124*, 3490–3499. [CrossRef]
31. Hodis, E.; Watson, I.R.; Kryukov, G.V.; Arold, S.T.; Imielinski, M.; Theurillat, J.-P.; Nickerson, E.; Auclair, D.; Li, L.; Place, C.; et al. A Landscape of Driver Mutations in Melanoma. *Cell* **2012**, *150*, 251–263. [CrossRef]
32. Ticha, I.; Hojny, J.; Michalkova, R.; Kodet, O.; Krkavcova, E.; Hajkova, N.; Nemejcova, K.; Bartu, M.; Jaksa, R.; Dura, M.; et al. A comprehensive evaluation of pathogenic mutations in primary cutaneous melanomas, including the identification of novel loss-of-function variants. *Sci. Rep.* **2019**, *9*, 17050. [CrossRef] [PubMed]
33. Shain, A.H.; Yeh, I.; Kovalyshyn, I.; Sriharan, A.; Talevich, E.; Gagnon, A.; Dummer, R.; North, J.P.; Pincus, L.B.; Ruben, B.S.; et al. The Genetic Evolution of Melanoma from Precursor Lesions. *N. Engl. J. Med.* **2015**, *373*, 1926–1936. [CrossRef]
34. Ross, A.L.; Sanchez, M.I.; Grichnik, J.M. Molecular Nevogenesis. *Dermatol. Res. Pract.* **2011**, *2011*, 463184. [CrossRef]
35. Ross, A.L.; Sanchez, M.I.; Grichnik, J.M. Nevogenesis: A Benign Metastatic Process? *ISRN Dermatol.* **2011**, *2011*, 813513. [CrossRef] [PubMed]
36. Fath, M.K.; Azargoonjahromi, A.; Soofi, A.; Almasi, F.; Hosseinzadeh, S.; Khalili, S.; Sheikhi, K.; Ferdousmakan, S.; Owrangi, S.; Fahimi, M.; et al. Current understanding of epigenetics role in melanoma treatment and resistance. *Cancer Cell Int.* **2022**, *22*, 313. [CrossRef]
37. Leonardi, G.C.; Falzone, L.; Salemi, R.; Zanghì, A.; Spandidos, D.A.; McCubrey, J.A.; Candido, S.; Libra, M. Cutaneous melanoma: From pathogenesis to therapy (Review). *Int. J. Oncol.* **2018**, *52*, 1071–1080. [CrossRef]
38. Silva-Rodríguez, P.; Fernández-Díaz, D.; Bande, M.; Pardo, M.; Loidi, L.; Blanco-Teijeiro, M.J. *GNAQ* and *GNA11* Genes: A Comprehensive Review on Oncogenesis, Prognosis and Therapeutic Opportunities in Uveal Melanoma. *Cancers* **2022**, *14*, 3066. [CrossRef] [PubMed]
39. Burns, D.; George, J.; Aucoin, D.; Bower, J.; Burrell, S.; Gilbert, R.; Bower, N. The Pathogenesis and Clinical Management of Cutaneous Melanoma: An Evidence-Based Review. *J. Med. Imaging Radiat. Sci.* **2019**, *50*, 460–469.e1. [CrossRef] [PubMed]
40. Haenssle, H.A.; Mograby, N.; Ngassa, A.; Buhl, T.; Emmert, S.; Schön, M.P.; Rosenberger, A.; Bertsch, H.P. Association of Patient Risk Factors and Frequency of Nevus-Associated Cutaneous Melanomas. *JAMA Dermatol.* **2016**, *152*, 291–298. [CrossRef]

41. Polak, M.E.; Borthwick, N.J.; Gabriel, F.G.; Johnson, P.; Higgins, B.; Hurren, J.; McCormick, D.; Jager, M.J.; Cree, I.A. Mechanisms of local immunosuppression in cutaneous melanoma. *Br. J. Cancer* **2007**, *96*, 1879–1887. [CrossRef]
42. Passarelli, A.; Tucci, M.; Mannavola, F.; Felici, C.; Silvestris, F. The metabolic milieu in melanoma: Role of immune suppression by CD73/adenosine. *Tumor Biol.* **2019**, *41*, 1010428319837138. [CrossRef] [PubMed]
43. Tang, L.; Wang, K. Chronic Inflammation in Skin Malignancies. *J. Mol. Signal.* **2016**, *11*, 2. [CrossRef] [PubMed]
44. Ohno, F.; Nakahara, T.; Kido-Nakahara, M.; Ito, T.; Nunomura, S.; Izuhara, K.; Furue, M. Periostin Links Skin Inflammation to Melanoma Progression in Humans and Mice. *Int. J. Mol. Sci.* **2019**, *20*, 169. [CrossRef] [PubMed]
45. Melnik, B.; John, S.; Carrera-Bastos, P.; Schmitz, G. MicroRNA-21-Enriched Exosomes as Epigenetic Regulators in Melanomagenesis and Melanoma Progression: The Impact of Western Lifestyle Factors. *Cancers* **2020**, *12*, 2111. [CrossRef] [PubMed]
46. Landsberg, J.; Tüting, T.; Barnhill, R.L.; Lugassy, C. The Role of Neutrophilic Inflammation, Angiotropism, and Pericytic Mimicry in Melanoma Progression and Metastasis. *J. Investig. Dermatol.* **2016**, *136*, 372–377. [CrossRef]
47. Trafford, A.; Parisi, R.; Kontopantelis, E.; Griffiths, C.E.M.; Ashcroft, D. Association of Psoriasis With the Risk of Developing or Dying of Cancer. *JAMA Dermatol.* **2019**, *155*, 1390–1403. [CrossRef]
48. Semaka, A.; Salopek, T.G. Risk of Developing Melanoma with Systemic Agents Used to Treat Psoriasis: A Review of the Literature. *J. Cutan. Med. Surg.* **2022**, *26*, 87–92. [CrossRef]
49. Bujoreanu, F.C.; Bezman, L.; Radaschin, D.S.; Niculet, E.; Bobeica, C.; Craescu, M.; Nadasdy, T.; Jicman, D.S.; Ardeleanu, V.; Nwabudike, L.C.; et al. Nevi, biologics for psoriasis and the risk for skin cancer: A real concern? (Case presentation and short review). *Exp. Ther. Med.* **2021**, *22*, 1354. [CrossRef] [PubMed]
50. Marasigan, V.; Morren, M.-A.; Lambert, J.; Medaer, K.; Fieuws, S.; Nijsten, T.; Garmyn, M. Inverse Association Between Atopy and Melanoma: A Case-control Study. *Acta Derm. Venereol.* **2017**, *97*, 54–57. [CrossRef] [PubMed]
51. Maru, G.B.; Gandhi, K.; Ramchandani, A.; Kumar, G. The Role of Inflammation in Skin Cancer. *Inflamm. Cancer* **2014**, *816*, 437–469. [CrossRef]
52. Neagu, M.; Constantin, C.; Caruntu, C.; Dumitru, C.; Surcel, M.; Zurac, S. Inflammation: A key process in skin tumorigenesis. *Oncol. Lett.* **2019**, *17*, 4068–4084. [CrossRef] [PubMed]
53. Neagu, M.; Constantin, C.; Dumitrascu, G.R.; Lupu, A.R.; Caruntu, C.; Boda, D.; Zurac, S. Inflammation markers in cutaneous melanoma—Edgy biomarkers for prognosis. *Discoveries* **2015**, *3*, e38. [CrossRef]
54. Pieniazek, M.; Matkowski, R.; Donizy, P. Macrophages in skin melanoma-the key element in melanomagenesis. *Oncol. Lett.* **2018**, *15*, 5399–5404. [CrossRef]
55. Kamiński, K.; Kazimierczak, U.; Kolenda, T. Oxidative stress in melanogenesis and melanoma development. *Contemp. Oncol. Współcz. Onkol.* **2022**, *26*, 1–7. [CrossRef] [PubMed]
56. Feller, L.; Khammissa, R.A.G.; Lemmer, J. A Review of the Aetiopathogenesis and Clinical and Histopathological Features of Oral Mucosal Melanoma. *Sci. World J.* **2017**, *2017*, 9189812. [CrossRef] [PubMed]
57. Emanuelli, M.; Sartini, D.; Molinelli, E.; Campagna, R.; Pozzi, V.; Salvolini, E.; Simonetti, O.; Campanati, A.; Offidani, A. The Double-Edged Sword of Oxidative Stress in Skin Damage and Melanoma: From Physiopathology to Therapeutical Approaches. *Antioxidants* **2022**, *11*, 612. [CrossRef] [PubMed]
58. Karki, P.; Angardi, V.; Mier, J.C.; Orman, M.A. A Transient Metabolic State in Melanoma Persister Cells Mediated by Chemotherapeutic Treatments. *Front. Mol. Biosci.* **2021**, *2*, 432154. [CrossRef] [PubMed]
59. Travnickova, J.; Muise, S.; Wojciechowska, S.; Brombin, A.; Zeng, Z.; Young, A.I.J.; Wyatt, C.; Patton, E.E. Fate mapping melanoma persister cells through regression and into recurrent disease in adult zebrafish. *Dis. Model. Mech.* **2022**, *15*, dmm049566. [CrossRef] [PubMed]
60. Davey, M.G.; Miller, N.; McInerney, N.M. A Review of Epidemiology and Cancer Biology of Malignant Melanoma. *Cureus* **2021**, *13*, e15087. [CrossRef] [PubMed]
61. Brożyna, A.A.; Hoffman, R.M.; Slominski, A.T. Relevance of Vitamin D in Melanoma Development, Progression and Therapy. *Anticancer. Res.* **2020**, *40*, 473–489. [CrossRef]
62. Scheau, C.; Draghici, C.; Ilie, M.; Lupu, M.; Solomon, I.; Tampa, M.; Georgescu, S.; Caruntu, A.; Constantin, C.; Neagu, M.; et al. Neuroendocrine Factors in Melanoma Pathogenesis. *Cancers* **2021**, *13*, 2277. [CrossRef] [PubMed]
63. Van Der Kooij, M.; Wetzels, M.; Aarts, M.; Berkmortel, F.V.D.; Blank, C.; Boers-Sonderen, M.; Dierselhuis, M.; De Groot, J.; Hospers, G.; Piersma, D.; et al. Age Does Matter in Adolescents and Young Adults versus Older Adults with Advanced Melanoma; A National Cohort Study Comparing Tumor Characteristics, Treatment Pattern, Toxicity and Response. *Cancers* **2020**, *12*, 2072. [CrossRef] [PubMed]
64. Paulson, K.G.; Gupta, D.; Kim, T.S.; Veatch, J.R.; Byrd, D.R.; Bhatia, S.; Wojcik, K.; Chapuis, A.G.; Thompson, J.A.; Madeleine, M.M.; et al. Age-Specific Incidence of Melanoma in the United States. *JAMA Dermatol.* **2020**, *156*, 57–64. [CrossRef] [PubMed]
65. Ribero, S.; Stucci, L.; Marra, E.; Marconcini, R.; Spagnolo, F.; Orgiano, L.; Picasso, V.; Queirolo, P.; Palmieri, G.; Quaglino, P.; et al. Effect of Age on Melanoma Risk, Prognosis and Treatment Response. *Acta Dermato-Venereologica* **2018**, *98*, 624–629. [CrossRef]
66. Rivera, A.; Nan, H.; Li, T.; Qureshi, A.; Cho, E. Alcohol Intake and Risk of Incident Melanoma: A Pooled Analysis of Three Prospective Studies in the United States. *Cancer Epidemiol. Biomark. Prev.* **2016**, *25*, 1550–1558. [CrossRef] [PubMed]
67. Sanzo, M.; Colucci, R.; Arunachalam, M.; Berti, S.; Moretti, S. Stress as a Possible Mechanism in Melanoma Progression. *Dermatol. Res. Pract.* **2010**, *2010*, 483493. [CrossRef]

68. Colucci, R.; Moretti, S. The role of stress and beta-adrenergic system in melanoma: Current knowledge and possible therapeutic options. *J. Cancer Res. Clin. Oncol.* **2016**, *142*, 1021–1029. [CrossRef]
69. Berge, L.A.M.; Andreassen, B.K.; Stenehjem, J.S.; Heir, T.; Karlstad, Ø.; Juzeniene, A.; Ghiasvand, R.; Larsen, I.K.; Green, A.C.; Veierød, M.B.; et al. Use of Immunomodulating Drugs and Risk of Cutaneous Melanoma: A Nationwide Nested Case-Control Study. *Clin. Epidemiology* **2020**, *12*, 1389–1401. [CrossRef]
70. Gong, C.; Xia, H. Resveratrol suppresses melanoma growth by promoting autophagy through inhibiting the PI3K/AKT/mTOR signaling pathway. *Exp. Ther. Med.* **2020**, *19*, 1878–1886. [CrossRef]
71. Ma, Y.; Xia, R.; Ma, X.; Judson-Torres, R.L.; Zeng, H. Mucosal Melanoma: Pathological Evolution, Pathway Dependency and Targeted Therapy. *Front. Oncol.* **2021**, *11*, 702287. [CrossRef]
72. Indini, A.; Roila, F.; Grossi, F.; Massi, D.; Mandalà, M. Molecular Profiling and Novel Therapeutic Strategies for Mucosal Melanoma: A Comprehensive Review. *Int. J. Mol. Sci.* **2022**, *23*, 147. [CrossRef] [PubMed]
73. Zito, P.M.; Brizuela, M.; Mazzoni, T. Oral Melanoma. In *StatPearls*; StatPearls Publishing: Treasure Island, FL, USA, 2022.
74. Lee Katie, J.; Janda, M.; Stark Mitchell, S.; Sturm Richard, A.; Peter, S.H. On Naevi and Melanomas: Two Sides of the Same Coin? *Front. Med.* **2021**, *8*, 635316. [CrossRef]
75. Damsky, W.; Bosenberg, M. Melanocytic nevi and melanoma: Unraveling a complex relationship. *Oncogene* **2017**, *36*, 5771–5792. [CrossRef]
76. Sondermann, W.; Utikal, J.S.; Enk, A.H.; Schadendorf, D.; Klode, J.; Hauschild, A.; Weichenthal, M.; French, L.E.; Berking, C.; Schilling, B.; et al. Prediction of melanoma evolution in melanocytic nevi via artificial intelligence: A call for prospective data. *Eur. J. Cancer* **2019**, *119*, 30–34, Epub in *Eur. J. Cancer* **2019**, *123*, 171. [CrossRef] [PubMed]
77. Eddy, K.; Shah, R.; Chen, S. Decoding Melanoma Development and Progression: Identification of Therapeutic Vulnerabilities. *Front. Oncol.* **2021**, *10*, 626129. [CrossRef]
78. Cymerman, R.M.; Shao, Y.; Wang, K.; Zhang, Y.; Murzaku, E.C.; Penn, L.A.; Osman, I.; Polsky, D. De Novo vs Nevus-Associated Melanomas: Differences in Associations With Prognostic Indicators and Survival. *Gynecol. Oncol.* **2016**, *108*, djw121. [CrossRef]
79. Tschandl, P.; Berghoff, A.S.; Preusser, M.; Burgstaller-Muehlbacher, S.; Pehamberger, H.; Okamoto, I.; Kittler, H. NRAS and BRAF Mutations in Melanoma-Associated Nevi and Uninvolved Nevi. *PLoS ONE* **2013**, *8*, e69639. [CrossRef]
80. Ulanovskaya, O.A.; Zuhl, A.M.; Cravatt, B.F. NNMT promotes epigenetic remodeling in cancer by creating a metabolic methylation sink. *Nat. Chem. Biol.* **2013**, *9*, 300–306. [CrossRef]
81. Ganzetti, G.; Sartini, D.; Campanati, A.; Rubini, C.; Molinelli, E.; Brisigotti, V.; Cecati, M.; Pozzi, V.; Campagna, R.; Offidani, A.; et al. Nicotinamide N-methyltransferase: Potential involvement in cutaneous malignant melanoma. *Melanoma Res.* **2018**, *28*, 82–88. [CrossRef]
82. Campagna, R.; Pozzi, V.; Sartini, D.; Salvolini, E.; Brisigotti, V.; Molinelli, E.; Campanati, A.; Offidani, A.; Emanuelli, M. Beyond Nicotinamide Metabolism: Potential Role of Nicotinamide *N*-Methyltransferase as a Biomarker in Skin Cancers. *Cancers* **2021**, *13*, 4943. [CrossRef]
83. Pampena, R.; Kyrgidis, A.; Lallas, A.; Moscarella, E.; Argenziano, G.; Longo, C. A meta-analysis of nevus-associated melanoma: Prevalence and practical implications. *J. Am. Acad. Dermatol.* **2017**, *77*, 938–945.e4. [CrossRef] [PubMed]
84. Martín-Gorgojo, A.; Nagore, E. Melanoma Arising in a Melanocytic Nevus. *Acta Dermosifiliogr.* **2018**, *109*, 123–132. (In English and Spanish) [CrossRef]
85. Pampena, R.; Pellacani, G.; Longo, C. Nevus-Associated Melanoma: Patient Phenotype and Potential Biological Implications. *J. Investig. Dermatol.* **2018**, *138*, 1696–1698. [CrossRef] [PubMed]
86. Sheen, Y.-S.; Liao, Y.-H.; Lin, M.-H.; Chen, J.-S.; Liau, J.-Y.; Liang, C.-W.; Chang, Y.-L.; Chu, C.-Y. Clinicopathological features and prognosis of patients with de novo versus nevus-associated melanoma in Taiwan. *PLoS ONE* **2017**, *12*, e0177126. [CrossRef] [PubMed]
87. Pandeya, N.; Kvaskoff, M.; Olsen, C.; Green, A.C.; Perry, S.; Baxter, C.; Davis, M.B.; Mortimore, R.; Westacott, L.; Wood, D.; et al. Factors Related to Nevus-Associated Cutaneous Melanoma: A Case-Case Study. *J. Investig. Dermatol.* **2018**, *138*, 1816–1824. [CrossRef] [PubMed]
88. Tas, F.; Erturk, K. De Novo and Nevus-Associated Melanomas: Different Histopathologic Characteristics but Similar Survival Rates. *Pathol. Oncol. Res.* **2020**, *26*, 2483–2487. [CrossRef] [PubMed]
89. Guo, W.; Wang, H.; Li, C. Signal pathways of melanoma and targeted therapy. *Signal Transduct. Target. Ther.* **2021**, *6*, 424. [CrossRef]
90. Conforti, C.; Zalaudek, I. Epidemiology and Risk Factors of Melanoma: A Review. *Dermatol. Pract. Concept.* **2021**, *11*, e2021161S. [CrossRef]
91. Bastian, B.C. The Molecular Pathology of Melanoma: An Integrated Taxonomy of Melanocytic Neoplasia. *Annu. Rev. Pathol. Mech. Dis.* **2014**, *9*, 239–271. [CrossRef]
92. Pizzimenti, S.; Ribero, S.; Cucci, M.A.; Grattarola, M.; Monge, C.; Dianzani, C.; Barrera, G.; Muzio, G. Oxidative Stress-Related Mechanisms in Melanoma and in the Acquired Resistance to Targeted Therapies. *Antioxidants* **2021**, *10*, 1942. [CrossRef]
93. Dantonio, P.M.; Klein, M.O.; Freire, M.R.V.; Araujo, C.N.; Chiacetti, A.C.; Correa, R.G. Exploring major signaling cascades in melanomagenesis: A rationale route for targetted skin cancer therapy. *Biosci. Rep.* **2018**, *38*, BSR20180511. [CrossRef] [PubMed]

94. Wilski, N.A.; Del Casale, C.; Purwin, T.J.; Aplin, A.E.; Snyder, C.M. Murine Cytomegalovirus Infection of Melanoma Lesions Delays Tumor Growth by Recruiting and Repolarizing Monocytic Phagocytes in the Tumor. *J. Virol.* **2019**, *93*, e00533-19. [CrossRef] [PubMed]
95. Carrera, C.; Marghoob, A.A. Discriminating Nevi from Melanomas. *Dermatol. Clin.* **2016**, *34*, 395–409. [CrossRef] [PubMed]
96. Rotaru, M.; Jitian, C.R.; Iancu, G.M. A 10-year retrospective study of melanoma stage at diagnosisin the academic emergency hospital of Sibiu county. *Oncol. Lett.* **2019**, *17*, 4145–4148. [CrossRef] [PubMed]
97. Liu, Y.; Sheikh, M.S. Melanoma: Molecular Pathogenesis and Therapeutic Management. *Mol. Cell. Pharmacol.* **2014**, *6*, 228.

Disclaimer/Publisher's Note: The statements, opinions and data contained in all publications are solely those of the individual author(s) and contributor(s) and not of MDPI and/or the editor(s). MDPI and/or the editor(s) disclaim responsibility for any injury to people or property resulting from any ideas, methods, instructions or products referred to in the content.

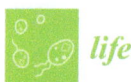 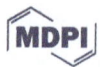

Article

The Many Roles of Dermoscopy in Melanoma Detection

Cristina-Raluca (Jitian) Mihulecea [1,2,*], Gabriela Mariana Iancu [2,3], Mihaela Leventer [4] and Maria Rotaru [1,2,3]

1. Doctoral Studies, Victor Babeș University of Medicine and Pharmacy of Timișoara, 300041 Timișoara, Romania
2. Dermatology Clinic, Emergency Clinical County Hospital of Sibiu, 550245 Sibiu, Romania
3. Dermatology Department, Faculty of Medicine, Lucian Blaga University of Sibiu, 550169 Sibiu, Romania
4. Dr Leventer Centre—Dermatology Clinic, 011216 Bucharest, Romania
* Correspondence: cristina.jitian@umft.ro

Abstract: Dermoscopy is a non-invasive method of examination that aids the clinician in many ways, especially in early skin cancer detection. Melanoma is one of the most aggressive forms of skin cancer that can affect individuals of any age, having an increasing incidence worldwide. The gold standard for melanoma diagnosis is histopathological examination, but dermoscopy is also very important for its detection. To highlight the many roles of dermoscopy, we analyzed 200 melanocytic lesions. The main objective of this study was to detect through dermoscopy hints of melanomagenesis in the studied lot. The most suspicious were 10 lesions which proved to be melanomas confirmed through histopathology. The second objective of this study was to establish if dermoscopy can aid in estimating the Breslow index (tumoral thickness) of the melanomas and to compare the results to the histopathological examination. We found that the tumoral thickness may be estimated through dermoscopy, but the histopathological examination is superior. To conclude, the aim of this study was to showcase the versatility and many roles of dermoscopy, besides being one of the most important tools for early melanoma diagnosis.

Keywords: nevi; melanoma; dermoscopy; melanomagenesis; tumoral thickness

Citation: (Jitian) Mihulecea, C.-R.; Iancu, G.M.; Leventer, M.; Rotaru, M. The Many Roles of Dermoscopy in Melanoma Detection. *Life* **2023**, *13*, 477. https://doi.org/10.3390/life13020477

Academic Editors: Alin Laurentiu Tatu and Paola Nieri

Received: 19 December 2022
Revised: 25 January 2023
Accepted: 6 February 2023
Published: 9 February 2023

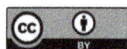

Copyright: © 2023 by the authors. Licensee MDPI, Basel, Switzerland. This article is an open access article distributed under the terms and conditions of the Creative Commons Attribution (CC BY) license (https:// creativecommons.org/licenses/by/ 4.0/).

1. Introduction

Dermoscopy is a non-invasive method of examination that aids the clinician in numerous ways, especially in the establishment of an early skin cancer diagnosis, significantly increasing the accuracy of melanoma detection. Besides the classification of melanocytic lesions, dermoscopy may also be used to predict the thickness of tumors based on specific dermoscopic criteria and colors, which could aid in choosing the right treatment option (dermoscopy is highly effective in skin cancer surgery, as it can help in preoperative marking and the selection of surgical margins) [1].

The main melanocytic lesions are nevi and melanoma. Melanocytic nevi can be classified as follows: acquired nevi (dysplastic—junctional/lentiginous, or compound, Spitz, and Reed), congenital nevi (superficial, superficial and deep, dermal—Miescher (located on the face), and Unna (located on the body)) [1]. The features of Spitz nevi often make them difficult to differentiate from melanomas [2]. They can affect individuals of all ages, but usually appear during childhood (mostly affecting children under 10 years old) or develop in young adults [2]. The management of these lesions is difficult due to their similarity to melanoma.

Melanoma is considered one of the most aggressive forms of skin cancer worldwide, affecting individuals of any age. It has a high potential to metastasize and is responsible for over 80% of deaths caused by skin cancers [3]. Cutaneous melanoma may be classified into the following subtypes: superficial spreading (considered to develop mostly on preexisting nevi), nodular, lentigo maligna, acral lentiginous (higher incidence in dark-skinned patients), amelanotic, and desmoplastic (rare subtype found in older individuals—formed by scant spindle cells with minimal cellular atypia) [1,4]. Tumoral thickness (Breslow index) is one of melanoma's most important prognostic factors [3]. The patients' prognosis is strongly related to the early diagnosis of melanoma, and their survival is inversely proportional to the tumoral thickness [3]. The Breslow index is measured through the histopathological examination, but an estimation of the tumoral thickness can also be made through dermoscopy (colors, dermoscopic structures). It may be difficult to differentiate thin melanomas from atypical nevi, as they can have similar clinical, dermoscopic, and even histopathologic characteristics. Certain studies attest to a linear progression, from nevi, atypical nevi, to melanoma, that may occur under mutational factors that are not yet fully understood [5]. This linear progression, although rare and controversial, is stated to apply to melanomas developing on preexisting nevi (20–30% are nevus-associated melanomas (NAM)), as the majority of melanomas develop de novo (approximately 70% are de novo melanomas (DNM)) [4,6–8]. Dermoscopy can help discover hints of melanomagenesis and may also aid in differentiating between DNM and NAM [6–8]. Besides the assessment of skin tumors (for patient monitoring, early skin cancer diagnosis, estimation of tumoral thickness), dermoscopy can also be used to examine perilesional skin (for example, for assessing solar damage), inflammatory conditions, and dermatoses (psoriasis, dermatitis—which can help differentiate these conditions from actinic keratoses or an in situ squamous cell carcinoma), hair and scalp (trichoscopy), skin infestations and infections (entomodermatoscopy), and nails [1].

The main objective of this study was to detect through dermoscopy hints of melanomagenesis in the studied melanocytic lesions and to showcase the versatility and many roles of dermoscopy, besides being one of the most important tools for early melanoma diagnosis. The second objective of this study was to establish if dermoscopy can aid in estimating the Breslow index (tumoral thickness) of the melanomas and to compare the results to the histopathological examination. We found that the tumoral thickness may be estimated through dermoscopy, but the histopathological examination remains superior. To conclude, dermatoscopy is an essential tool for dermatologists, helping them read the "messages" left by skin cancers and many other dermatological conditions.

2. Materials and Methods

We examined 200 melanocytic lesions (dermoscopic images) of dermatologically monitored patients between 2017 and 2022 at the Emergency Clinical County Hospital of Sibiu and a private dermatology office from Sibiu, Romania. We assessed the dermoscopic images to detect any hints of melanoma. The most suspicious lesions were either excised or proposed for excision. Out of all the studied lesions, 10 proved to be melanomas, which were histopathologically confirmed. We also tried to determine the tumoral thickness of the melanomas to establish if dermoscopy can be used in this regard, and we compared our findings with the histopathological results. The main objective of this study was to detect through dermoscopy hints of melanomagenesis in the studied melanocytic lesions and to showcase the versatility and many roles of dermoscopy, besides being one of the most important tools for early melanoma diagnosis. The study has the approval of the Ethics Committee of Sibiu's County Clinical Hospital (Sibiu, Romania).

Statistical analysis: This was a retrospective and descriptive study. Data were collected and tabulated on Microsoft Excel spreadsheets for statistical analysis [calculation of the prevalence of the variables (%)]. The variables were expressed in numbers and percentages to simplify the statistical process.

3. Results

The results of the present study will be separated into two categories: melanoma (main dermoscopic criteria, dermoscopic prediction of melanoma thickness) and nevi dermoscopic classification (pattern analysis, atypical nevi—dermoscopic key findings of melanomagenesis). The Seven-Point Checklist dermoscopic algorithm [1] (major criteria—atypical pigment network, blue-white veil, atypical vascular pattern—2 points each;

minor criteria—irregular streaks (or pseudopods), irregular dots/globules, eccentric hyperpigmentation region (irregular pigmentation), regression structures—1 point each; ≥3 points = melanoma, <3 = nevi) and pattern analysis (reticular, globular, homogenous, starburst patterns, parallel furrow, parallel ridge, lattice-like and fibrillar) were used to analyze the selected lesions for this study [1,9]. While assessing the melanocytic nevi, we highlighted the main dermoscopic criteria that are usually found in melanomas to showcase the similarity between nevi and melanomas. As for the confirmed melanoma lesions, the tumoral thickness was assessed through dermoscopic colors and specific criteria and compared to the histopathological results.

3.1. Melanoma—Main Dermoscopic Criteria

Cutaneous melanoma may be classified into the following subtypes: superficial spreading, nodular, lentigo maligna, acral lentiginous, amelanotic, and desmoplastic (rare subtype formed by scant spindle cells with minimal cellular atypia) [4]. The dermatoscopic diagnosis of melanoma is based on the recognition of its chaotic appearance and morphological asymmetry and/or one or more of the following characteristics: atypical network, irregular blotch, irregular dots/globules, irregular streaks/pseudopods, regression structures, white shiny streaks, blue-white veil, atypical vascular pattern, irregular hyperpigmented areas, prominent skin markings, and polygons/angulated lines [10]. Other dermoscopic criteria that may be found in melanomas are the rainbow pattern (a sign of invasive melanoma) [11], rosettes (unknown mechanism) [12], and crusts/erosions (a sign of advanced lesions) [8].

We will list the main dermoscopic criteria that were found while examining the selected melanoma lesions from this study, and they will also be assessed with the Seven-Point Checklist dermoscopic algorithm.

- **Superficial Spreading Melanoma (SSM)**

Five out of the ten melanoma lesions selected for this study were superficial spreading melanomas. All the tumors had morphological asymmetry and the following dermoscopic criteria: regression structures—80%, irregular hyperpigmented areas, atypical network, blue-white veil—60%, pseudopods, polygons/angulated lines, white shiny streaks, irregular dots/globules, crusts/erosions, rosettes—40%, prominent skin markings, rainbow pattern—20%. As for the Seven-Point Checklist dermoscopic algorithm, one of them had 2 points, while four out of five tumors had over 3 points (confirmed melanomas), with one tumor having the highest score of 8 points.

- **Nodular Melanoma (NM)**

Only one tumor was a nodular melanoma. Conventional melanoma dermoscopic findings are typically not found in nodular melanomas as these criteria are specific for this type of tumor: blue and black color (blue-black rule), atypical vascular pattern (linear irregular vessels/more than two types of vessels), milky-red color [10]. The studied tumor had a symmetrical shape and the following dermoscopic criteria: blue-white veil, white shiny streaks, and crusts/erosions. While performing the Seven-Point Checklist dermoscopic algorithm, we obtained a score of 2 points for this lesion.

- **Lentigo Maligna Melanoma (LMM)**

Four out of ten melanomas corresponded to the lentigo maligna subtype. All tumors had an asymmetric morphology, and out of the conventional melanoma dermoscopic criteria, the following were more specific for LMM: irregular hyperpigmented areas, irregular dots/globules, white shiny streaks, regression structures—100%, irregular blotch, polygons/angulated lines, blue-white veil—75%, rosettes—50%, atypical vascular pattern—25%. All tumors had 3 points or more after being assessed with the Seven-Point Checklist dermoscopic algorithm, with 5 points being the highest score, see Table 1—Melanoma—Dermoscopic findings, and Figure 1—Main melanoma subtypes.

Table 1. Melanoma—Dermoscopic findings. "-" = no dermoscopic findings; "+" = positive dermoscopic findings.

Dermoscopic Findings	SSM (Percentage of Dermoscopic Criteria)	NM (Percentage of Dermoscopic Criteria)	LMM (Percentage of Dermoscopic Criteria)
Morphological asymmetry	100%	-	100%
Irregular streaks/pseudopods	40%	-	0%
Atypical network	60%	-	0%
Polygons/angulated lines	40%	-	75%
Blue-white veil	60%	+	75%
Irregular hyperpigmented areas	60%	-	100%
Irregular blotch	0%	-	50%
White shiny streaks	40%	+	100%
Irregular dots/globules	40%	-	100%
Rosettes	40%	-	50%
Regression structures	80%	-	100%
Prominent skin markings	20%	-	0%
Rainbow pattern	20%	-	0%
Crusts/erosions	40%	+	0%
Atypical vascular pattern	0%	-	25%

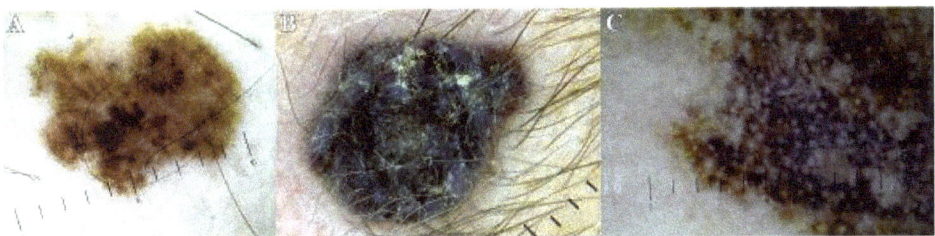

Figure 1. Main melanoma subtypes. (**A**). Superficial spreading melanoma (SSM). (**B**) Nodular melanoma (NM). (**C**). Lentigo maligna melanoma (LMM).

- **Dermoscopic prediction of melanoma thickness**

Dermoscopy helps increase the diagnostic accuracy of melanoma and may be of help in estimating the tumoral thickness [13]. Each dermoscopic color has a histopathological correspondent that can help estimate the depth of the pigments and the tumoral thickness: black—melanin found in the stratum corneum, dark/light brown—melanin found in the epidermis or the dermal/epidermal junction, grey—melanin found in the dermis (mostly superficial dermis), blue—melanin found in the deep dermis, yellow/orange—serum/keratin in the epidermis, white—fibrosis, collagen located in the dermis, red—blood found in the vessels in the superficial dermis, purple—low oxygen levels in the blood vessels (the color of blood varies from red to purple/blue, depending on the degree of oxygenation)—located in the deep dermis [1,10]. One of the most important prognostic factors for melanoma is the Breslow index (IB) [3]. To estimate it, we used the correlation of the Clark staging to the IB [14] based on the dermoscopic criteria listed in Table 1. As a correlation of Clark–Breslow index staging (which may vary according to the localization of the tumor and the thickness of the skin of different anatomical sites), we will refer to it as Clark Level 1 (epidermis)—IB $\leq$ 1.00 mm, Clark Level 2 (papillary dermis)—IB 1.00–2.00 mm, Clark Level 3 (papillary dermis-reticular junction)—IB 2.00–4.0 mm, Clark Level IV (reticular dermis)—IB > 4.0 mm, Clark Level V (subcutaneous invasion). We also assessed the dermatoscopic colors (black, brown, blue, grey, yellow/orange, red, violet) of the studied melanomas, and the following results were obtained:

- **Superficial spreading melanoma (SSM)**

The most frequently encountered dermoscopic colors in this subtype were: black and brown—100%, white—80%, grey and blue—60%, and yellow/orange—40%. To estimate the Breslow index, we assessed the melanomas that had five colors (black, brown, grey, blue, and white) and the highest score (8 points) at the Seven-Point Checklist algorithm. The black/brown colors encountered in this tumor are associated with melanin located in the epidermis, whereas the blue color is associated with melanin found in the deep dermis [1,10]. As for the dermoscopic structures, this tumor had: atypical pigmented network/eccentric hyperpigmentation—mostly correlated with elongated rete ridges with melanin found at the dermal-epidermal junction (DEJ) [15]; blue-white veil—typical to an elevated part of the lesion and its histologic correspondent are extremely pigmented atypical melanocytes/melanophages located in the dermis; pseudopods—associated with heavily pigmented nests of melanocytes mostly located in the DEJ or superficial dermis; irregular dots/globules—melanin located in the epidermis [15]; regression structures—associated with fibrosis located in the dermis [15]. If we were to consider the dermoscopic colors, with blue meaning melanin located in the dermis, the tumor would have a Clark Level IV—IB > 4.0 mm [1,10,14,15]. As for the dermoscopic structures, the tumors should be located somewhere between the epidermis and superficial dermis, meaning a Clark Level of I-II—IB $\leq$ 1.00, 1.1–2.00 mm [12,13]. The histopathological results of this tumor showed the following: Clark Level II, IB = 0.5 mm, with a pT1a stage.

- **Nodular melanoma (NM)**

We observed the following colors in the assessed nodular melanoma: black, brown, blue, yellow/orange, and white. The correspondents of the tumor's colors were: black/brown—associated with melanin located in the epidermis, yellow/orange—serum/keratin in the epidermis, blue—melanin found in the deep dermis, white—fibrosis, collagen located in the dermis. The blue-white veil dermoscopic criterion is associated with atypical melanocytes/melanophages in the dermis [15]. Based on these dermoscopic findings, the tumoral thickness should correspond to a Clark Level I-II (epidermis, papillary dermis) = IB 1.00–2.00 mm. The histopathological results showed: Clark Level II, IB of 1.2 mm, and a pT2a stage.

- **Lentigo maligna melanoma (LMM)**

The main colors found in these tumors were black, brown, grey, white—100%, and blue—66.66%. We assessed the tumor with the most colors (five) and the highest score (5 points) on the Seven-Point Checklist algorithm. This tumor had the following colors: black/brown—melanin found in the epidermis, grey—melanin in the superficial dermis, blue—correlated with the deep dermis, and white—fibrosis, collagen located in the dermis [1,10]. Dermoscopic structures: blue-white veil—associated with atypical melanocytes/melanophages located in the dermis [13], irregular dots/globules—melanin located in the epidermis [15], eccentric hyperpigmentation—melanin found at the dermal-epidermal junction (DEJ) [15], regression structures—fibrosis located in the dermis. Based on the dermoscopic findings, the tumor should be located somewhere between the epidermis and the dermis, with a Clark Level of I-II—IB $\leq$ 1.00–2.00 mm. The histopathological exam showed: Clark Level I, IB = 0.37 mm, see Figure 2—Dermoscopic and histopathological aspects of melanoma.

After we performed the Seven-Point Checklist, according to the algorithm, we had a median of 4.1 points for the confirmed melanomas, with 8 points being the highest score obtained for a superficial spreading melanoma.

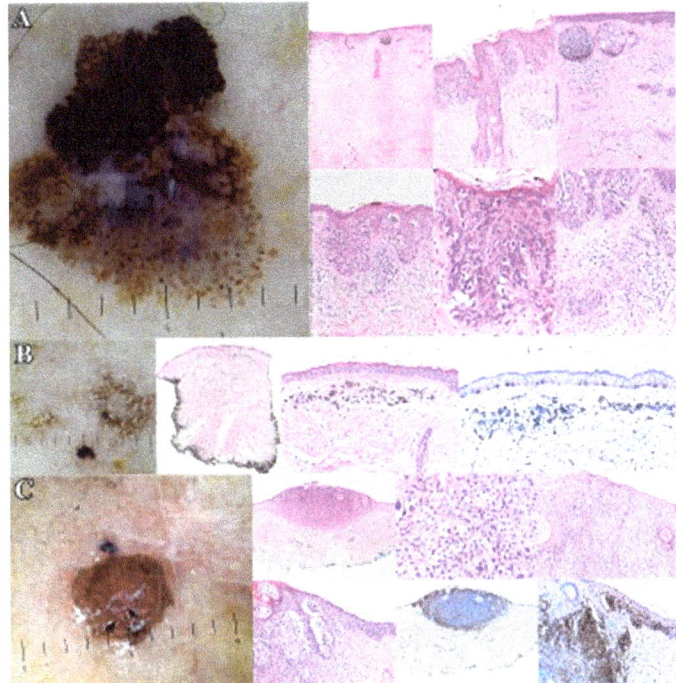

Figure 2. Dermoscopic and histopathologic aspects of melanoma. (**A**). Superficial spreading melanoma (SSM)—Main dermoscopic criteria—asymmetrical melanocytic lesion, with atypical network, eccentric hyperpigmented areas, irregular dots/globules, irregular streaks/pseudopods, central blue-white veil, regression structures. Histopathologic description—SSM without ulceration, BI (Breslow index) = 0.5 mm (pT1a), Clark level II, developed on a preexisting nevus—atypical melanocytes located in the dermal-epidermal junction, with pagetoid ascension. (**B**). Lentigo maligna melanoma (initial lesion)—Main dermoscopic criteria—asymmetrical melanocytic lesions with irregular dots/globules, eccentric hyperpigmented area, and regression structures. Histopathologic description: complete regression of the lentiginous component of a lentigo maligna melanoma—flattened epidermis, severe dermal solar elastosis, melanophages deposited in a band-like in the papillary dermis. Immunohistochemistry—Melan A and SOX 10—melanocytes with quasi-normal characteristics and disposition in the basal layer of the epidermis. (**C**). Lentigo maligna melanoma (vertical growth phase, recurrence after 8 months on the post-operative scar)—Main dermoscopic criteria—atypical vascular pattern, eccentric hyperpigmented area, regression structures. Histopathologic description—LMM (vertical growth phase) without ulceration, BI = 2.2 mm (pT3a), Clark level IV—atypical melanocytes arranged lentiginously and in nests at the dermo-epidermal junction, with pagetoid invasion in the epidermis. Immunohistochemistry—Melan A and Tyrosinase—positive. Histopathologic images—provided through the courtesy of Dr. Tiberiu Tebeică, Dr. Leventer Centre—Bucharest, Romania.

3.2. Nevi—Dermoscopic Classification

Melanocytic nevi can be classified into the following categories: acquired nevi (dysplastic—junctional/lentiginous, or compound, Spitz, and Reed), congenital nevi (superficial, superficial, and deep, dermal—Miescher (face), and Unna (body) [1]. We classified most of the nevi selected for this study based on their dermoscopic patterns (pattern analysis): reticular, globular, homogenous, and starburst [9].

Two of the selected nevi were acral melanocytic lesions, for which we used the following patterns for analysis: parallel furrow, parallel ridge, lattice-like, and fibrillar; these lesions had a mainly parallel furrow pattern. After the pattern analysis for the rest of the nevi, 48.42% of the tumors (92 nevi) had only one pattern, with the reticular pattern being the most frequent—20%. There were also nevi with two patterns (46.31%, 88 lesions), out of which, the reticular and homogenous nevi were the most encountered—25.78%. Only 4.21% of the nevi (8 lesions) had three patterns (reticular, globular, and homogenous nevi).

- **Atypical nevi—dermoscopic key findings of melanomagenesis?**

Atypical nevi are benign tumors that some studies consider to be precursors of melanoma [16], and it is believed that there could be a linear progression from common to dysplastic nevi that may eventually transform into melanoma under different internal/external factors [16]. It is often difficult to differentiate an atypical nevus from a thin melanoma, due to their clinical and dermoscopic similarities, which is why it is necessary to have an early diagnosis to make the right therapeutic decision (to perform an excision or not, since approximately 30% of this skin cancer is nevus-associated melanomas) [16,17]. To determine if there were any hints of a nevus possibly transforming into a melanoma (hints of melanomagenesis) we assessed the nevi based on the Seven-Point Checklist dermoscopic algorithm (<3 points = nevi, $\geq$3 points = melanoma—we correlated the results with the lesion possibly being an atypical nevus/candidate for excision). After performing this algorithm, we obtained a median of 0.90 points (compared to the 4.1 median obtained for the confirmed melanomas). We obtained a score of $\geq$3 points for 21 out of 190 nevi (11.05%), with 4 points being the highest score, whereas most of the nevi had <3 points (169 out of 190 lesions—approximately 88.95%). The lesions that had $\geq$ 3 points were considered atypical nevi and we further analyzed them to see if any other melanoma-specific dermoscopic criteria (white shiny streaks, prominent skin markings, polygons/angulated lines) were present. We obtained the following results: 12 out of 21 lesions (57.14%) presented at least one of the criteria listed above, with polygons/angulated lines being the most predominant criterion (11 out of 21 lesions).

4. Discussion

Dermoscopy is an essential tool for the clinician that helps increase the accuracy of melanoma diagnosis, leading to its early detection, and increasing the patient's chances of survival [3]. Melanoma is an aggressive skin cancer that can arise de novo or on a preexisting nevus [6]. The morphologic heterogeneity of this neoplasm oftentimes makes it difficult to differentiate, especially in its early stages, from certain nevi, as they may have clinical, dermoscopic, or histopathological similarities [16]. For example, in a study by C. Longo et al., there are reports of a rare type of melanoma, nevoid melanoma, that is difficult to differentiate from a nevus, but dermoscopy may provide clues to help identify it [18]. This type of melanoma can be classified as nevus-like, amelanotic, or multi-component type [18]. The most common dermoscopic criteria found in nevoid melanomas are atypical vessels and irregular dots/globules [18].

Melanoma can affect all ages. There are studies that report the occurrence of melanoma at very young ages which are based on both the mutations of certain genes and the expression of carcinogenic risk factors (from intense and unprotected exposure to natural UV radiation, exposure to artificial UV sources, lack of photoprotection, phototype I and II, a high number of nevi, the presence of atypical nevi, and outdoor occupations, to certain oncogenic genotypes of human papillomaviruses) [19].

According to a study by Bernard Ackerman [20], all primary cutaneous melanomas arise in the epidermis, under a sequence of events, with the proliferation of melanocytes that at first extend horizontally along the basal layer and later on extend deeper and deeper into the dermis. Whereas some studies report that nevi are not precursors of melanoma [21], others attest that this is a controversial matter and that a small number of nevi could eventually transform into melanomas through a linear progression influenced by a series of mutagenic factors [22,23]. This linear progression would lead to the occurrence of nevus-associated melanomas (on preexisting nevi) that are reported to develop with a frequency of 20–30%, as the majority of melanomas develop de novo (approximately 70–80%) [4,6–8,17,22,23]. However, several studies reported that the histology of nevus-associated melanomas may present an abrupt histologic transition between the benign (nevus) and malignant (melanoma) components [24–26]. This may contradict the linear progression theory (the evolution from common/atypical nevi to melanoma). A nevus-associated melanoma is histologically defined by the coexistence of nevus and melanoma components. Two of the main histopathological features of nevi are nesting (melanocytes forming clusters of cells within a tissue) and maturation (progressive change in nest architecture/melanocyte cytology)—characteristics that are usually lost in melanomas [17]. Furthermore, some studies attest that definitive histological features of common and atypical nevi are not observed in the same lesion (nevus-associated melanoma), which suggests that a progression from common to atypical nevi, and later on to melanoma, is probably rare [17]. This theory is strengthened by studies that attest that the risk of a nevus transforming into melanoma over the course of 80 years has been estimated at 0.03% in men and 0.009% in women [7]. A study by Alendar et al. also rejected the theory about tumor progression from common nevi to atypical nevi and then to melanoma, as it was found that melanomas usually develop from a "superficial"/"superficial and deep" congenital nevus, and not from an atypical nevus evolved from a common nevus [27].

As for the results of the study, to analyze the lesions, the Seven-Point Checklist and the pattern analysis algorithms were used. We found the Seven-Point Checklist algorithm to be a very useful tool in distinguishing between nevi and melanomas, as most of the analyzed nevi (169 out of 190 nevi—approximately 88.95%) had under 3 points (benign tumors/nevi), whereas most of the histopathologically confirmed melanomas (8 out of 10 melanomas—80%) had ≥3 points (malignant tumor/melanoma). In a study by Schweizer et al., the Seven-Point Checklist algorithm had an accuracy of 63.9–83.6%, being the second best after the ABCDE rule [28]. Similarly, a study by Argenziano et al. shows that the Seven-Point Checklist has a high sensitivity for melanoma diagnosis [29].

We found the pattern analysis algorithm to be an important tool in classifying nevi, which also draws attention to the atypical morphology of some lesions, especially to those that had two (46.31%) or three patterns (4.21%). In a study by Wolner et al., pattern analysis showed superior diagnostic performance, helping assess the heterogeneity and pattern of the studied lesions [30]. In a study by Seidenari et al., the following dermoscopic criteria were found to be more specific to melanoma in situ, as opposed to atypical nevi: an atypical network that involved more than 75% of the lesion, with more than a type of network, reticular grey-blue areas (78%—MIS vs. 48%—atypical nevi), focal thickening of the network, and a black network [31]. In our study, the most encountered criteria in the atypical nevi population were the polygons/angulated lines (11 out of 21 lesions). The evolution of nevi is a complex process that involves intrinsic and extrinsic factors. Among the different types of nevi, the Spitz nevus is one of the most difficult types to differentiate from melanoma, as it may present itself as a pink-red plaque or nodule (similar to amelanotic melanoma), or it can be pigmented (Reed nevus) [32]. For Spitz nevi/spitzoid lesions, there is yet to be an established consensus regarding their management. As it is oftentimes difficult to differentiate a melanoma from a spitzoid lesion, the following was proposed: for typical Spitz nevi in children under 12 years, the recommendation is for regular clinical follow-up, whereas for lesions that occur after 12 years, they should be excised or digitally monitored until stabilized [33]. All atypical spitzoid lesions, regardless of the age of the patient, should be excised [33].

Regarding the estimation of tumoral thickness, for the studied melanomas, we used dermoscopic colors and specific criteria, and we compared the results to the histopathological examination. The dermoscopic color assessment was not a very accurate criterion for this study as it did not help to establish the exact depth of the tumors; for example, one of the analyzed SSMs had blue colors, which means melanin located in the deep dermis, but the tumor had a histopathologically confirmed Breslow index of 0.5 mm (though it may vary according to the examined situs of the tumor and the experience and knowledge of the pathologist). Our study showed that dermoscopy may not be a very accurate tool for assessing tumoral thickness, but at large, it may help orient the clinician in making the right therapeutic decision. In a study by Martinez-Piva et al., it was reported that dermoscopy is useful in estimating preoperative Breslow thickness in melanoma [13]. In a different study by Sgouros et al., not enough evidence was found regarding dermoscopy estimating the IB of nodular melanoma, but it seems that it may assist in the early recognition of this melanoma subtype [34]. According to a study by Rodriguez-Lomba et al., the accuracy of the combination of dermoscopic colors and structures is yet to be established, but dermoscopy may help in the discrimination between thin and invasive melanomas [35].

Some of the most encountered dermoscopic criteria in the studied melanomas were: polygons (75%—LMM, 40%—SSM), white shiny streaks (100% in LMM, 40%—SSM), blue-white veil (60%—SSM, 75%—LMM), regression structures (80%—SSM, 100%—LMM), rosettes (40%—SSM, 50%—LMM), and irregular hyperpigmented areas (60%—SSM, 100%—LMM). A study by González-Álvarez et al. states that rosettes may be an indicator of incipient melanomas [36], and this may be correct as one of the studied tumors that had rosettes had an IB of 0.37 mm. Concerning the polygons, we found them to be more specific to LMM (75%), similar to a study by Iznardo et al. that highlights that polygons/angulated lines are more frequently seen in lentigo maligna located on the face [37]. All the LMM tumors had white shiny streaks, with them being present in 40% of the studied SSM too, showing that it is a specific dermoscopic structure for melanoma, similar to a study by Verzi et al. that states that white shiny streaks are very specific for melanoma [38]. Blue-white veil and regression structures were some of the most encountered dermoscopic structures that are specific to melanoma. In a study by Martins da Silva, the blue-white veil is mostly found in invasive melanomas [39]. Bassoli et al. stated that identifying regression structures in a tumor is helpful in the diagnosis of early melanoma [40]. In our study, none of the studied tumors that had a blue-white veil or regression structures were invasive melanomas. As for the identification of irregular hyperpigmented areas, in our study, they were found in all the LMM tumors, none of which were invasive melanomas. In a paper published by Lallas et al., irregular hyperpigmented areas seemed to be an indicator of in situ melanoma [41].

One of the article's limitations is the relatively low number of melanomas which may limit the study's accuracy. However, we consider this paper to be important as it highlights dermoscopy's versatility and the many ways in which it can help the clinician, besides being one of the most important tools in skin cancer detection. Another limitation is the research design, which could raise confusion for the audience as it may seem like a mix between a review and an original research article. The intent was to build an original research article, but some aspects had to be discussed (for example, the utility of dermoscopy, Spitz nevi, and various aspects of melanoma) to raise awareness regarding the importance of early melanoma detection and skin cancer prevention. It is very important to diagnose melanoma in its early stages as it is easier to treat, with lower morbidity and mortality rates, as opposed to diagnosing and treating advanced melanomas. In a study by Rotaru et al., most of the studied tumors were diagnosed as advanced melanomas, with an IB of over 2 mm, making the treatment of the patients much more difficult, and associated with low survival rates [42].

Dermoscopy is undoubtedly one of the main tools in early melanoma diagnosis which helps the clinician to better the patient's prognosis and chances of survival. It is also a great tool for monitoring the patient, especially for individuals with a high risk for melanoma (atypical mole syndrome) [43]. Aside from aiding in diagnosing early skin cancer, dermoscopy also reduces the rates of unnecessary excisions, which leads to cost savings, lower morbidity rates, and less pain and scarring for the patient—facts highlighted in a study by Plüddemann et al. [44]. Moreover, dermoscopy can be used for examining perilesional skin, inflammatory conditions, dermatoses (psoriasis, dermatitis), hair and scalp (trichoscopy), skin infestations and infections (entomodermatoscopy), and nails [1].

5. Conclusions

Dermoscopy is a non-invasive and useful tool in the establishment of an early melanoma diagnosis. In addition to classifying melanocytic lesions, it may roughly predict the thickness of tumors based on dermoscopic colors and structures, which may help in choosing the right treatment option. Though tumoral thickness/the Breslow index may be estimated through dermoscopy, the histopathological examination remains superior in this matter. To ease the diagnostic process, the clinician may use certain dermoscopic algorithms, such as the Seven-Point Checklist or pattern analysis. In this study, the Seven-Point Checklist and the pattern analysis algorithms proved to be useful tools for the classification of melanocytic nevi and for differentiating them from melanoma. Early melanoma diagnosis is the key to a better prognosis for the patient as dermoscopy remains an essential tool for dermatologists, with many roles and applications, which helps them read the "messages" left by skin cancers and many other dermatological conditions.

Author Contributions: C.-R.M.—conceptualization, data curation, formal analysis, investigation, methodology, validation, visualization, writing—original draft, project administration, writing—review, and editing. G.M.I.—conceptualization, supervision, validation, visualization, project administration, writing—review and editing. M.L.—conceptualization, resources, validation, visualization, supervision, writing—review and editing, M.R.—conceptualization, data curation, investigation, methodology, resources, supervision, validation, visualization, project administration, writing—review and editing. All authors have read and agreed to the published version of the manuscript.

Funding: This research received no external funding.

Institutional Review Board Statement: The study was conducted in accordance with the Declaration of Helsinki and approved by the Ethics Committee of the Emergency Hospital of Sibiu County (approval no. 6001/09.03.2022).

Informed Consent Statement: Not applicable.

Data Availability Statement: The datasets used and/or analyzed during the present study are available from the corresponding author upon reasonable request.

Acknowledgments: Tiberiu Tebeică—Dr Leventer Centre—Dermatology clinic, Bucharest, Romania—for providing valuable data to the article (histopathological images).

Conflicts of Interest: The authors declare no conflict of interest.

References

1. Rosendahl, C.; Marozava, A. Dermatoscopy and Skin Cancer. In *A Handbook for Hunters of Skin Cancer and Melanoma*; Scion Publishing Ltd.: Banbury, UK, 2019.
2. Sainz-Gaspar, L.; Sánchez-Bernal, J.; Noguera-Morel, L.; Hernández-Martín, A.; Colmenero, I.; Torrelo, A. Spitz Nevus and Other Spitzoid Tumors in Children—Part 1: Clinical, Histopathologic, and Immunohistochemical Features. *Actas Dermosifiliogr (Engl. Ed.)* **2020**, *111*, 7–19, (In English, Spanish). [CrossRef] [PubMed]
3. Trindade, F.M.; de Freitas, M.L.P.; Bittencourt, F.V. Dermoscopic evaluation of superficial spreading melanoma. *An. Bras. De Dermatol.* **2021**, *96*, 139–147. [CrossRef]
4. Ward, W.H.; Lambreton, F.; Goel, N.; Jian, Q.Y.; Farma, J.M. Clinical Presentation and Staging of Melanoma. In *Cutaneous Melanoma: Etiology and Therapy [Internet]*; Ward, W.H., Farma, J.M., Eds.; Codon Publications: Brisbane, Australia, 2017; Chapter 6. Available online: https://www.ncbi.nlm.nih.gov/books/NBK481857/ (accessed on 12 December 2022). [CrossRef]
5. Shain, A.H.; Bastian, B.C. From melanocytes to melanomas. *Nat. Rev. Cancer* **2016**, *16*, 345–358, Erratum in: *Nat. Rev. Cancer* **2020**, *20*, 355. [CrossRef] [PubMed]
6. Pampena, R.; Kyrgidis, A.; Lallas, A.; Moscarella, E.; Argenziano, G.; Longo, C. A meta-analysis of nevus-associated melanoma: Prevalence and practical implications. *J. Am. Acad. Dermatol.* **2017**, *77*, 938–945.e4. [CrossRef] [PubMed]
7. Martín-Gorgojo, A.; Nagore, E. Melanoma Arising in a Melanocytic Nevus. *Actas Dermosifiliogr. (Engl. Ed.)* **2018**, *109*, 123–132. (In English, Spanish) [CrossRef] [PubMed]
8. Seebacher, N.A. Melanoma. 2022. Available online: https://dermnetnz.org/topics/melanoma (accessed on 12 December 2022).
9. Soyer, H.P.; Argenziano, G.; Hofmann-Wellenhof, R.; Zaludek, I. *Dermoscopy The Essentials*, 3rd ed.; Elsevier: Amsterdam, The Netherlands, 2020.
10. Lallas, A.; Apalla, Z.; Lazaridou, E.; Ioannides, D. *Dermatoscopy A-Z*; CRC Press: Boca Raton, FL, USA; Taylor & Fancis Group: Abingdon, UK, 2020.

11. Rodríguez-Lomba, E.; García-Piqueras, P.; Lozano-Masdemont, B.; Nieto-Benito, L.M.; Hernández de la Torre, E.; Parra-Blanco, V.; Suárez-Fernández, R.; Lázaro-Ochaita, P.; Avilés-Izquierdo, J.A. 'Rainbow pattern': A dermoscopic sign of invasive melanoma. *Clin. Exp. Dermatol.* **2022**, *47*, 529–533. [CrossRef] [PubMed]
12. Ishida, M.; Iwai, M.; Yoshida, K.; Kagotani, A.; Okabe, H. A distinct histopathological variant of a malignant melanoma with perivascular pseudorosettes: A case report. *Oncol. Lett.* **2013**, *6*, 673–675. [CrossRef]
13. Martínez-Piva, M.M.; Vacas, A.S.; Rodríguez Kowalczuk, M.V.; Gallo, F.; Rodrígues Vasconcelos, M.; Mazzuoccolo, L.D. Dermoscopy as a Tool for Estimating Breslow Thickness in Melanoma. *Actas Dermosifiliogr. (Engl. Ed.)* **2021**, *112*, 434–440. (In English, Spanish) [CrossRef] [PubMed]
14. Hasney, C.; Butcher, R.B., 2nd; Amedee, R.G. Malignant melanoma of the head and neck: A brief review of pathophysiology, current staging, and management. *Ochsner. J.* **2008**, *8*, 181–185.
15. Massone, C.; Hofman-Wellenhof, R.; Chiodi, S.; Sola, S. Dermoscopic Criteria, Histopathological Correlates and Genetic Findings of Thin Melanoma on Non-Volar Skin. *Genes* **2021**, *12*, 1288. [CrossRef]
16. Jitian, C.-R.; Frățilă, S.; Rotaru, M. Clinical-dermoscopic similarities between atypical nevi and early stage melanoma. *Exp. Ther. Med.* **2021**, *22*, 854. [CrossRef]
17. Damsky, W.E.; Bosenberg, M. Melanocytic nevi and melanoma: Unraveling a complex relationship. *Oncogene* **2017**, *36*, 5771–5792. [CrossRef]
18. Longo, C.; Piana, S.; Marghoob, A.; Cavicchini, S.; Rubegni, P.; Cota, C.; Ferrara, G.; Cesinaro, A.M.; Baade, A.; Bencini, P.L.; et al. Morphological features of naevoid melanoma: Results of a multicentre study of the International Dermoscopy Society. *Br. J. Dermatol.* **2015**, *172*, 961–967. [CrossRef] [PubMed]
19. Rotaru, M.; Iancu, G.; Mihalache, M.; Anton, G.; Morariu, S. α-HPV positivity analysis in a group of patients with melanoma and non-melanoma skin cancer. *Rev. Romana Med. Lab.* **2014**, *22*, 471–478. [CrossRef]
20. Ackerman, A.B. Malignant melanoma: A unifying concept. *Hum. Pathol.* **1980**, *11*, 591–595. [CrossRef]
21. Ackerman, A.B.; Mihara, I. Dysplasia, dysplastic melanocytes, dysplastic nevi, the dysplastic nevus syndrome, and the relation between dysplastic nevi and malignant melanomas. *Hum. Pathol.* **1985**, *16*, 87–91. [CrossRef]
22. Cymerman, R.M.; Shao, Y.; Wang, K.; Zhang, Y.; Murzaku, E.C.; Penn, L.A.; Osman, I.; Polsky, D. De Novo vs Nevus-Associated Melanomas: Differences in Associations With Prognostic Indicators and Survival. *J. Natl. Cancer Inst.* **2016**, *108*, djw121. [CrossRef]
23. Sondermann, W.; Utikal, J.S.; Enk, A.H.; Schadendorf, D.; Klode, J.; Hauschild, A.; Weichenthal, M.; French, L.E.; Berking, C.; Schilling, B.; et al. Prediction of melanoma evolution in melanocytic nevi via artificial intelligence: A call for prospective data. *Eur. J. Cancer* **2019**, *119*, 30–34, Erratum in: *Eur. J. Cancer* **2019**, *123*, 171. [CrossRef] [PubMed]
24. Longo, C.; Rito, C.; Beretti, F.; Cesinaro, A.M.; Piñeiro-Maceira, J.; Seidenari, S.; Pellacani, G. De novo melanoma and melanoma arising from pre-existing nevus: In vivo morphologic differences as evaluated by confocal microscopy. *J. Am. Acad. Dermatol.* **2011**, *65*, 604–614. [CrossRef] [PubMed]
25. Loghavi, S.; Curry, J.L.; Torres-Cabala, C.A.; Ivan, D.; Patel, K.P.; Mehrotra, M.; Bassett, R.; Prieto, V.G.; Tetzlaff, M.T. Melanoma arising in association with blue nevus: A clinical and pathologic study of 24 cases and comprehensive review of the literature. *Mod Pathol.* **2014**, *27*, 1468–1478. [CrossRef] [PubMed]
26. Ferrara, G.; Improta, G. The Histopathological Diagnosis and Reporting of Melanoma: A New Look at an Old Challenge. *Austin. J. Dermatolog.* **2016**, *3*, 1044.
27. Alendar, T.; Kittler, H. Morphologic characteristics of nevi associated with melanoma: A clinical, dermatoscopic and histopathologic analysis. *Dermatol. Pract. Concept.* **2018**, *8*, 104–108. [CrossRef]
28. Schweizer, A.; Fink, C.; Bertlich, I.; Toberer, F.; Mitteldorf, C.; Stolz, W.; Enk, A.; Kilian, S.; Haenssle, H.A. Differentiation of combined nevi and melanomas: Case-control study with comparative analysis of dermoscopic features. *J. Dtsch Dermatol. Ges.* **2020**, *18*, 111–118. [CrossRef] [PubMed]
29. Argenziano, G.; Zalaudek, I. Recent Advances in Dermoscopic Diagnostic Technologies. *Dermatol. Cancer—Eur. Oncol. Dis.* **2007**, *1*, 104–106. [CrossRef]
30. Wolner, Z.J.; Yélamos, O.; Liopyris, K.; Marghoob, A.A. Dermoscopy of Melanocytic Lesions. In *Melanoma*; Riker, A., Ed.; Springer: Cham, Switzerland, 2018. [CrossRef]
31. Seidenari, S.; Ferrari, C.; Borsari, S.; Bassoli, S.; Cesinaro, A.M.; Giusti, F.; Pellacani, G.; Ponti, G.; Zalaudek, I.; Argenziano, G. The dermoscopic variability of pigment network in melanoma in situ. *Melanoma Res.* **2012**, *22*, 151–157. [CrossRef] [PubMed]
32. Argenziano, G.; Agozzino, M.; Bonifazi, E.; Broganelli, P.; Brunetti, B.; Ferrara, G.; Fulgione, E.; Garrone, A.; Zalaudek, I. Natural evolution of Spitz nevi. *Dermatology* **2011**, *222*, 256–2600. [CrossRef] [PubMed]
33. Sainz-Gaspar, L.; Sánchez-Bernal, J.; Noguera-Morel, L.; Hernández-Martín, A.; Colmenero, I.; Torrelo, A. Spitz Nevus and Other Spitzoid Tumors in Children. Part 2: Cytogenetic and Molecular Features. Prognosis and Treatment. *Actas Dermosifiliogr. (Engl. Ed.)* **2020**, *111*, 20–25, (In English, Spanish). [CrossRef] [PubMed]
34. Sgouros, D.; Lallas, A.; Kittler, H.; Zarras, A.; Kyrgidis, A.; Papageorgiou, C.; Puig, S.; Scope, A.; Argenziano, G.; Zalaudek, I.; et al. Dermatoscopic features of thin (≤2 mm Breslow thickness) vs. thick (>2 mm Breslow thickness) nodular melanoma and predictors of nodular melanoma versus nodular non-melanoma tumours: A multicentric collaborative study by the International Dermoscopy Society. *J. Eur. Acad. Dermatol. Venereol.* **2020**, *34*, 2541–2547. [CrossRef]

35. Rodríguez-Lomba, E.; Lozano-Masdemont, B.; Nieto-Benito, L.M.; Hernández de la Torre, E.; Suárez-Fernández, R.; Avilés-Izquierdo, J.A. Dermoscopic Predictors of Tumor Thickness in Cutaneous Melanoma: A Retrospective Analysis of 245 Melanomas. *Dermatol. Pract. Concept.* **2021**, *11*, e2021059. [CrossRef]
36. González-Álvarez, T.; Armengot-Carbó, M.; Barreiro, A.; Alarcón, I.; Carrera, C.; García, A.; Malvehy, J.; Puig, S. Dermoscopic rosettes as a clue for pigmented incipient melanoma. *Dermatology* **2014**, *228*, 31–33. [CrossRef] [PubMed]
37. Iznardo, H.; Garcia-Melendo, C.; Yélamos, O. Lentigo Maligna: Clinical Presentation and Appropriate Management. *Clin. Cosmet. Investig. Dermatol.* **2020**, *13*, 837–855. [CrossRef]
38. Verzi, A.E.; Quan, V.L.; Walton, K.E.; Martini, M.C.; Marghoob, A.A.; Garfield, E.M.; Kong, B.Y.; Isales, M.C.; VandenBoom, T.; Zhang, B.; et al. The diagnostic value and histologic correlate of distinct patterns of shiny white streaks for the diagnosis of melanoma: A retrospective, case-control study. *J. Am. Acad. Dermatol.* **2018**, *78*, 913–919. [CrossRef]
39. Silva, V.P.; Ikino, J.K.; Sens, M.M.; Nunes, D.H.; Di Giunta, G. Dermoscopic features of thin melanomas: A comparative study of melanoma in situ and invasive melanomas smaller than or equal to 1 mm. *An. Bras. Dermatol.* **2013**, *88*, 712–717. [CrossRef]
40. Bassoli, S.; Borsari, S.; Ferrari, C.; Giusti, F.; Pellacani, G.; Ponti, G.; Seidenari, S. Grey-blue regression in melanoma in situ-evaluation on 111 cases. *J. Skin Cancer* **2011**, *2011*, 180980. [CrossRef]
41. Lallas, A.; Longo, C.; Manfredini, M.; Benati, E.; Babino, G.; Chinazzo, C.; Apalla, Z.; Papageorgiou, C.; Moscarella, E.; Kyrgidis, A.; et al. Accuracy of Dermoscopic Criteria for the Diagnosis of Melanoma In Situ. *JAMA Dermatol.* **2018**, *154*, 414–419. [CrossRef]
42. Rotaru, M.; Jitian, C.R.; Iancu, G.M. A 10-year retrospective study of melanoma stage at diagnosis in the academic emergency hospital of Sibiu county. *Oncol. Lett.* **2019**, *17*, 4145–4148. [CrossRef]
43. Rotaru, M.; Nati, A.E.; Avrămoiu, I.; Grosu, F.; Mălăescu, G.D. Digital dermoscopic follow-up of 1544 melanocytic nevi. *Rom J. Morphol. Embryol.* **2015**, *56*, 1467–1472. [PubMed]
44. Plüddemann, A.; Heneghan, C.; Thompson, M.; Wolstenholme, J.; Price, C.P. Dermoscopy for the diagnosis of melanoma: Primary care diagnostic technology update. *Br. J. Gen. Pract.* **2011**, *61*, 416–417. [CrossRef]

Disclaimer/Publisher's Note: The statements, opinions and data contained in all publications are solely those of the individual author(s) and contributor(s) and not of MDPI and/or the editor(s). MDPI and/or the editor(s) disclaim responsibility for any injury to people or property resulting from any ideas, methods, instructions or products referred to in the content.

 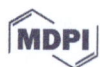

Article

Basal Cell Carcinoma—A Retrospective Descriptive Study Integrated in Current Literature

Carmen Giuglea [1,2,†], Andrei Marin [1,2,*,†], Iulia Gavrila [1,2], Alexandra Paunescu [3], Nicoleta Amalia Dobrete [4] and Silviu Adrian Marinescu [1,5,†]

1. Pastic Surgery Department, Faculty of Medicine, "Carol Davila" University of Medicine and Pharmacy, 020021 Bucharest, Romania
2. Plastic Surgery Department, "St. John" Hospital, 042122 Bucharest, Romania
3. Pathology Department, "St. John" Hospital, 042122 Bucharest, Romania
4. Hematology Department, Ploiesti County Hospital, 100576 Ploiesti, Romania
5. Plastic Surgery Department, "Bagdasar Arseni" Hospital, 041915 Bucharest, Romania
* Correspondence: andrei.marin@umfcd.ro
† These authors contributed equally to this work.

Abstract: Basal cell carcinoma (BCC) is considered to be the most common cancer in humans. It has a slow growth rhythm, and for this reason, metastases are rare. For our retrospective study, we selected 180 patients from those who underwent surgery for a variety of skin tumours between January 2019 and August 2022 and whose histopathological examination revealed basal cell carcinoma. All surgeries were performed by plastic surgeons at the "St. John" hospital in Bucharest. The aim of this article is to provide observational data regarding BCC—in terms of histopathology and diagnostic and therapeutic management and to integrate these data into the current knowledge of this pathology.

Keywords: skin cancer; basal cell carcinoma; skin surgery

1. Introduction

Basal cell carcinoma is considered to be the most common malignancy in the white population [1]. This pathology has different incidences around the world—depending on race and geographic influences—with the highest incidence in Australia and the lowest in Africans from Kenya [2].

The pathogenesis of BCC involves the activation of the hedgehog intracellular signalling pathway, which is responsible for cell growth and division. There are several mutations which can occur in different genes: some with suppressive/inhibiting roles (PTCH1, SUFU, p53) and others which activate tumour formation (SMOm) [3].

However, this type of cancer has a slow growth rate, usually resulting in a local invasion of surrounding tissue, with very few metastases [4].

BCC has a predominance in male patients according to Asgari et al. [5]. The major risk factor is considered to be sun exposure (UVA and UVB radiation), with a predilection for exposed skin areas (head and neck) and a fair skin complexion (Fitzpatrick types 1 and 2) [3,5]. Immunosuppression is also a significant risk factor, as patients with organ transplants are 5 to 10 times more likely to develop BCC [3]. Other risk factors that deserve mention are a family history of skin cancer, artificial tanning, photosensitising drugs, childhood sunburn, ionising radiation and chemicals [6–10].

According to WHO Classification of skin tumours, BCC includes the following histopathological subtypes: superficial BCC, nodular (solid) BCC, micronodular BCC, infiltrating BCC, sclerosing/morphoeic BCC, fibroepithelial BCC, BCC with adnexal differentiation, basosquamous carcinoma, BCC with sarcomatoid differentiation and pigmented BCC [11].

There are several diagnostic tools, which include dermoscopy, as well as clinical microscopy [12] and confocal microscopy [13]; nonetheless, the final diagnosis is provided from the histopathology examination. Other diagnostic tools include high-resolution ultrasonography, optical coherence tomography, Raman spectroscopy, terahertz pulse imaging and reflectance confocal microscopy [14,15].

2. Materials and Methods

The inclusion criteria for the patients in our study were represented by a positive diagnosis for BCC, taken from histopathology reports of patients that were operated on in St. John's Hospital between January 2019 and August 2022. All patients that were operated on in this time frame for skin lesions with a positive histopathologic result for BCC were selected for this study (including patients that were operated on for multiple lesions in which at least one turned out to be a BCC). Exclusion criteria were represented by operated skin lesions for which there was no histopathologic report and singular skin lesions which had other results on the histopathologic report (SCC, melanoma).

The variables extracted from these reports were represented by age and sex of the patient, experience of the operator, tumour localisation, date of the operation, size of the excised specimen (length, width and depth), largest diameter of the BCC, markings of the specimen for orientation, histopathological type (infiltrative/nodular/micronodular/superficial/basosquamouspigmented), if the tumour was ulcerated, if the margins were clear of tumour, if more tumours were excised during the same operation (and if those were benign or malignant).

From the medical file of the patients with BCC, we extracted the following data: type of surgery (direct closure/skin graft/flap), if the patient came for a relapse or for a BCC at the first excision, patients which were re-excised for incomplete first excision and personal medical history for each patient.

The data were processed by using IBM Statistical Package for Social Science 25 (SPSS).

3. Results

Our study included a total of 180 patients with a total of 211 basal cell carcinomas operated (155 patients had 1 BCC, 22 patients had 2 BCC, 2 patients had 3 BCC and 1 patient had 5 BCC). The sex distribution in our group was 88 women (48.9%) and 92 men (51.1%). The median age of the women's group was 73 years, while for men the median was 73.5 years. Age/sex distribution is represented in the following histogram (Figure 1).

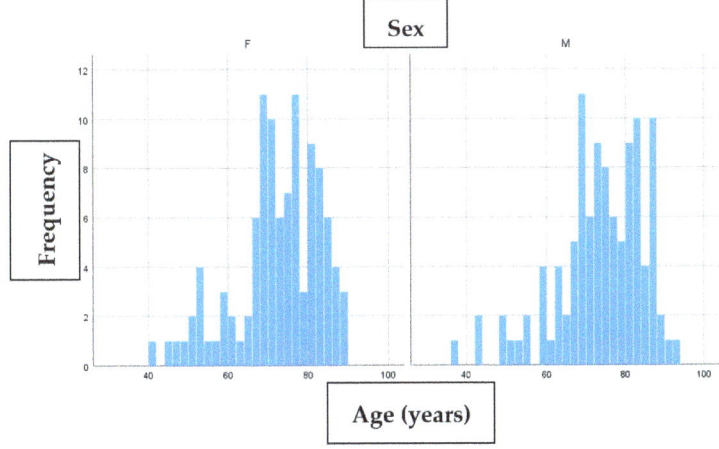

Figure 1. Age/sex distribution for BCC.

Between January 2019 and August 2022, there were 180 patients operated for BCC in our hospital. Figure 2 shows the percentage of patients operated each year.

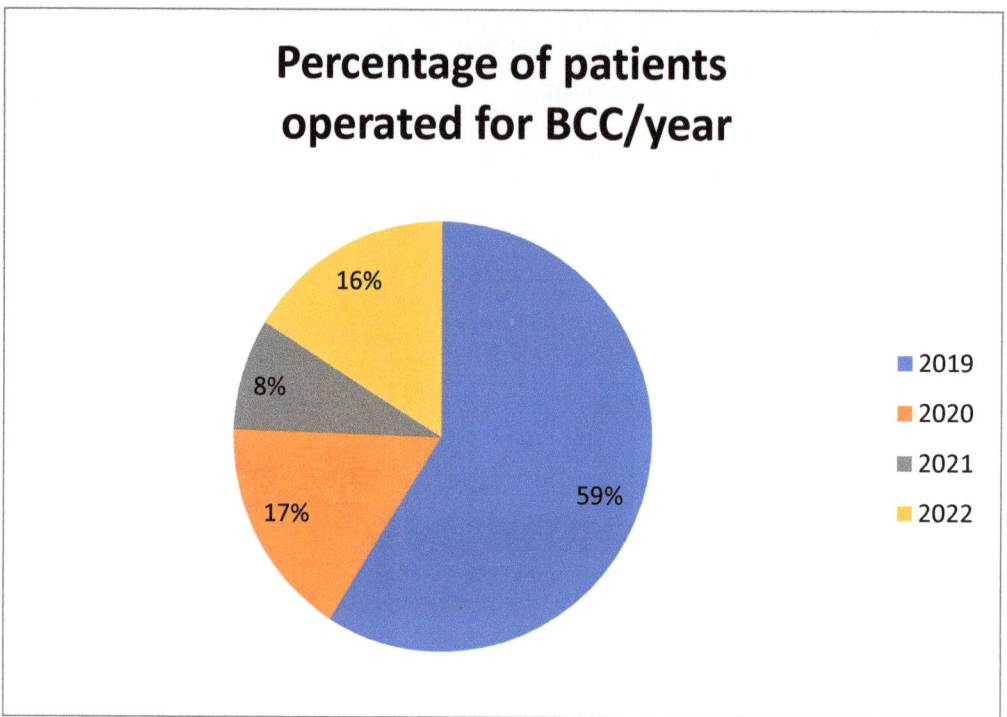

Figure 2. The percentage of patients operated each year.

Table 1 reflects the distribution of BCC related to age. Only 5.6% of the total number of patients with BCC was under the age of 50.

Table 1. Distribution of BCC related to age.

	Percentage of Patients </> 50 Years Old	
Patient's Age	**No. of Patients**	**%**
≤50 years	10	5.6
>50 years	170	94.4
Total	180	100.0

The 211 BCC lesions were classified based on localisation according to the following table (Table 2).

Out of the 211 lesions with BCC, 206 of them had recordings of the surface area. The median surface area of the lesions was 2.81 cm^2, with the following difference between the 2 genders: 2.341 cm^2 (IQR: 3.32 cm^2) for women and 3.42 cm^2 (IQR: 4.09 cm^2) for men.

Although our study revealed a difference between men and women in terms of the median surface area of the lesions (3.42 cm^2 for men and 2.341 cm^2 for women), this result lacked statistical power ($p = 0.094$). We also analysed whether the surgeon opted to excise the tumour in one single piece or if he/she excised the tumour and the margins separately (in order to evaluate if there are residual tumour cells). In 27 cases out of 211 (12.8%), the margins were separately excised, while for the 184 remaining cases, the tumours were excised entirely without separate margins.

Table 2. Localisation of BCC.

Localisation	Number	Percentage
Nose	65	30.8
Scalp	14	6.6
Fronto-temporal area	25	11.8
Genio-maseterian area	27	12.8
Periocular region	20	9.5
Perioral/mental region	7	3.3
Auricular	13	6.2
Neck	18	8.5
Trunk	14	6.6
Upper limbs	6	2.8
Lower limbs	2	0.9
Total	211	100.0

Another aspect which we took into consideration was the marking of the tumour for histopathology orientation. Of the lesions, 144 (68.2%) were not marked, 15 (7.1%) were marked in one extremity and 52 (24.6%) had 2 different extremities marked for proper orientation.

The BCC subtypes were also noted—the lesions were described as infiltrative, nodular, micronodular, superficial, pigmented and basosquamous. The other subtypes were not found in our histopathological results. In 11 cases, there was no mention of a histopathological subtype. In most cases, these histopathological subtypes were mixed (2 or more subtypes were present in a single BCC lesion). In Table 3, we presented the total number of each subtype found (either alone or mixed with other subtypes), and in Table 4, we analysed the mixed subtypes separate from the lesions which had only a single histopathological subtype.

Table 3. BCC subtypes (absolute values).

Histopathological Subtype	Present	Absent/ Not Mentioned	Total
Infiltrative	170 (80.6%)	41 (19.4%)	
Nodular	157 (74.4%)	54 (25.6%)	
Micronodular	8 (3.8%)	203 (6.2%)	211 (100%)
Superficial	10 (4.7%)	201 (95.3%)	
Basosquamous	6 (2.8%)	205 (97.2%)	
Pigmented	3 (1.4%)	208 (98.6%)	

Table 4. BCC subtypes (isolated and combined).

Histopathological Subtype	Number and Percentage
Infiltrative only	28 (13.27%)
Nodular only	17 (8.06%)
Micronodular only	2 (0.95%)
Superficial only	4 (1.9%)
Basosquamous only	2 (0.95%)
Mixt (2 or more of the above)	147 (69.67%)
Missing	11 (5.21%)
Total	211 (100%)

Ulceration of the BCC in evolution was also analysed; 132 of 211 (62.6%) lesions presented ulceration. The results are presented in Tables 3 and 4.

One more aspect which was taken into consideration was whether the same patient that was operated for a BCC had other skin tumours which were operated at the same time of the BCC excision. In 139 cases (65.9%), there were no other tumours other than a single BCC. In 49 cases (23.2%), there were other benign tumours excised, while in 23 cases (10.9%), there were other malignant tumours excised simultaneously with the BCC. The separate benign tumours which were excised together with the BCC lesions were one of the following: haemangiomas, sebaceous nevi, sebaceous keratosis, papillomas or simple tissue fragments that presented histological modifications. The other malignant/premalignant tumours included squamous cell carcinoma, actinic keratosis or at least one other BCC lesion on the same patient.

The T value in the TNM system was also analysed, with the results presented in Table 5.

Table 5. T values for BCC lesions.

T Value	Number of Lesions	Percentage
0	2	0.9
1	131	62.1
2	25	11.8
3	8	3.8
Total present	166	78.7
Missing	45	21.3
Total	211	100.0

We also divided the 211 excisions based on the type of surgery performed, and the results are depicted in Table 6.

Table 6. Type of surgery.

Operation Type	Number	Percentage
Direct suture	149	70.6
Skin graft	22	10.4
Local flap	35	16.6
Regional flap	5	2.4
Total	211	100.0

In terms of tumour margins, we noticed that 36 patients (17.1%) had positive margins. (Table 7).

Table 7. Tumour margins.

Margin Type	Number	Percentage
Negative margins	175	82.9%
Positive margins	36	17.1%
Total	211	100%

Of the operated patients, 17 presented themselves for a recurrence for BCC, while 194 had a primary BCC (Table 8).

Table 8. Type of tumour.

Type of Tumour	Recurrence	
	Number	Percentage
Primary tumour	194	91.9%
Recurrent tumour	17	8.1%
Total	211	100%

We analysed the group of patients with BCC recurrence to see whether a consultant with more than 10 years of experience had less cases of BCC recurrence compared to a specialist with less than 10 years of experience. Out of 87 patients, 4 patients (4.6%) had a BCC recurrence in the specialist group, while in the consultant group, 13 (10.4%) patients out of 124 had a recurrence. There was no statistical difference between the two types of doctors ($X^2 = 2.39$, $p = 0.112$) (Tables 9 and 10).

Table 9. Recurrence related to operator experience.

	Recurrence Rate in Relation to Operator's Experience			
			Specialist	Consultant
Recurrence	Without recurrence	Count	83	111
		Percentage	95.4%	89.6%
	With recurrence	Count	4	13
		Percentage	4.6%	10.4%
	Total	Count	87	124
		Percentage	100%	100%

Table 10. Association between tumour marking and surface area.

	Case Processing Summary					
	Valid		Missing Cases		Surface Area (cm^2)	
Tumour marking	N	Percentage	N	Percentage	Median	IQR
Unmarked	142	98.6%	2	1.4%	2.23	2.97
1 marked pole	13	86.7%	2	13.3%	3.5	3.11
2 marked poles	51	98.1%	1	1.9%	4.68	5.35

Each row tests the null hypothesis that the Sample 1 and Sample 2 distributions are the same. Asymptotic significances (2-sided tests) are displayed. The significance level is 0.05. Significance values have been adjusted by the Bonferroni correction for multiple tests.

We analysed whether the surface area of the excised tumours correlated with the marking decision of the specimen. Table 10 reflects this decision; tumour marking was performed for BCC with a higher surface area. The marking of the tumour was statistically significantly associated with the median surface area ($X^2 = 2.8, p < 0.001$).

We compared the difference between the specialist and consultant in terms of the median surface area of the operated BCC. A total of 206 BCC lesions had recordings of the surface, with a median of 2.81 cm². The specialists operated a total of 87 BCC lesions; 2 of them had no recordings of surface area, while the remaining 85 lesions had a median surface area of 2.55 cm² (IQR = 3.58). The consultants operated a total of 124 lesions; 3 of them had no recordings of the surface area, and the remaining 121 BCCs had a median surface area of 3.2 cm² (IQR = 3.53). There was no statistical difference between the surface areas of the lesions operated by the specialists and those operated by the consultants ($X^2 = 2.81, p = 0.203$).

We also analysed whether the depth of the tumour could be associated with the recurrence incidence. Table 11 reflects these results; the tumour depth could not be associated with the cases in which recurrence occurred ($X^2 = 5, p = 0.665$).

Table 11. Association between recurrence and tumour depth.

Recurrence	Case Processing Summary				Depth	
	Valid		Missing			
	N	Percentage	N	Percentage	Depth Median	IQR
Cases without recurrence	164	84.5%	30	15.5%	5 mm	4 mm
Cases with recurrence	15	88.2%	2	11.8%	5 mm	5 mm

We also evaluated if the surface area of the lesions can be associated with the positive/negative margins. The median surface area for negative margins was 2.85 cm² (IQR 3.78 cm²) and the mean: 4.73 cm², SD 6.5 cm². The median surface area for positive margins was 2.54 cm² (IQR 3.29 cm²) and the mean 4.39 cm², SD 5.5 cm². Therefore, the surface area of the lesion could not be associated with either type of margins ($X^2 = 2.81, p = 0.463$).

The cases with recurrence were analysed to see whether they had positive margins. A higher percentage of relapse was observed in the cases in which the margins were positive ($p = 0.003$). These results are presented in Table 12.

Table 12. Association between tumours with invaded margins and relapses.

			Relapsed Lesions		Total
			No Relapse	Relapsed	
Margins	No tumoral invasion	Count	166	9	175
		% within Margins	94.9%	5.1%	100.0%
	Tumoral invasion	Count	28	8	36
		% within Margins	77.8%	22.2%	100.0%
	Total	Count	194	17	211
		% within Margins	91.9%	8.1%	100.0%

Finally, all comorbidities of the patients were noted and analysed in Table 13.

Table 13. Personal history of patients with BCC.

Complications	Number (Percentage)		
	Without	Present	Total
Cardiovascular	70 (33.2%)	141 (66.8%)	
Diabetes	168 (79.6%)	43 (20.4%)	
Infectious	204 (96.7%)	7 (3.3%)	
Pulmonary	198 (93.8%)	13 (6.2%)	211 (100%)
Digestive	172 (81.5%)	39 (18.5%)	
Hematologic	205 (97.2%)	6 (2.8%)	
Renal	177 (83.9%)	34 (16.1%)	

4. Discussion

Although the female/male ratio inclined the balance in favour of men in our study, there was only a small difference between sexes (the male:female ratio in our study was 1.045:1). The age distribution indicated that BCC appeared frequently in the 7th decade (with over 90% of all BCC that were excised being in the case of patients above 50 years old), with the median age being slightly higher in the male patients.

The number of patients was significantly smaller in 2020 compared to 2019 due to the COVID-19 pandemic, but this number was still higher compared that of 2021 (when the hospital was declared a COVID hospital, and no other pathologies were allowed for treatment). The year 2022 showed a mild comeback (taken into consideration that the first few months were still under strict COVID regulation and that the results of the study were only until August 2022). This is due to the fact that during the COVID pandemic, many patients with chronic pathologies have delayed seeking medical care [14].

Almost 1/3 of the operated BCC were located on the nose, with more than 75% of all BCC being located at the level of the head. This clearly suggests a higher frequency of this type of malignancy at the more sun exposed regions and is consistent with the research presented by Costache et al. and Asilian et al. [16,17].

BCC is a tumour that can vary in size: from small lesions to giant ones, with giant BCC being over 5 cm in diameter [18]. Although we did not have a significant statistical difference between men and women in term of the size of the lesions, the men presented with higher surface-area BCC. This could be explained by the fact that men generally seek professional healthcare later than women (allowing such tumours to grow larger). Based on the size of the tumour according to the TNM scale, almost 80% of the patients were included in T1, and more than 95% are below T2, which indicates that most of these tumours are excised before an important local invasion.

Tumour markings and tumour margins are extremely important in the management of BCC; our study showed that while separate margins were taken in only 12.8% of the cases, almost 1/3 of all excised tumours were marked for orientation. Tullet et al. questioned whether the marking sutures for orientation were useful for further management of BCC, and in his study, only one case was re-operated based on those margins (0.2%). They concluded that routine marking is not necessary and should be performed in case of ill-defined lesions or for histopathological types with high risk [19].

In our study, a positive correlation between surface area and tumour marking was shown; this indicates that tumour marking was performed for BCC with higher surface area due to the operator's suspicion that the bigger tumours might not be completely excised, and a new surgical intervention might be needed.

According to Costache et al., there are five subtypes of BCC based on histopathology: nodular, infiltrative/morpheaform, superficial, pigmented and fibroepithelioma of Pinkus [16]. Our study is consistent with the frequencies of these histopathology subtypes in this article, with the nodular type reaching 75% of all cases and the infiltrative type reaching more than 80% of all cases. In our study, all histopathological subtypes were present, both alone and mixed, except for the pigmented subtype, which appeared only in mixed subtype lesions. The majority of the CBC lesions (69.67%) had mixed histopathological subtypes.

Another study conducted by Fung-Soon Lim et al. divided the histopathological subtypes of BCC based on the risk of subclinical extension into two categories: high risk (morpheaform, infiltrative, metatypical, mixed and superficial) and low risk (basosquamous, micronodular, nodular and unspecified) [20]. These aspects are important for a clinician to evaluate the relapse risk after tumour excision.

There are two aspects which can be researched and improved when considering BCC: one is represented by the diagnostic tools, and the other is represented by the therapeutic options. The limitation of our study is represented by the diagnostic and therapeutic options. We used clinical diagnosis and classical surgical excision for all lesions. There are, however, more modern diagnostic tools and therapeutic options which can achieve good results.

With the development of modern medical engineering, the correct diagnosis and the appropriate size of the BCC (in terms of depth and surface area) can now be evaluated even before the surgical excision. This has a major advantage due to the fact that it can reduce significantly the relapse rate in case of BCC (thus improving the quality of life of patients, who will undergo only one operation instead of two or more). Niculet et al. consider that the combination of optical coherence tomography (OCT) and reflectance confocal microscopy (RCM) can provide useful information for both depth and horizontal extension of a tumour and could be used prior to surgery in order to explore subclinical extension [21]. This is especially useful in the case of high risk histopathological subtypes of BCC, where due to an incomplete excision, relapse is a major concern.

RCM offers information about blood vessels at the level of the BCC in terms of density, size, and flow intensity. BCC, compared to benign tumours or normal skin, presents a peripheral stroma which has a higher density of microvessels [22].

From a histopathological perspective, the differential diagnosis of basal cell carcinoma includes both benign and malignant lesions. Trichoepithelioma and trichoblastoma represent the main benign tumours with a basaloid morphology that need to be taken into consideration. These tumours, however, only rarely present immunoexpression for BerEp4 and CD10, with the latter being more frequently positive in the peritumoural stroma of trichoepithelioma [23]. A microcystic or pseudoglandular morphology of BCC may also pose differential diagnosis problems with microcystic schwannoma, from which it can be easily differentiated by using an immunohistochemical panel containing S100, SOX10 and BerEP4 [24]. From the malignant category, one should always have in mind the option of a cutaneous metastasis. A basosquamous carcinoma must be differentiated from a basaloid squamous cell carcinoma (SCC), a keratoacanthoma or an adenoid cystic carcinoma. Both SCC and BCC can express p63; however, SCC usually expresses EMA, while BCC characteristically expresses BerEP4 [25,26].

In terms of therapeutic options, the surgical excision with negative margins represents the treatment of choice for plastic surgeons. In our study, the majority of the operated tumours were closed directly, which supports the idea that BCC is a slow-growing tumour and the surgical management can be performed in most cases under local anaesthesia without complications. While it is generally known that a skin graft may be easier to perform, the aesthetic result after a skin graft is inferior to the local flap. With 16% of all operations performed being a local flap (compared to 10% for skin graft), one can observe the tendency of the plastic surgeons to achieve coverage by using more aesthetic methods. This option could be influenced by the fact that the majority of the operations were performed at the level of the head, where good aesthetic results are expected.

An important surgical option is Mohs micrographic surgery (MMS), which is considered to be the standard of care for BCC and skin cancers in general. Although this technique is conservative and preserves as much as possible from the surrounding tissue, due to its high costs, it has some indications when MMS is considered appropriate: cases with risk of disfigurement; large malignant tumours; tumours with aggressive histopathological subtype or with poorly defined margins; recurrent tumours and skin cancers caused by genetic predisposition [27].

There are also some alternative options to surgery which can be used in the case of BCCs. However, it is mandatory that a correct selection of patients is performed when choosing these alternative options in order not to risk a recurrence. Among the non-surgical treatments which can be used, cryosurgery, ablative CO_2 laser, 5-fluorouracil and imiquimod are the most frequently used therapies, which are performed specifically in dermatology practices. The advantages of these options are represented by the following arguments: they are non-invasive/minimally invasive; they achieve a better aesthetic result; and they can be used at the same time in case of multiple tumours. The disadvantages consist in the fact that they may be useful only for small tumours; they may have a higher risk of recurrence; and in some cases, more than one treatment session might be needed (compared to surgical excision, when all is performed in a single, more invasive stage).

Scurtu et al. reported superior cosmetic results from using these types of treatments compared to surgery, with a recurrence rate of under 1% [28]. Thompson et al. sustain the idea that although surgical excision has lower recurrence rates, non-surgical treatments have superior aesthetic results with acceptable recurrence rates [29]. For unresectable BCC or metastatic BCC, vismodegib—a kinase inhibitor—remains the primary option for treatment [30].

Among our operated patients, ~34% of them presented other skin tumours which were operated at the same time of the surgical excision of the BCC (23% benign and 11% malignant). This percentage of patients who had other skin tumours could be significantly higher (because not all patients want all their tumours operated in one surgery).

There was no association between the experience of the surgeon and the recurrence rate. Paradoxically, the consultants (doctors with over 10 years of experience) seemed to have more cases of recurrent BCC compared with specialists (doctors with less than 10 years of experience). This could be due to the fact that the consultants had more cases (124 cases vs. 87 cases), and these cases were more difficult compared to the cases solved by specialists (the median surface area of the BCC lesions was 2.55 cm^2 in the case of specialists compared to 3.2 cm^2 in the case of consultants).

In our study, the positive/negative margins of the specimen could not be associated with the surface area of the tumour, and neither could the recurrence rate with the tumour depth. This proved that even though large tumours (in size or depth) could theoretically be more susceptible to incomplete excision followed by recurrence (as most tumours are located at the level of the face, where the surgeon tries to be as conservative as possible), this was not the case in our study. However, an incomplete excision with positive margins has been statistically proven to cause a recurrent BCC more frequently, which would need a new surgical intervention. For this reason, either MMS or an extemporaneous histopathological examination could reduce the risk of an incomplete excision with positive margins.

With regard to comorbidities, 66.8% of all patients presented some type of cardiovascular pathology. This high percentage is, however, explicable due to the median age of the patients in our study, as the seventh decade has a high probability of having such comorbidities. The hematologic, pulmonary and infectious comorbidities were not so frequently seen in the personal history of the patients with BCC; renal comorbidities, diabetes and digestive comorbidities were, however, found in over 15% of all patients. Renal transplant is frequently associated in the literature with BCC, which could explain the high incidence of BCC in patients with renal comorbidities [31,32].

The future management of BCC is probably based on gene analysis and biomarkers that influence the prognosis of BCC, with p16 being one of the genes involved in the pathogenesis of human BCC [33,34].

5. Conclusions

BCC is a pathology which should be approached in a multidisciplinary team. Our study reveals aspects related to margins, surface areas and surgical treatment approach used in our clinic.

Author Contributions: A.M., I.G., S.A.M., A.P. and C.G. contributed to the conception, analysis and interpretation of data and drafted the manuscript. N.A.D. conceived the study, analysed the data, interpreted the results and critically revised the manuscript. C.G. critically reviewed and revised the manuscript. S.A.M. was responsible for the work and supervised the study. All authors have read and agreed to the published version of the manuscript.

Funding: This research received no external funding.

Institutional Review Board Statement: Not applicable.

Informed Consent Statement: Not applicable.

Data Availability Statement: The datasets used and/or analyzed during the present study are available from the corresponding author upon reasonable request.

Acknowledgments: Publication of this paper was supported by the University of Medicine and Pharmacy Carol Davila, through the institutional program Publish not Perish.

Conflicts of Interest: The authors declare no conflict of interest.

References

1. Peris, K.; Fargnoli, M.C.; Garbe, C.; Kaufmann, R.; Bastholt, L.; Seguin, N.B.; Bataille, V.; Del Marmol, V.; Dummer, R.; Harwood, C.A.; et al. Diagnosis and treatment of basal cell carcinoma: European consensus-based interdisciplinary guidelines. *Eur. J. Cancer* **2019**, *118*, 10–34. [CrossRef]
2. Tanese, K. Diagnosis and Management of Basal Cell Carcinoma. *Curr. Treat Options Oncol.* **2019**, *20*, 13. [CrossRef] [PubMed]
3. Kim, D.P.; Kus, K.J.B.; Ruiz, E. Basal Cell Carcinoma Review. *Hematol. Oncol. Clin. North Am.* **2019**, *33*, 13–24. [CrossRef] [PubMed]
4. McDaniel, B.; Badri, T.; Steele, R.B. Basal cell carcinoma. In *StatPearls*; StatPearls Publishing: Treasure Island, FL, USA, 2022.
5. Asgari, M.M.; Moffet, H.H.; Ray, G.T.; Quesenberry, C.P. Trends in Basal Cell Carcinoma Incidence and Identification of High-Risk Subgroups, 1998–2012. *JAMA Dermatol.* **2015**, *151*, 976–981. [CrossRef] [PubMed]
6. Martinez, V.D.; Vucic, E.A.; Becker-Santos, D.D.; Gil, L.; Lam, W.L. Arsenic exposure and the induction of human cancers. *J. Toxicol.* **2011**, *2011*, 431287. [CrossRef]
7. Gallagher, R.P.; Hill, G.B.; Bajdik, C.D.; Fincham, S.; Coldman, A.J.; McLean, D.I.; Threlfall, W.J. Sunlight exposure, pigmentary factors, and risk of nonmelanocytic skin cancer. *Arch. Dermatol.* **1995**, *131*, 157. [CrossRef]
8. Karagas, M.R.; Stannard, V.A.; Mott, L.A.; Slattery, M.J.; Spencer, S.K.; Weinstock, M.A. Use of tanning devices and risk of basal cell and squamous cell skin cancers. *J. Natl. Cancer Inst.* **2002**, *94*, 224–226. [CrossRef]
9. Karagas, M.R.; McDonald, J.A.; Greendberg, E.R.; Stukel, T.A.; Weiss, J.E.; Baron, J.A.; Stevens, M.M.; Skin Cancer Prevention Study Group. Risk of basal cell and squamous cell skin cancers after ionizing radiation therapy. *J. Natl. Cancer Inst.* **1996**, *88*, 1848–1853. [CrossRef] [PubMed]
10. Robinson, S.N.; Zens, M.S.; Perry, A.E.; Spencer, S.K.; Duell, E.J.; Karagas, M.R. Photosensitizing agents and the risk of non-melanoma skin cancer: A population-based case—Control study. *J. Investig. Dermatol.* **2013**, *133*, 1950–1955. [CrossRef]
11. Elder, D.E.; Massi, D.; Scolyer, R.A.; Willemze, R. *WHO Classification of Skin Tumours*; International Agency for Research on Cancer: Lyon, France, 2018.
12. Heath, M.S.; Bar, A. Basal Cell Carcinoma. *Dermatol. Clin.* **2023**, *41*, 13–21. [CrossRef]
13. Lupu, M.; Popa, I.M.; Voiculescu, V.M.; Caruntu, A.; Caruntu, C. A Systematic Review and Meta-Analysis of the Accuracy of in VivoReflectance Confocal Microscopy for the Diagnosis of Primary Basal Cell Carcinoma. *J. Clin. Med.* **2019**, *8*, 1462. [CrossRef]
14. Niculet, E.; Craescu, M.; Rebegea, L.; Bobeica, C.; Nastase, F.; Lupasteanu, G.; Stan, D.J.; Chioncel, V.; Anghel, L.; Lungu, M.; et al. Basal cell carcinoma: Comprehensive clinical and histopathological aspects, novel imaging tools and therapeutic approaches (Review). *Exp. Ther. Med.* **2022**, *23*, 60. [CrossRef] [PubMed]
15. Chen, K.L.; Brozen, M.; Rollman, J.E.; Ward, T.; Norris, K.C.; Gregory, K.D.; Zimmerman, F.J. How is the COVID-19 pandemic shaping transportation access to health care? *Transp. Res. Interdiscip. Perspect.* **2021**, *10*, 100338. [CrossRef] [PubMed]
16. Costache, M.; Georgescu, T.A.; Oproiu, A.M.; Costache, D.; Naie, A.; Sajin, M.A.; Nica, A.E. Emerging concepts and latest advances regarding the etiopathogenesis, morphology and immunophenotype of basal cell carcinoma. *Rom. J. Morphol. Embryol.* **2018**, *59*, 427–433. [PubMed]
17. Asilian, A.; Tamizifar, B. Aggressive and neglected basal cell carcinoma. *Dermatol. Surg.* **2005**, *31*, 1468–1471. [PubMed]

18. Oudit, D.; Pham, H.; Grecu, T.; Hodgson, C.; Grant, M.E.; Rashed, A.A.; Allan, D.; Green, A.C. Reappraisal of giant basal cell carcinoma: Clinical features and outcomes. *J. Plast. Reconstr. Aesthet. Surg.* **2020**, *73*, 53–57. [CrossRef] [PubMed]
19. Tullett, M.; Whittaker, M.; Walsh, S. Marking sutures to orientate specimens of basal cell carcinoma: Do they really make a difference? *Br. J. Oral Maxillofac. Surg.* **2016**, *54*, 682–685. [CrossRef] [PubMed]
20. Lim, G.F.; Perez, O.A.; Zitelli, J.A.; Brodland, D.G. Correlation of basal cell carcinoma subtype with histologically confirmed subclinical extension during Mohs micrographic surgery: A prospective multicenter study. *J. Am. Acad. Dermatol.* **2022**, *86*, 1309–1317. [CrossRef]
21. Niculet, E.; Tatu, A.L. Comment on "Correlation of basal cell carcinoma subtype with histologically confirmed subclinical extension during Mohs micrographic surgery: A prospective multicenter study". *J. Am. Acad. Dermatol.* **2022**, *87*, e49–e50. [CrossRef]
22. Lupu, M.; Caruntu, C.; Popa, M.I.; Voiculescu, V.M.; Zurac, S.; Boda, D. Vascular patterns in basal cell carcinoma: Dermoscopic, confocal and histopathological perspectives. *Oncol. Lett.* **2019**, *17*, 4112–4125. [CrossRef]
23. Bhambri, A.; Prieto, V.G. Immunohistochemistry helps distinguish hamartomatous basal cell carcinoma from trichoepithelioma. *Am. J. Dermatopathol.* **2010**, *32*, 404.
24. Georgescu, T.A.; Dumitru, A.V.; Oproiu, A.M.; Nica, A.E.; Costache, D.; Pătraşcu, O.M.; Lăzăroiu, A.M.; Chefani, A.E.; Sajin, M.; Costache, M. Cutaneous microcystic/reticular schwannoma: Case report and literature review of an exceedingly rare entity with an unusual presentation. *Rom. J. Morphol. Embryol.* **2018**, *59*, 303–309.
25. Georgescu, T.A.; Oproiu, A.M.; Rădăşan, M.G.; Dumitru, A.V.; Costache, D.; Patrascu, O.M.; Lazaroiu, A.M.; Chefani, A.E.; Sajin, M.; Costache, M. Keratoacanthoma centrifugum marginatum: An unusual clinical and histopathological diagnostic pitfall. *Rom. J. Morphol. Embryol.* **2017**, *58*, 561–565.
26. Wick, M.R.; Swanson, P.E. Primary adenoid cystic carcinoma of the skin. A clinical, histological, and immunocytochemical comparison with adenoid cystic carcinoma of salivary glands and adenoid basal cell carcinoma. *Am. J. Dermatopathol.* **1986**, *8*, 2–13. [CrossRef]
27. Golda, N.; Hruza, G. Mohs Micrographic Surgery. *Dermatol. Clin.* **2023**, *41*, 39–47. [CrossRef]
28. Scurtu, L.G.; Petrica, M.; Grigore, M.; Avram, A.; Popescu, I.; Simionescu, O. A Conservative Combined Laser Cryoimmunotherapy Treatment vs. Surgical Excision for Basal Cell Carcinoma. *J. Clin. Med.* **2022**, *11*, 3439. [CrossRef] [PubMed]
29. Thomson, J.; Hogan, S.; Leonardi-Bee, J.; Williams, H.C.; Bath-Hextall, F.J. Interventions for basal cell carcinoma of the skin. *Cochrane Database Syst. Rev.* **2020**, *11*, CD003412. [CrossRef] [PubMed]
30. Vismodegib. In *LiverTox: Clinical and Research Information on Drug-Induced Liver Injury*; National Institute of Diabetes and Digestive and Kidney Diseases: Bethesda, MD, USA, 2018.
31. Kanitakis, J.; Ducroux, E.; Hoelt, P.; Cahen, R.; Jullien, D. Basal-Cell Carcinoma With Matrical Differentiation: Report of a New Case in a Renal-Transplant Recipient and Literature Review. *Am. J. Dermatopathol.* **2018**, *40*, e115–e118. [CrossRef]
32. Tsironi, T.; Gaitanis, G.; Pappas, C.; Koutlas, V.; Dounousi, E.; Bassukas, I.D. Immunocryosurgery is a safe and feasible treatment for basal cell carcinoma and Bowen disease in renal transplant recipients. *Dermatol. Ther.* **2022**, *35*, e15405. [CrossRef]
33. Lupu, M.; Caruntu, C.; Ghita, M.A.; Voiculescu, V.; Voiculescu, S.; Rosca, A.E.; Caruntu, A.; Moraru, L.; Popa, I.M.; Calenic, B.; et al. Gene Expression and Proteome Analysis as Sources of Biomarkers in Basal Cell Carcinoma. *Dis. Markers* **2016**, *2016*, 9831237. [CrossRef]
34. Eshkoor, S.A.; Ismail, P.; Rahman, S.A.; Oshkour, S.A. p16 gene expression in basal cell carcinoma. *Arch. Med. Res.* **2008**, *39*, 668–673. [CrossRef] [PubMed]

Disclaimer/Publisher's Note: The statements, opinions and data contained in all publications are solely those of the individual author(s) and contributor(s) and not of MDPI and/or the editor(s). MDPI and/or the editor(s) disclaim responsibility for any injury to people or property resulting from any ideas, methods, instructions or products referred to in the content.

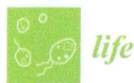

Brief Report

Immunohistochemical Analysis of Adhesion Molecules E-Selectin, Intercellular Adhesion Molecule-1, and Vascular Cell Adhesion Molecule-1 in Inflammatory Lesions of Atopic Dermatitis

Sandra Marinović Kulišić [1], Marta Takahashi [2,*], Marta Himelreich Perić [3], Vedrana Mužić Radović [4] and Ružica Jurakić Tončić [1]

1. Department of Dermatology and Venereology, University Hospital Centre Zagreb, 10000 Zagreb, Croatia
2. Department of Communicology, Catholic University of Croatia, 10000 Zagreb, Croatia
3. Health Center Zagreb West, 10000 Zagreb, Croatia; marta.himelreich-peric@dzz-zapad.hr
4. Hospital for Medical Rehabilitation of the Health and Lung Diseases and Rheumatism "Thalassotherapia-Opatija", 51410 Opatija, Croatia
* Correspondence: marta.takahashi@unicath.hr

Abstract: E-selectin, ICAM-1 (intercellular adhesion molecule-1), and VCAM-1 (vascular cell adhesion molecule-1) play a role in atopic dermatitis (AD). This study aimed to evaluate their expression in skin biopsy specimens of patients diagnosed with AD using an optimized computer program. A descriptive analysis and comparison of digitally measured surface area and cell number were performed. The number of E-selectin-positive cells did not vary between the groups. In patients with AD, decreases of 1.2-fold for ICAM-1- and 1.3-fold for VCAM-1- positive cells were observed. The E-selectin-positive epidermal surface area increased ($p < 0.001$), while ICAM1 and VCAM1 decreased 2.5-fold and 2-fold, respectively, compared to controls. In the AD-affected skin, the E-selectin-positive endothelial area was 3.5-fold larger ($p < 0.001$), and the ICAM1-positive area was almost 4-fold larger ($p < 0.001$). E-selectin and ICAM-1 were expressed in the control dermis moderately and weakly, respectively. A strong E-selectin signal was detected in the AD-affected skin macrophages and a strong ICAM-1 signal in the dermal vessel endothelium. In the endothelial cells of AD-affected skin, no VCAM-1 signal could be found. E-selectin, ICAM-1, and VCAM-1 expression show significant disease-specific changes between AD-affected and control skin. The combination of digital analysis and a pathologist's evaluation may present a valuable follow-up of AD activity parameters.

Keywords: atopic dermatitis; E-selectin; ICAM-1; VCAM-1

Citation: Marinović Kulišić, S.; Takahashi, M.; Himelreich Perić, M.; Mužić Radović, V.; Jurakić Tončić, R. Immunohistochemical Analysis of Adhesion Molecules E-Selectin, Intercellular Adhesion Molecule-1, and Vascular Cell Adhesion Molecule-1 in Inflammatory Lesions of Atopic Dermatitis. *Life* **2023**, *13*, 933. https://doi.org/10.3390/life13040933

Academic Editor: Alin Laurentiu Tatu

Received: 2 March 2023
Revised: 29 March 2023
Accepted: 31 March 2023
Published: 2 April 2023

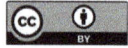

Copyright: © 2023 by the authors. Licensee MDPI, Basel, Switzerland. This article is an open access article distributed under the terms and conditions of the Creative Commons Attribution (CC BY) license (https:// creativecommons.org/licenses/by/ 4.0/).

1. Introduction

Atopic dermatitis (AD) is a chronic inflammatory disease mediated by type I and IV immunologic mechanisms in its pathogenesis [1]. A wide variation in the prevalence of AD is present in different populations of the world [2] but overall, it appears to be increasing [3–5]. AD is a skin disease with significant morbidity and quality-of-life impairment [6,7] and represents a healthcare burden. In 1980, Hanifin and Rajka proposed major and minor diagnostic criteria for AD [8] based on the history and clinical picture, determining the basis of the diagnostic criteria worldwide which has been re-evaluated since then [9–11].

The etiopathogenesis of AD includes the interplay of environmental and genetic factors that cause derangements in the structure and function of the epidermal barrier and immune system [12,13] and even non-lesional skin seems to bear ultrastructural changes [14]. The main types of AD are extrinsic and intrinsic, differentiated by IgE levels, prevalence, clinical features, role of the filaggrin gene, and cytokine expression [15]. Extrinsic (or allergic) AD is burdened by high serum IgE levels, the presence of environment- or food-specific IgEs, and has a high prevalence. Meanwhile, intrinsic (or non-allergic) AD shows normal IgE values, the absence of specific IgE, and has a relatively low prevalence (20%) with female predominance and a late onset, milder clinical features, and higher interferon-γ expression [16]. Many studies focus on the complexity of cytokines and chemokines involved in the immune response of AD patients and the function of various cell types and epidermal barriers, which is perturbed in the extrinsic type of AD [4,13]. One of the crucial proteins in epidermal differentiation, filaggrin, facilitates the skin barrier formation [17,18] and a variety of *FLG* gene mutations were found in many patients with extrinsic AD. Cellular markers and adhesion molecules play a significant role in AD pathogenesis [19] via endothelial–leukocyte interactions, lymphocyte circulation, enhanced vascularization, and inflow of immunocompetent cells [20]. The two main types of AD are differentiated by higher expression of interleukin (IL) -4, IL-5, and IL-13, and the lower expression of interferon-γ in the extrinsic type [15]. IL-13 contributes to the pathogenesis of AD, although IL-4 is necessary for the Th2 cell polarization [21]. Defining the molecular cocktail typical for the AD type is crucial in the treatment decision. For example, inhibition of IL-4 and IL-13 is the main goal of dupilumab, an IgG monoclonal antibody used in the treatment of inadequately controlled AD, targeting the IL-4 receptor alpha subunit, thus inhibiting the IL-4 and IL-13 pathways [22].

Adhesion molecules, such as intercellular adhesion molecule–1 (ICAM-1), ICAM-3, E-selectin, and L-selectin, are highly expressed in lesions of patients with AD and play an essential role in the AD etiopathogenesis [23–28]. Intercellular adhesion molecule-1 (ICAM-1, CD54) is a 90 kDa member of the immunoglobulin (Ig) superfamily. It is critical for the transmigration of leukocytes from blood vessels to tissues, and is constitutively present on endothelial cells and increases in expression in response to pro-inflammatory cytokines. ICAM-1 acts as a leukocyte adhesion molecule and contributes to inflammatory responses by increasing endothelial cell activation [29]. Vascular cell adhesion molecule-1 (VCAM-1, CD 56), an adhesion molecule with Ig domains mainly expressed in endothelial cells, is strongly induced by inflammatory cytokines and plays a critical role in mediating leukocyte adhesion on endothelial cells, and activation of signaling pathways to facilitate leukocyte passage from blood to tissue. [30]. E-selectin (CD62E, endothelial–leukocyte adhesion molecule 1, leukocyte–endothelial cell adhesion molecule 2) is mainly expressed after inflammatory stimulation by activated endothelial cells, and is also expressed in bone marrow and skin. E-selectin binds to ligands expressed in polymorphonuclear and mononuclear leukocytes during inflammation [31].

These adhesion molecules stimulate selective migration of memory cutaneous leukocyte-associated antigen, as well as lymphocyte, monocyte, and granulocyte diapedesis in both skin and blood in AD. Studies have shown that adhesion molecules E-selectin, VCAM-1, and ICAM-1 are highly expressed on vascular endothelial cells in the skin of patients suffering from AD [20,25,26,28]. E-selectin is synthesized and expressed on the endothelium after stimulation by inflammatory cytokines. ICAM-1 and VCAM-1, as essential adhesion molecules in the migration of lymphocytes, correlate with the degree of dermal lymphocyte inflammation [32] and the latter is also significant in vasculogenesis in adults [33]. The determination of inflammation markers in the serum of patients with AD seems to be a valuable indicator of AD activity [23–27,34–37].

We aimed to determine the expression and topography of adhesion molecules E-selectin, ICAM-1, and VCAM-1 in the epidermis and dermis of atopic skin compared to healthy skin by comparing measurements by pathologists and a method of digital analysis. This correlation would present a valuable tool for disease assessment and follow-up of AD activity due to its simplicity and clinical value.

2. Materials and Methods

2.1. Biopsy Specimens (Patients)

This retrospective case–control study (level of evidence 2B) [38] included 30 patients aged 28–45 (mean age 32 years) (Table 1) who were diagnosed with AD using the clinical diagnostic criteria [8]. The patients had a diagnostic lesional skin biopsy performed earlier that confirmed the diagnosis and were not treated for at least two weeks prior to the study to eliminate any potential effect of corticosteroids or other immunosuppressive drugs. The specimens were archived at the Referral Centre for Contact Dermatitis, Department of Dermatology and Venereology, University Hospital Centre Zagreb. Skin biopsy specimens (punch biopsy technique provided full-thickness 4 mm skin specimens) were also obtained from the same site [39] from 10 healthy age-matched donors (Table 1) who had a regular appointment for benign skin lesion excision and were used as the control group. Informed consent for performing the biopsy, participating in this research, and data publication for this study was obtained from all included patients. Exclusion criteria for patients suffering from AD and controls are shown in Figure 1. All patient-related data were fully anonymized in the analysis within the study. The study protocol followed the EU guidelines and was approved by the ethical committee of the School of Medicine, University of Zagreb.

Table 1. Demographic data of patients included in the study. N = number.

	Patients with Atopic Dermatitis	Controls
N	30	10
N females	21	5
N males	9	5
age	28–45	24–32
mean age	32	28

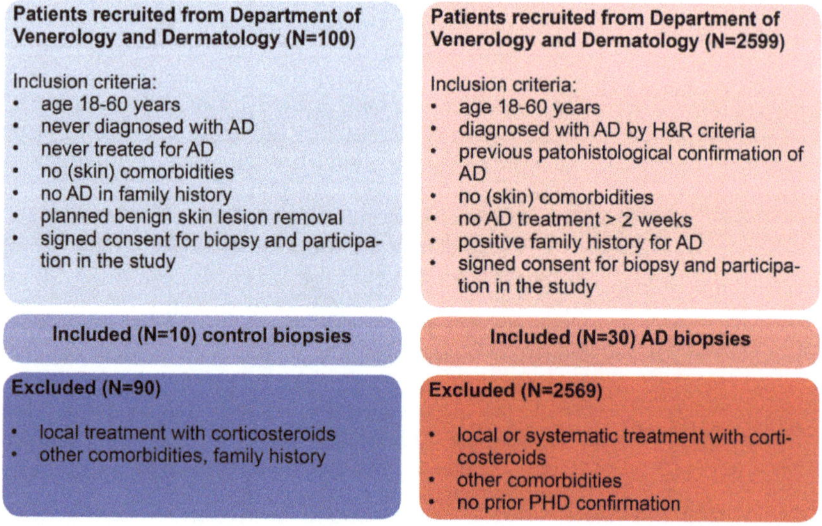

Patients recruited from Department of Venerology and Dermatology (N=100)

Inclusion criteria:
- age 18-60 years
- never diagnosed with AD
- never treated for AD
- no (skin) comorbidities
- no AD in family history
- planned benign skin lesion removal
- signed consent for biopsy and participation in the study

Included (N=10) control biopsies

Excluded (N=90)
- local treatment with corticosteroids
- other comorbidities, family history

Patients recruited from Department of Venerology and Dermatology (N=2599)

Inclusion criteria:
- age 18-60 years
- diagnosed with AD by H&R criteria
- previous patohistological confirmation of AD
- no (skin) comorbidities
- no AD treatment > 2 weeks
- positive family history for AD
- signed consent for biopsy and participation in the study

Included (N=30) AD biopsies

Excluded (N=2569)
- local or systematic treatment with corticosteroids
- other comorbidities
- no prior PHD confirmation

Figure 1. Flowchart of control patients (blue) and patients with atopic dermatitis (red) included in the study. N = number, AD = atopic dermatitis, H&R = Hanifin and Rajka atopic dermatitis clinical criteria [8].

2.2. Immunohistochemistry

Biopsy specimens were formalin-fixed, paraffin-embedded, and sectioned with a microtome. The 4 μm thick skin sections from healthy participants and patients with AD were deparaffinized at 56 °C and immunohistochemically stained with E-selectin, ICAM-1, and VCAM-1 antibodies (Dako Animal Research Kit, Peroxidase; Dako, Code No. K3954, Dako,

Glostrup, Denmark), following the manufacturer's instructions and using the standard avidin–biotin immunoperoxidase staining method. Endogenous peroxidase activity was blocked with 0.3% hydrogen peroxide in Tris-buffered saline (TBS) for 15 min at room temperature (RT). The slides were then incubated with primary antibodies for E-selectin (clone 4.5a2 No M2063), ICAM-1 (clone 6.5b5, No M7063), and VCAM-1 (clone 1.4C3, No M7106), all diluted 1:80 with antibody dilution solution (No S2022) for 1 h at RT. The sections were incubated with a biotinylated secondary antibody (Dako LSAB Kit, No K678) for 30 min and streptavidin–peroxidase (No K678) for 30 min, also at RT. 3.3-diaminobenzidine tetrachloride (DAB) was used to visualize the staining. Between incubations, the slides were washed three times with TBS and counterstained with hematoxylin, washed in tap water, dehydrated through grades of alcohols to xylene, and covered with mounting media (Faramount media, DAKO) and a coverslip at RT.

2.3. Quantitative and Qualitative Staining Measurements

The expression of adhesion molecules in the epidermis and dermis of control and patients with AD was analyzed by evaluating the incidence and intensity of positively stained areas in the tissue sections. This descriptive analysis was used to determine the topographical scatter of molecular expression by classifying the staining intensity as negative, weak, moderate, or strong and was performed by two pathologists.

To quantify changes in the expression of adhesion molecules, the number of epidermal ICAM-1, VCAM-1, and E-selectin positive cells was measured digitally [40]. The number of positively stained cells was expressed as a percentage of positive epidermal or endothelial cells in all epidermal or endothelial cells per microscopical field, respectively.

Positive ICAM-1, VCAM-1, and E-selectin epidermal surface area in control and AD-affected skin, as well as endothelial surface areas in the dermal blood vessel wall, were measured using the method of digital image analysis described previously [41]. The data were expressed as the percentage of E-selectin-, ICAM-1-, and VCAM-1-positive epidermal/endothelial surface area, respectively, in the whole analyzed epidermal or endothelial surface area in a microscopical field, depending on where the measurement was performed.

All measurements and staining analysis were performed on digital images of skin tissues (Nikon Eclipse E600 light microscope and Nikon DXM1200 digital camera (Nikon, Kingston-upon-Thames, UK)) using the Imaging Software Lucia G 4.80 (Laboratory Imaging Ltd., Prague, Czech Republic). These measurements were performed on six fields per section at $1000\times$ magnification.

2.4. Biopsy Specimens (Patients)

The sample size was determined in a pilot study, performed prior to the main data collection, and supported by data obtained from the literature. The data were statistically analyzed using the Statistica 6.0 software package (StatSoft, Tulsa, OK, USA). Descriptive analysis was performed for all data. Statistical significance of the difference in the percentage and the overall number of the immunostained tissue area was tested using the Student's t-test. Tables and graphs show the mean values and standard errors of the mean. The statistical significance level was $p < 0.05$.

3. Results

3.1. E-Selectin

Immunohistochemical analysis of skin from healthy controls and lesional skin from patients with AD showed expression of E-selectin in both the epidermis and dermis.

In the epidermis of healthy control skin, E-selectin was expressed in most cells of the basal layer and some cells of the suprabasal layer. The strongest staining was observed in the cytoplasm around the nucleus. In the epidermis of AD-affected skin, E-selectin expression was also found in the cells of the basal and suprabasal layer. However, the staining was weaker than in the control group (Figure 2).

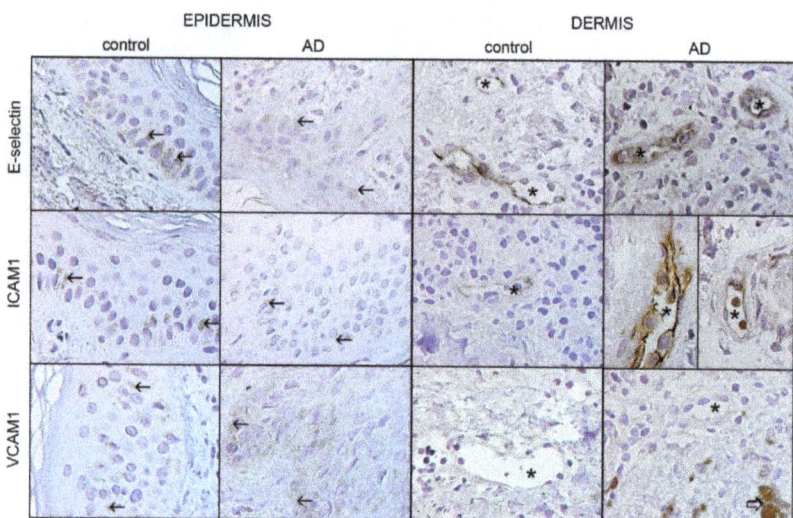

Figure 2. Representative images of immunohistochemical staining in the epidermis and dermis in controls and skin affected by atopic dermatitis. The staining of E-selectin, ICAM1, and VCAM1 showed differences in expression. Arrows (→) mark the DAB-positive signal in the cell cytoplasm, asterisks (*) show the vascular lumen, and the thick arrow (⇨) shows macrophages. DAB, hematoxylin counterstain, 1000× magnification.

Quantitative staining analysis revealed that the number of E-selectin-positive epidermal cells in control ($p = 0.097$) and AD-affected ($p = 0.091$) skin did not significantly differ (Figure 3). In contrast, the positive epidermal area was significantly increased ($p < 0.001$) in patients with AD (Figure 4) compared to controls ($p = 0.064$). In the dermis, E-selectin expression was found in the endothelial cells of blood vessels as a moderately stained reaction. However, the staining was much stronger in AD-affected skin than in control skin, with a strong granular signal in macrophages (Figure 2). The quantification also revealed significant changes in the endothelial expression in the form of an enlarged positive endothelial area in the vessel wall, which was 3.5 times higher ($p < 0.001$) in AD-affected skin compared to control skin ($p = 0.073$) (Figure 5).

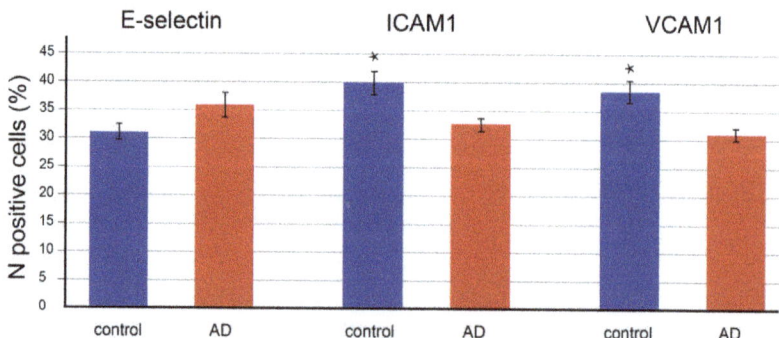

Figure 3. The number of DAB-positive epidermal cells in controls and skin affected by atopic dermatitis. The number is expressed as the percentage of immunostained epidermal cells in the overall epidermal cell number. The number did not significantly change for the E-selectin-positive signal; it decreased by 1.2× in AD patients compared to controls ($p = 0.005$) for ICAM-1-positive epidermal cells and decreased by 1.3× in AD patients ($p < 0.001$) for VCAM-1-positive cells. Data are presented as mean ± SEM. Student's t-test, two-tailed; * $p < 0.001$.

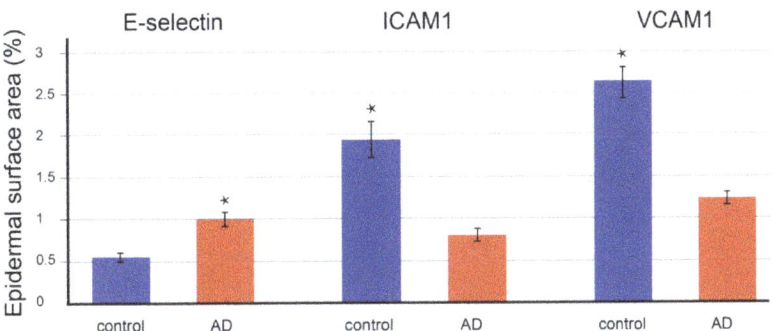

Figure 4. The epidermal surface area in controls and skin affected by atopic dermatitis. The area surface is expressed as a percentage of immunostained epidermal area in the overall epidermal area. The E-selectin-positive epidermal area was significantly increased ($p < 0.001$) in AD patients, while ICAM1- and VCAM1-positive epidermal areas were decreased in AD patients compared to controls: ICAM1 2.5× ($p < 0.001$) and VCAM1 2× ($p < 0.001$). Data are presented as mean ± SEM. Student's t-test, two-tailed; * $p < 0.001$.

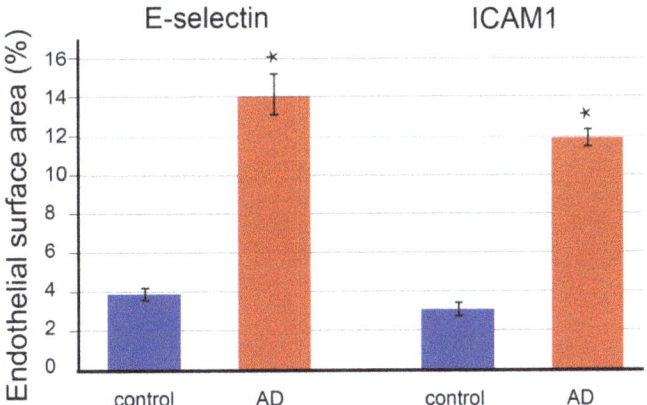

Figure 5. The endothelial surface area in controls and skin affected by atopic dermatitis. The area surface is expressed as a percentage of the immunostained endothelial vessel wall area in the overall endothelial area. The E-selectin-positive endothelial area was significantly larger (3.5×, $p < 0.001$) in AD skin and the ICAM1-positive area was almost 4× larger ($p < 0.001$) in AD skin. Data are presented as mean ± SEM. Student's t-test, two-tailed; ª $p < 0.001$.

3.2. ICAM-1

In the epidermis of control skin, ICAM-1 was expressed in most cells of the basal layer and some cells of the suprabasal layer. The strongest staining was found around the nucleus. In the skin of patients with AD, ICAM-1 expression showed a similar topographical pattern, although with weaker intensity (Figure 2). The quantitative analysis showed a significant decrease in epidermal expression in patients with AD. The number of positive cells decreased 1.2 times ($p = 0.005$ vs. $p = 0.055$, Figure 3), and the positive epidermal area decreased 2.5 times compared to the control group ($p < 0.001$ vs. $p = 0.67$, Figure 4).

In the dermis of control skin, ICAM-1 was weakly expressed only in vascular endothelial cells. On the contrary, in AD-affected skin, the staining was very strong in almost all endothelial cells (Figure 2).

The quantitative staining analysis also revealed a significant increase in endothelial expression of ICAM-1 in the vessel wall in the form of an enlarged positive endothelial area, which was 3.8 times larger ($p < 0.001$, Figure 5) than that in control skin ($p = 0.077$).

3.3. VCAM-1

VCAM-1 was expressed almost in all layers of the epidermis, with the strongest staining observed in the suprabasal layer cells. However, the expression was significantly weaker in AD-affected skin than in control skin (Figure 2).

Quantifying the immunostained area revealed a significant decrease in epidermal expression in AD-affected skin. The number of positive cells decreased 1.3 times ($p < 0.001$ vs. $p = 0.121$, Figure 3) and the positive area decreased by half compared to the control ($p < 0.001$ vs. $p = 0.095$, Figure 4).

In the dermis of control and AD-affected skin, VCAM-1 expression was found only in the macrophage-like cells of AD-affected skin (Figure 2), and therefore, no quantitative analysis of endothelial expression could be performed.

4. Discussion

This study showed a detailed spatial arrangement of E-selectin, ICAM-1, and VCAM-1 expression and the difference in the molecular scatter in healthy and AD-affected skin. We found E-selectin to have a moderate expression in basal and suprabasal epidermal layers of controls and weak expression in the case of patients with AD. In the dermis, AD-affected skin showed an intense E-selectin signal in the vascular endothelium and macrophages with a weak signal in the endothelium of controls. ICAM-1 was weakly expressed in the basal and suprabasal epidermal layers of healthy and AD-affected skin. The vascular endothelium in the dermis showed a strong signal for ICAM-1 in patients with AD and a weak one in controls. VCAM-1 expression was found in all epidermal layers of controls but not the dermis. In patients with AD, VCAM-1 expression was scarce in the epidermal basal and suprabasal layers, strong in dermal macrophages, and non-existent in the vascular endothelium.

In this study of adhesion molecules in AD, we confirmed their presence and proved their importance as immunological factors involved in the pathogenesis of AD. There has been evidence of expression of adhesion molecules E-selectin, VCAM-1, and ICAM-1 in the skin of patients with AD [23–26]. These molecules are important in the allergic inflammation in AD because they stimulate the migration of cutaneous memory T-lymphocytes with cutaneous leukocyte-associated antigen, as well as lymphocyte, monocyte, and granulocyte diapedesis in skin and blood [20,28,32]. Soluble E-selectin and soluble ICAM-1 are a marker of the activity of AD in children [28]. Our results also agree with those of an earlier study [42] showing that adhesion molecules play a crucial role in allergic inflammation because they induce selective migration of T-lymphocytes expressing CLA, thereby enabling diapedesis of cells such as monocytes and granulocytes [37]. Increased levels of endothelial leukocyte adhesion molecules ICAM-1 and VCAM-1 have been found in the tissue and serum samples obtained from patients with AD [23–28].

Although studies in patients suffering from AD showed evidence supporting a contributing role of ICAM-1 and VCAM-1 in AD by proof of higher dermal vascular expressions of these two molecules, there has been evidence of adhesion molecule ICAM-1 in the endothelium, in cells surrounding blood vessels, and in the (supra)basal layer of the epidermis [19,20,24,28]. ICAM-1 is a critical adhesion molecule in lymphocyte migration into the dermis, which is in correlation with the stage of dermal lymphocyte inflammation, and it is considered the most crucial adhesion molecule in the etiopathogenesis of AD. ICAM-1 expression was identified in the epidermis's basal and suprabasal layers and the walls of blood vessels in the dermis. These findings are consistent with the findings of Wüthrich et al., who proved the expression of ICAM-1 on keratinocytes, fibroblasts, lymphocytes, and perivascular cells [24].

Some inconsistencies were found when comparing our results with the work of other researchers saying that VCAM-1 is an adhesion molecule expressed in endothelial cells and perivascular dermis-infiltrating cells, presenting an essential parameter for estimating inflammation activity in AD [23,24]. Our results demonstrated that VCAM-1, much more than ICAM-1, contributes to developing skin inflammation in AD.

This study's data contribute to the understanding of the etiopathogenesis of AD. Our study led us to conclude that E-selectin might be the most sensitive parameter for estimation of the clinical course of AD. This study demonstrated the presence of changes in organization and topographical scatter of adhesion molecules in the skin that are specific for AD. These findings further support the hypothesis that adhesion molecules play a vital role in the pathogenesis of AD.

In order to maximally avoid bias caused by different scoring categories, non-standardized approaches, and variability of visual analysis, a digital image analysis method was used, which was described previously as an optimal method when the dataset is not too large and the analyzed tissue is histologically homogenous [40,41].

Further studies might include a comparison of adhesion molecule expression in lesional and non-lesional AD-affected skin [14] on the T-cell receptor repertoire.

Despite many different studies on the etiopathogenesis of atopic dermatitis, this issue remains an unsolved puzzle for further investigations of immunological factors responsible for inflammation in this disease.

In conclusion, AD-affected skin expressed E-selectin, ICAM-1, and VCAM-1 in a disease-specific way. E-selectin may be the most sensitive parameter for estimation of the clinical course of AD. The topographical scatter and specific changes in the organization of adhesion molecules in the skin that are specific for AD further support the hypothesis that adhesion molecules play a vital role in the pathogenesis of AD.

Author Contributions: Conceptualization, S.M.K. and R.J.T.; methodology, M.T.; formal analysis, M.H.P.; investigation, V.M.R.; resources, S.M.K.; data curation, M.T.; writing—original draft preparation, S.M.K. and M.T.; writing—review and editing, M.T.; visualization, R.J.T.; supervision, R.J.T.; project administration, V.M.R.; funding acquisition, M.H.P. All authors have read and agreed to the published version of the manuscript.

Funding: This research was funded by the School of Medicine, University of Zagreb, as part of the project "Immunologic factors in pathogenesis of atopic dermatitis, seborrheic dermatitis and psoriasis" (# 0108166).

Institutional Review Board Statement: The study was conducted according to the guidelines of the Declaration of Helsinki and was approved by the Ethics Committee of the University of Zagreb, School of Medicine (approved 4 January 2010), protocol code 218-00/00-000-3657.

Informed Consent Statement: Informed consent was obtained from all subjects involved in the study.

Data Availability Statement: Not applicable.

Conflicts of Interest: The authors declare no conflict of interest.

References

1. Weidinger, S.; Novak, N. Atopic dermatitis. *Lancet* **2016**, *387*, 1109–1122. [CrossRef] [PubMed]
2. Silverberg, J.I.; Patel, N.; Immaneni, S.; Rusniak, B.; Silverberg, N.B.; Debashis, R.; Fewkes, N.; Simpson, E.L. Assessment of atopic dermatitis using self-report and caregiver report: A multicentre validation study. *Br. J. Dermatol.* **2015**, *173*, 1400–1404. [CrossRef]
3. Lugović, L.; Lipozenčić, J.C.A. Are respiratory allergic diseases related to atopic dermatitis? *Coll. Antropol.* **2000**, *24*, 11.
4. Sohn, A.; Frankel, A.; Patel, R.V.; Goldenberg, G. Eczema. *Mt. Sinai J. Med.* **2011**, *78*, 730–739. [CrossRef] [PubMed]
5. Chiesa Fuxench, Z.C.; Block, J.K.; Boguniewicz, M.; Boyle, J.; Fonacier, L.; Gelfand, J.M.; Grayson, M.H.; Margolis, D.J.; Mitchell, L.; Silverberg, J.I.; et al. Atopic dermatitis in America study: A cross-sectional study examining the prevalence and disease burden of atopic dermatitis in the US adult population. *J. Investig. Dermatol.* **2019**, *139*, 583–590. [CrossRef] [PubMed]
6. Silverberg, J.I. Public health burden and epidemiology of atopic dermatitis. *Dermatol. Clin.* **2017**, *35*, 283–289. [CrossRef] [PubMed]
7. Schmitt, J.; Langan, S.; Deckert, S.; Svensson, A.; von Kobyletzki, L.; Thomas, K.; Spuls, P. Assessment of clinical signs of atopic dermatitis: A systematic review and recommendation. *J. Allergy Clin. Immunol.* **2013**, *132*, 1337–1347. [CrossRef]
8. Hanifin, J.M.; Rajka, G. Diagnostic features of atopic dermatitis. *Acta Derm. Venereol.* **1980**, *92*, 4. [CrossRef]
9. Kim, K.H. Overview of atopic dermatitis. *Asia Pac. Allergy* **2013**, *3*, 79–87. [CrossRef]
10. Gu, H.; Chen, X.S.; Chen, K.; Yan, Y.; Jing, H.; Chen, X.Q.; Shao, C.G.; Ye, G.Y. Evaluation of diagnostic criteria for atopic dermatitis: Validity of the criteria of Williams et al. in a hospital-based setting. *Br. J. Dermatol.* **2001**, *145*, 428–433. [CrossRef]

11. Eichenfield, L.F.; Tom, W.L.; Chamlin, S.L.; Feldman, S.R.; Hanifin, J.M.; Simpson, E.L.; Berger, T.G.; Bergman, J.N.; Cohen, D.E.; Cooper, K.D.; et al. Guidelines of care for the management of atopic dermatitis: Section 1. Diagnosis and assessment of atopic dermatitis. *J. Am. Acad. Dermatol.* **2014**, *70*, 338–351. [CrossRef]
12. Jurakić Tončić, R.; Marinović, B. The role of impaired epidermal barrier function in atopic dermatitis. *Acta Dermatovenerol. Croat.* **2016**, *24*, 95–109.
13. Bin, L.; Leung, D.Y.M. Genetic and epigenetic studies of atopic dermatitis. *Allergy Asthma Clin. Immunol.* **2016**, *12*, 52. [CrossRef]
14. Brunner, P.M.; Emerson, R.O.; Tipton, C.; Garcet, S.; Khattri, S.; Coats, I.; Krueger, J.G.; Guttman-Yassky, E. Nonlesional atopic dermatitis skin shares similar T-cell clones with lesional tissues. *Allergy* **2017**, *72*, 2017–2025. [CrossRef] [PubMed]
15. Tokura, Y. Extrinsic and intrinsic types of atopic dermatitis. *J. Dermatol. Sci.* **2010**, *58*, 6. [CrossRef]
16. Fölster-Holst, R.; Pape, M.; Buss, Y.L.; Christophers, E.; Weichenthal, M. Low prevalence of the intrinsic form of atopic dermatitis among adult patients. *Allergy* **2006**, *61*, 629–632. [CrossRef] [PubMed]
17. Drislane, C.; Irvine, A.D. The role of filaggrin in atopic dermatitis and allergic disease. *Ann. Allergy Asthma Immunol.* **2020**, *124*, 36–43. [CrossRef]
18. Palmer, C.N.; Irvine, A.D.; Terron-Kwiatkowski, A.; Zhao, Y.; Liao, H.; Lee, S.P.; Goudie, D.R.; Sandilands, A.; Campbell, L.E.; Smith, F.J.; et al. Common loss-of-function variants of the epidermal barrier protein filaggrin are a major predisposing factor for atopic dermatitis. *Nat. Genet.* **2006**, *38*, 441–446. [CrossRef]
19. Lugović, L.; Cupić, H.; Lipozencić, J.; Jakić-Razumović, J. The role of adhesion molecules in atopic dermatitis. *Acta Dermatovenerol. Croat.* **2006**, *14*, 2–7. [PubMed]
20. Sigurdsson, V.; de Vries, I.J.; Toonstra, J.; Bihari, I.C.; Thepen, T.; Bruijnzeel-Koomen, C.A.; van Vloten, W.A. Expression of VCAM-1, ICAM-1, E-selectin, and P-selectin on endothelium in situ in patients with erythroderma, mycosis fungoides and atopic dermatitis. *J. Cutan. Pathol.* **2000**, *27*, 436–440. [CrossRef]
21. Tatu, A.L.; Nadasdy, S.T.; Arbune, S.A.; Chioncel, S.V.; Bobeica, S.C.; Niculet, E.; Iancu, S.A.V.; Dumitru, C.; Popa, V.T.; Kluger, S.N.; et al. Interrelationship and sequencing of interleukins 4, 13, 31, and 33: An integrated systematic review: Dermatological and multidisciplinary perspectives. *J. Inflamm. Res.* **2022**, *15*, 5163–5184. [CrossRef] [PubMed]
22. Foti, C.; Romita, P.; Ambrogio, F.; Manno, C.; Filotico, R.; Cassano, N.; Vena, G.A.; De Marco, A.; Cazzato, G.; Mennuni, B.G. Treatment of severe atopic dermatitis with dupilumab in three patients with renal diseases. *Life* **2022**, *12*, 2002. [CrossRef] [PubMed]
23. Shimizu, Y.; Newman, W.; Gopal, T.V.; Horgan, K.J.; Graber, N.; Beall, L.D.; van Seventer, G.A.; Shaw, S. Four molecular pathways of T-cell adhesion to endothelial cells: Roles of LFA-1, VCAM-1, and ELAM-1 and changes in pathway hierarchy under different activation conditions. *J. Cell Biol.* **1991**, *113*, 1203–1212. [CrossRef] [PubMed]
24. Wüthrich, B.; Joller-Jemelka, H.; Kägi, M.K. Levels of soluble ICAM-1 in atopic dermatitis. A new marker for monitoring the clinical activity? *Allergy* **1995**, *50*, 88–89. [CrossRef]
25. Jung, K.; Linse, F.; Heller, R.; Moths, C.; Goebel, R.; Neumann, C. Adhesion molecules in atopic dermatitis: VCAM-1 and ICAM-1 expression is increased in healthy-appearing skin. *Allergy* **1996**, *51*, 452–460. [CrossRef]
26. Koide, M.; Furukawa, F.; Tokura, Y.; Shirahama, S.; Takigawa, M. Evaluation of soluble cell adhesion molecules in atopic dermatitis. *J. Dermatol.* **1997**, *24*, 88–93. [CrossRef]
27. Yusuf-Makagiansar, H.; Anderson, M.E.; Yakovleva, T.V.; Murray, J.S.; Siahaan, T.J. Inhibition of LFA-1/ICAM-1 and VLA-4/VCAM-1 as a therapeutic approach to inflammation and autoimmune diseases. *Med. Res. Rev.* **2002**, *22*, 146–167. [CrossRef]
28. Wolkerstorfer, A.; Savelkoul, H.F.; de Waard van der Spek, F.B.; Neijens, H.J.; van Meurs, T.; Oranje, A.P. Soluble E-selectin and soluble ICAM-1 levels as markers of the activity of atopic dermatitis in children. *Pediatr. Allergy Immunol.* **2003**, *14*, 302–306. [CrossRef]
29. Lawson, C.; Wolf, S. ICAM-1 signaling in endothelial cells. *Pharmacol. Rep.* **2009**, *61*, 22–32. [CrossRef]
30. Chen, Q.; Massagué, J. Molecular Pathways: VCAM-1 as a potential therapeutic target in metastasis. *Clin. Cancer Res.* **2012**, *18*, 5520–5525. [CrossRef]
31. Telen, M.J. Cellular adhesion and the endothelium: E-selectin, L-selectin, and pan-selectin inhibitors. *Hematol. Oncol. Clin. N. Am.* **2014**, *28*, 341–354. [CrossRef]
32. Yamashita, N.; Kaneko, S.; Kouro, O.; Furue, M.; Yamamoto, S.; Sakane, T. Soluble E-selectin as a marker of disease activity in atopic dermatitis. *J. Allergy Clin. Immunol.* **1997**, *99*, 410–416. [CrossRef]
33. Käßmeyer, S.; Plendl, J.; Custodis, P.; Bahramsoltani, M. New insights in vascular development: Vasculogenesis and endothelial progenitor cells. *Anat. Histol. Embryol.* **2009**, *38*, 1–11. [CrossRef] [PubMed]
34. Wierenga, E.A.; Snoek, M.; Jansen, H.M.; Bos, J.D.; van Lier, R.A.; Kapsenberg, M.L. Human atopen-specific types 1 and 2 T helper cell clones. *J. Immunol.* **1991**, *147*, 2942–2949. [CrossRef] [PubMed]
35. Bos, J.D.; Kapsenberg, M.L.; Smitt, J.H. Pathogenesis of atopic eczema. *Lancet* **1994**, *343*, 1338–1341. [CrossRef] [PubMed]
36. Chen, L.; Lin, S.X.; Amin, S.; Overbergh, L.; Maggiolino, G.; Chan, L.S. VCAM-1 blockade delays disease onset, reduces disease severity and inflammatory cells in an atopic dermatitis model. *Immunol. Cell Biol.* **2010**, *88*, 334–342. [CrossRef] [PubMed]
37. Antiga, E.; Volpi, W.; Torchia, D.; Fabbri, P.; Caproni, M. Effects of tacrolimus ointment on Toll-like receptors in atopic dermatitis. *Clin. Exp. Derm.* **2011**, *36*, 235–241. [CrossRef] [PubMed]

38. Howick, J.; Chalmers, I.; Glasziou, P.; Greenhalgh, T.; Heneghan, C.; Liberati, A.; Moschetti, I.; Philips, B.; Thornton, H. *The 2011 Oxford CEBM Evidence Levels of Evidence (Introductory Document)*; Oxford Centre for Evidence-Based Medicine: Oxford, UK, 2011; Available online: http://www.cebm.net/index.aspx?o=5653 (accessed on 18 January 2022).
39. Kamp, S.; Balkert, L.S.; Stenderup, K.; Rosada, C.; Pakkenberg, B.; Kemp, K.; Jemec, G.B.; Dam, T.N. Stereological estimation of epidermal volumes and dermo-epidermal surface area in normal skin. *Dermatology* **2011**, *223*, 131–139. [CrossRef]
40. Fedchenko, N.; Reifenrath, J. Different approaches for interpretation and reporting of immunohistochemistry analysis results in the bone tissue—A review. *Diagn. Pathol.* **2014**, *9*, 221. [CrossRef]
41. Zou, Z.; Liu, S.; An, J.; Huang, Y.; Sun, D.; Shen, H. Stereological study of epidermis in human skin grafts on nude athymic mice. *Anal. Quant. Cytol. Histol.* **2017**, *39*, 7.
42. Caproni, M.; Volpi, W.; Giomi, B.; Torchia, D.; Del Bianco, E.; Fabbri, P. Cellular adhesion molecules in chronic urticaria: Modulation of serum levels occurs during levocetirizine treatment. *Br. J. Dermatol.* **2006**, *155*, 1270–1274. [CrossRef] [PubMed]

Disclaimer/Publisher's Note: The statements, opinions and data contained in all publications are solely those of the individual author(s) and contributor(s) and not of MDPI and/or the editor(s). MDPI and/or the editor(s) disclaim responsibility for any injury to people or property resulting from any ideas, methods, instructions or products referred to in the content.

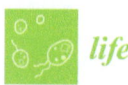

Article

Niosomal Curcumin Suppresses IL17/IL23 Immunopathogenic Axis in Skin Lesions of Psoriatic Patients: A Pilot Randomized Controlled Trial

Hanieh Kolahdooz [1,2], **Vahid Khori** [3], **Vahid Erfani-Moghadam** [4], **Fatemeh Livani** [5,6], **Saeed Mohammadi** [6,7,*] and **Ali Memarian** [2,8,*]

1. Student Research Committee, Golestan University of Medical Sciences, Gorgan 49341-74515, Iran
2. Department of Immunology, Faculty of Medicine, Golestan University of Medical Sciences, Gorgan 49341-74515, Iran
3. Ischemic Disorders Research Center, Golestan University of Medical Sciences, Gorgan 49341-74515, Iran
4. Medical Cellular and Molecular Research Center, Golestan University of Medical Sciences, Gorgan 49341-74515, Iran
5. Clinical Research Development Unit (CRDU), Sayyad Shirazi Hospital, Golestan University of Medical Sciences, Gorgan 49341-74515, Iran
6. Infectious Diseases Research Center, Golestan University of Medical Sciences, Gorgan 49341-74515, Iran
7. Stem Cell Research Center, Golestan University of Medical Sciences, Gorgan 49341-74515, Iran
8. Rheumatology Research Center, Golestan University of Medical Sciences, Gorgan 49341-74515, Iran
* Correspondence: s.mohammadi@goums.ac.ir (S.M.); alimemarian@goums.ac.ir (A.M.)

Citation: Kolahdooz, H.; Khori, V.; Erfani-Moghadam, V.; Livani, F.; Mohammadi, S.; Memarian, A. Niosomal Curcumin Suppresses IL17/IL23 Immunopathogenic Axis in Skin Lesions of Psoriatic Patients: A Pilot Randomized Controlled Trial. *Life* **2023**, *13*, 1076. https://doi.org/10.3390/life13051076

Academic Editor: Alin Laurentiu Tatu

Received: 20 March 2023
Revised: 10 April 2023
Accepted: 20 April 2023
Published: 24 April 2023

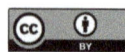

Copyright: © 2023 by the authors. Licensee MDPI, Basel, Switzerland. This article is an open access article distributed under the terms and conditions of the Creative Commons Attribution (CC BY) license (https:// creativecommons.org/licenses/by/ 4.0/).

Abstract: Psoriasis (PS) is characterized by hyperplasia of epidermis and infiltration of immune cells in the dermis. A negligible susceptibility of hypodermic permeation for local anti-inflammatory remedies is one of the major causes of medication failures. Although curcumin (CUR) has indicated effectiveness in treatment of inflammation, its successful permeation through the stratum corneum is yet a challenging issue. Therefore, niosome (NIO) nanoparticles were used as curcumin carriers to enhance its delivery and anti-inflammatory effects. Curcumin-niosome (CUR-NIO) formulations were constructed by the thin-film-hydration (TFH) technique and were added to hyaluronic acid and Marine-collagen gel-based formulation. Five mild-to-moderate PS patients (18–60 years) with PASI scores < 30 with symmetrical and similar lesions were included in the study. The prepared formulation (CUR 15 µM) was topically administered for 4 weeks on the skin lesions, in comparison to the placebo. Clinical skin manifestations were monitored and skin punches were obtained for further gene expression analyses. There was a significant reduction in redness, scaling, and an apparent improvement in CUR-NIO-treated group in comparison to the placebo-treated counterpart. The gene expression analyses resulted in significantly downregulation of IL17, IL23, IL22, and TNFα, S100A7, S100A12, and Ki67 in CUR-NIO-treated lesions. Consequently, CUR-NIO could provide therapeutic approaches for the patients with mild-to-moderate PS by suppressing the IL17/IL23 immunopathogenic axis.

Keywords: curcumin; IL17; IL23; IL22; Ki67; niosome; psoriasis; S100A7; S100A12; TNFα

1. Introduction

Psoriasis (PS) is a systemic inflammatory autoimmune disorder described by the formation of skin plaques with an inflammatory, painful or itchy surface, limiting the quality of life among involved patients [1]. These skin rashes form pink to red patches on white (Type 1 and 2 Fitzpatrick skin type) skins with silvery to white scales, while forming brown to dark patches with grey scales on dark (Type 5 and 6 Fitzpatrick skin type) skins [2]. Psoriasis is reported in all age and gender groups, mostly demonstrated in adults between 45–64 years [3]. PS patients may develop a rheumatologic state called *"psoriatic arthritis* (PsA)" which leads to inflamed, painful and swollen joints, mostly in fingertips and spine [4]. According to recent epidemiological studies, PS involves 2–3% of the world's population [5]. The PsA condition has been reported in 25–30 percent of PS patients, with varying clinical symptoms [6].

The diagnosis of PS typically involves laboratory and clinical assessments; however, histological analyses of the lesions reveal an accelerated renewal of the epidermis, characterized by hyperkeratosis, parakeratosis, and acanthosis, as well as vasodilation and lymphocytic infiltration. Additionally, ki67 overexpression has been observed [7–9].

Although the hyperproliferation of keratinocytes is the most remarkable characteristic of PS, the underlying mechanism of the loss of control is not well studied. Environmental factors, genetic background, and immune responses may be involved in the pathogenesis of PS [10]. Although the immunopathological mechanisms underlying this disease with defective immune responses are not yet fully understood, research has highlighted the significant roles played by immune cells located in the dermis and epidermis, such as dendritic cells (DCs) and T lymphocytes (T cells) [11,12]. Activated DCs produce high levels of TNFα and IL23, boosting the differentiation of naïve T cells into the Th17 cells. IL17 and TNFα activate keratinocytes, cultivating epidermal hyperplasia and recruiting other inflammatory cells, especially neutrophils [12]. TNFα-dependent pathways along with the IL23/IL17 axis represent a cross-talk between innate and adaptive immunity which are known as the most important immunological factors in PS pathogenesis [13,14].

Recent evidence has highlighted the role of keratinocytes, particularly in their production of IL23, in both the onset and progression of chronic PS. [15]. Moreover, both IL17 and IL23 induce IL22 production, by Th22 cells, which is also known as a key factor in PS development [16,17]. IL22 stimulates epidermal keratinocyte proliferation and activation, and induces epithelial cells to produce antimicrobial peptides that are synergistically upregulated on the side of IL17 [18–20].

S100 family of proteins are small calcium-binding proteins known as inflammatory antimicrobial peptides (AMPs) [21]. In particular, IL17A could induce production of some AMP components including S100A7 (psoriasin) and S100A12 (calgranulin c) from keratinocytes [22,23]. AMPs not only recruit leukocytes such as neutrophils (PMNs), Th17 cells, DCs, and macrophages, [24] but also induce TNFα production [25]. Furthermore, S100A12 could be considered as the most promising biomarker for PS [26].

Although several therapeutic approaches are currently prescribed or under investigation for PS, corticosteroid topical therapy is still applied as the first option of treatment for mild-to-moderate PS [27,28]. Corticosteroids not only have several side effects, but also do not prompt satisfactory clinical impacts [29]. Medication alternatives to corticosteroids include methotrexate, cyclosporine, and small molecule biologicals such as adalimumab (Humira), a TNF-alpha-blocking antibody, and brodalumab (Siliq), a human antibody against interleukins (IL12/23 inhibitors, IL17 inhibitors, IL23 inhibitors) [30,31].

Evidence shows that the effects of some topical herbal remedies may contribute considerably to the healing process and reduce inflammation [32]. Natural products that have been associated with some success include aloe vera, omega-3 fatty acids, turmeric (curcumin), and Oregon grape [33]. Curcumin (CUR) is a derivative of Curcuma longa which has therapeutic and immunomodulatory properties [34]. Several clinical investigations showed that CUR could be beneficial against different cancer types [35,36], cardiovascular diseases (CVDs) [37], and inflammatory and skin diseases [38,39]. It efficiently relieves clinical manifestations, reduces the level of inflammatory markers, slows down disease progression, and prevents disease relapse [40]. Although the role of CUR in PS has not been well described, it was studied in human and experimental animal studies [41,42]. Previous findings have shown that CUR has the potential to suppress inflammatory cytokines including IL23 and IL17, which have major roles in PS pathogenesis and chronic inflammation [43].

Despite promising therapeutic properties, the use of CUR might be limited because of low bioavailability and solubility, insufficient pharmacokinetics, and rapid degradation [44,45]. On the other side, there is an evidence suggesting that nanoparticles encapsulation can enhance its delivery and stability [11]. The encapsulation of lipophilic compositions into the nanoemulsion intensifies their infiltration into the deep skin layers for local delivery, and may increase their efficacy [46]. Niosomes, as non-ionic surfactant-based vesicles, are obtained by hydration of single-chain surfactants and could be stable at 10 to 1000 nm in size. They have the ability to preserve both lipophilic and hydrophilic drugs by encapsulating them in an aqueous compartment and distributing them within the bilayer [47]. The application of niosomes as carriers for local drug delivery could improve the effectiveness and safety of some drugs, including CUR [48,49]. The use of niosomes has been reported in the cosmetics industry [50]. Additionally, several investigations have revealed that the widespread application of gel-based hyaluronic acid and marine collagen in nano-drug delivery structures improve the stability, release, and absorption of the drugs via epidermis in the skin lesions [51]. The excellent solubility of hyaluronic acid has led to its development as one of the most remarkable carriers for topical delivery of medications to the skin, especially in combination with the nano-carriers [52].

Our current clinical trial evaluated the IL17/IL23 immunopathogenic axis besides healing process in skin lesions of PS patients who treated by a topical formulation containing curcumin-niosomes (CUR-NIO) within a hyaluronic acid and marine collagen gel.

2. Materials and Methods

2.1. Preparing the CUR-NIO Formulation

CUR-NIO was constructed by thin-film hydration (TFH) method, as described previously [53,54]. Briefly, accurately-weighed quantities of Tween80 and Squalene (Sigma, St. Louis, MO, USA) were dissolved in 2 mL of chloroform and methanol in a round bottom flask (2:1 ratio). Then, 10 mL of CUR 1 mg/mL in methanol was added to the combination and mixed gently with a magnet stirrer (25 °C for 15 min). The dissolved mixture was subsequently evaporated (45 °C for 20 min), using a rotary evaporator, under vacuum and constant rotation to obtain a thin film. By utilizing the hand-shaking process, the thin film was hydrated with 5 mL of isotonic phosphate buffer saline (PBS: pH 7.4) at room temperature (RT) to form the CUR-NIO suspension. This suspension was sonicated within an ultrasonic water bath for 20 min, purified using a 0.2 μm membrane filter, and kept in −80 °C for 2 h. Finally, it was lyophilized in a vacuum freeze-dryer (Crisp Beta 2-8LD plus, Osterode am Harz, Germany) for 24 h in −50 °C.

2.2. Characterizing the CUR-NIO Composition

2.2.1. Size, Distribution and Zeta Potential

The size and distribution of constructed niosomes were specified by measuring the vesicles in each preparation using Dynamic Light Scattering (DLS). The lyophilized nanoparticles were dispersed in PBS (pH 7.4) using an ultrasonic water bath for 5 min at 25 °C and the parameters were evaluated. The zeta potential, size, and polydispersity index (PDI) of each preparation was assessed by DLS (Zetasizer Nano ZS; Malvern Instruments, Malvern, UK) utilizing an argon laser beam at 633 nm and a 90° scattering angle. Each sample was measured in triplicates and results were expressed as means ± standard deviation (SD).

2.2.2. Encapsulation Efficiency (EE%) and Loading Capacity of Vesicles

The encapsulation efficiency (EE%) and loading capacity (LC) was assessed and quantified by the direct method through the following formulations. We dissolved 1 mg of lyophilized CUR-NIO in 1 mL of methanol and evaluated by UV–VIS spectrophotometry at 425 nm (Shimadzu, Japan). The amount of entrapped CUR was assessed using the CUR standard curve.

$$EE\% = \frac{\text{Amounts of encapculated curcumin} * 100}{\text{Initial amount of curcumin}}$$

$$LC\% = \frac{\text{Amounts of encapculated curcumin} * 100}{\text{Initial amount of nanoparticle}}$$

2.2.3. Preparing the of CUR-NIO Loaded Topical Cream

Topical formulations should contain adequate viscosity to be suitable for administration to the skin. Hyaluronic acid (0.1%) and marine-collagen (2.5%) (formulated by Kimia Golestan Green Chemical Company, Gorgan, Iran) were selected as the matrix of the CUR-NIO gel. Hyaluronic acid and collagen were added into the lyophilized CUR-NIO in a drop-wise fashion, with gentle, but constant stirring in darkness for 2 h. The concentration of CUR-NIO was 0.1% (w/w) in the gel.

2.3. Patients and Sample Selection

2.3.1. Criteria

Five patients, aged 18 to 60 years, with mild-to-moderate PS (PASI < 30, based on the PS area severity index [55]) and at least two symmetrical and/or similar skin lesions were enrolled in this study. Patients were not pregnant or breastfeeding and were not taking any kind of corticosteroids or topical treatments in the last two months or during the trial. They were not suffering from metabolic syndrome, hepatic, renal or other autoimmune diseases. The key demographic and clinical characteristics of the psoriasis patients included in the study are presented in Table S1. We also used peripheral blood samples from five healthy controls. Written informed consents were signed by all participants. This study was approved by the committee of research ethics at Golestan University of Medical Sciences (IR.GOUMS.REC.1397.275) and registered in the Iranian Registry of Clinical Trials (IRCT20181217042030N1).

2.3.2. Ex-Vivo Study

At first, for ex vivo evaluation including cell cytotoxicity and gene expression assessments, we isolated peripheral blood mononuclear cells (PBMCs) from blood samples of healthy donors and patients using Ficoll-Paque density gradient centrifugation, as described [56]. 10^6 live cells were treated with CUR, CUR-NIO, NIO, and a vehicle control (DMSO), in separate wells for 6 h. They were subsequently stimulated by anti-CD3 (1 µg/mL; Sinabiotech, Tehran, Iran), as described previously [57]. After four days, treated PBMCs were collected for cell apoptosis and gene expression analyses.

2.3.3. Intervention

Instructions on application of the formulation were given to the patients, in which they were instructed to apply a thin layer of the 0.1% CUR-NIO gel and the placebo twice a day for four weeks onto their eligible skin lesions, in the manner of a placebo-controlled clinical trial. Specifically, each patient used CUR-NIO gel for one lesion and placebo for the counterpart. The placebo was only composed of gel-based hyaluronic acid and marine-collagen. After four weeks of treatment, the drug- and placebo-treated psoriatic lesions were assessed by a dermatologist and skin punches were obtained from both lesions of each patient for further gene expression evaluation.

2.4. Apoptosis Assessment of CUR-NIO

Flow cytometry measurements were conducted using FITC-conjugated Annexin V and PI staining kits (BioLegend, San Diego, CA, USA) for apoptosis. Isolated PBMCs from healthy donors were cultured as described above and treated with three concentrations of CUR (5, 10 and 15 mM). After four days, cultured cells were harvested and prepared for assessment following the manufacturer's directions. Finally, each tube was immediately evaluated using BD accuri C6 flow cytometer (BD PharMingen, San Diego, CA, USA). The data were analyzed using the BD Accuri™ C6 software version 1.0.264.21 (Accuri Cytometers, Ann Arbor, MI, USA).

2.5. Quantitative Real-Time PCR

Total RNA was isolated from homogenized samples in RNX-Plus (Sinacolon, Tehran, Iran) for RNA extraction and then reverse transcribed into cDNA using Yekta-Tajhiz cDNA synthesis

Kit (Tehran, Iran), according to the manufacturer's protocols. The primers of genes including IL17A, IL22, IL23, TNF-α, S100A7, S100A12, ki67, and 18sRNA (as internal control) were synthesized by *Takapuzist* Gene Molecular Biotechnology Co. (Tehran, Iran), listed in the Table 1. Real-time qPCR amplifications were performed using Master Mix SYBR green kit (Parstous, Mashhad, Iran), which was used for each mRNA on a Real-time PCR detection system (Bioer Technology, Hangzhou, China). The cycle of threshold (Ct) for every gene and the internal control were determined for each sample. The relative mRNA expression was quantified, using 2^{-dct} method. Each sample was tested in triplicate [58].

Table 1. The list of primers sequences used in real-time PCR.

	Gene	Plus (5′ > 3′)	Minus (5′ > 3′)	Product (bp)	T_m
1	IL23A	TCAGGCTCAAAGCAAGTGGA	AGCAGCAACAGCAGCATTAC	128	60
2	IL17A	CGCAATGAGGACCCTGAGAG	TAGTCCACGTTCCCATCAGC	92	60
3	IL22	AGCCCTATATCACCAACCGC	TCTCCCCAATGAGACGAACG	87	60
4	TNFα	CATCCAACCTTCCCAAACGC	CTGTAGGCCCCAGTGAGTTC	246	60
5	S100A7	CACTCAAGCTGAGAGGTCCAT	AAAGACATCGGCGAGGTAATTTG	169	60
6	S100A12	ACCACTGCTGGCTTTTTGCT	GGGTGTCAAAATGCCCCTTC	150	60
7	Ki67	TCTGTTATTGATGAGCCTGTA	GTTGACTTCCTTCCATTCTG	107	58
8	18srRNA	ACCCGTTGAACCCCATTCGTGA	GCCTCACTAAACCATCCAATCGG	159	60

2.6. Statistical Analyses

Statistical analyses of the obtained data and graphs were prepared using SPSS 16.0 and GraphPad Prism 5.04 statistical software (GraphPad, Boston, MA, USA). One-way ANOVA or the equivalent non-parametric Kruskal–Wallis test was utilized to obtain the differences of means between two groups, while Tukey's post hoc test was performed to confirm the significant differences. In addition, independent samples *t*-test or Mann–Whitney U test were used to compare the means between two groups. *p*-values smaller than 0.05 were considered to be significant.

3. Results

3.1. Characterizing NIO Nanoparticles

CUR was effectively encapsulated in niosome particles by the single emulsion solvent evaporation technique. The average diameter of nanoparticles (13 ± 2.20 nm), polydispersity index (PDI) (less than 0.2), mean zeta (ξ) potential (2.40 ± 0.602 mV), encapsulation efficacy (86%), and loading efficiency (7.35%) of these NPs were evaluated.

3.2. The CUR-NIO Suspension Exerted Low Toxic Effects on PBMCs

The apoptosis assay was used to confirm that the CUR-NIO suspension has trace cytotoxicity. PBMCs from healthy donors were treated with CUR, CUR-NIO, NIO and DMSO; CUR had three different concentrations (5, 10, 15 μM) (Figure 1). In all three concentrations the survival rate of the PBMC was almost the same. The highest expected concentration (15 μM) was selected for further analyses.

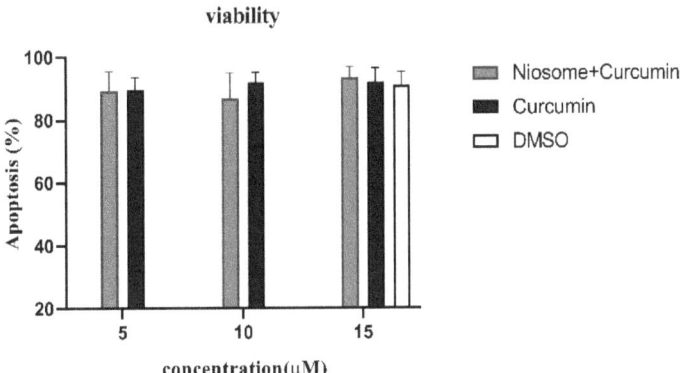

Figure 1. Cytotoxicity assessment by apoptosis. PBMCs from healthy volunteers ($n = 5$) were cultured with CUR, CUR-NIO, and DMSO; curcumin concentrations were 5, 10, and 15 µM. After 4 days, apoptosis was analyzed by flow cytometry.

3.3. Effect of CUR on IL17 Gene Expression in PBMCs from Healthy Donors and PS Patients

Despite the higher expression levels of IL17 among PS patients in all treatment groups and the CUR effect on reducing IL17 gene expression, our results demonstrated no significant change in the PBMCs from patients or from healthy donors for any treatment (Figure 2). Comparisons between patients and normal subjects within similar combinations, however, showed significantly higher levels of IL17 in patients' cells ($p < 0.05$).

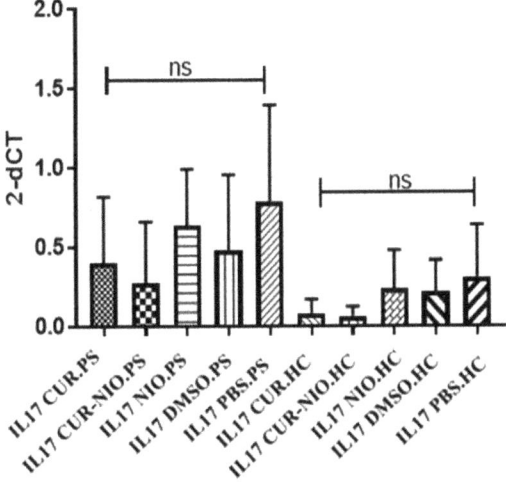

Figure 2. Relative gene expression of IL17 in treated PBMCs with different CUR combinations from PS patients ($n = 5$) and healthy donors ($n = 5$). Although CUR was observed to reduce IL17 gene expression and higher levels of IL17 were detected among psoriasis patients in all treatment groups, our results did not reveal any significant changes across the different treatments in PBMCs from the patient and healthy donor groups. Bars depict relative gene expression of IL17 in stimulated PBMCs by anti-CD3 following treatment with CUR, CUR-NIO, NIO, and DMSO as vehicle control, for 4 days. The results are demonstrated as the mean (±SEM) of the measured gene expression (2^{-dCT}). Statistical significance was determined by one-way ANOVA, with Mann Whitney test to compare treatment groups against the control group (ns: non-significance). CUR: curcumin, CUR-NIO: curcumin-niosome, NIO: noisome, PS: psoriasis, HC: healthy control.

3.4. CUR-NIO Gel Reduces Inflammatory Cytokines in Psoriatic Lesions

As demonstrated in Figure 3A, the mRNA expressions of IL17, IL23, IL22, and TNFα in skin lesions of PS patients were significantly decreased following treatment by CUR-NIO gel in comparison to the placebo ($p < 0.05$).

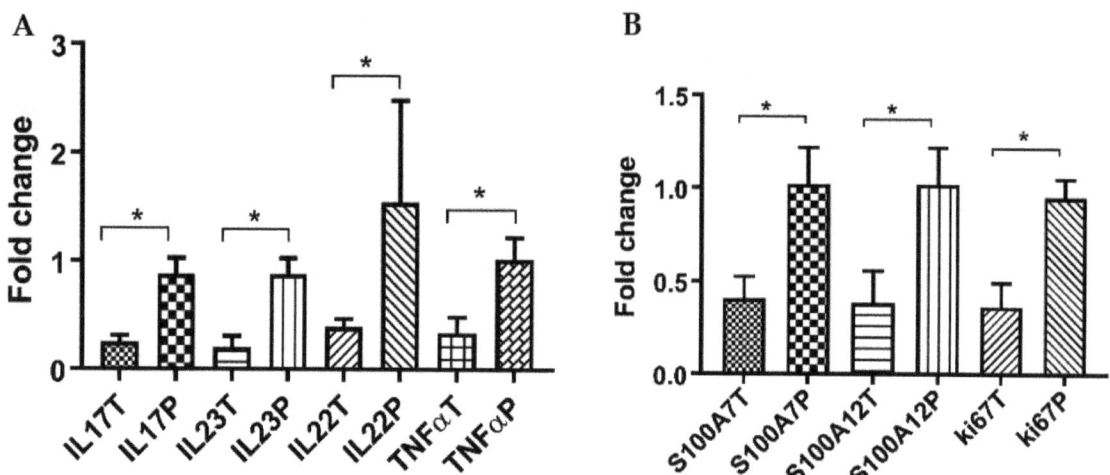

Figure 3. Relative expression of IL17, IL23, IL22 and TNFα genes (**A**) and S100A7, S100A12 and Ki67 genes (**B**) after CUR-NIO gel treated (T) versus placebo (P) in psoriatic skin lesions. mRNA expression was assessed by qPCR in skin tissues from CUR-NIO and placebo groups following 4 weeks of topical administration. The C_t values were normalized to 18s RNA. All mRNA expressions were significantly decreased in CUR-NIO group, compared with the placebo. The asterisk marks indicate significant differences, which are shown on the brackets in the figures (* for $p < 0.05$). Data show mean ± SEM.

3.5. Effects of CUR-NIO Gel on S100A7, S100A12 and ki67

There were also significant downregulations in expression of all S100A7, S100A12, and ki67 genes in skin lesions among CUR-NIO gel treated PS patients compared to the placebo counterparts ($p < 0.05$) (Figure 3B).

3.6. Clinical Observation of the Skin of PS Patients

Figure 4 illustrates the skin of a selected PS patient before and after treatment with the CUR-NIO gel versus placebo. Similar to our quantitative evaluation, we observed that employing CUR-NIO gel had positive clinical effects on the patients' lesions, including reduced redness, levels of PS plaques, and scaling in patients. Furthermore, itching and skin dryness as annoying manifestations of PS declined in lesions following treatment by CUR-NIO gel, in comparison to placebo. Moreover, redness and inflammatory margin in skin lesions were shrunken and considerably ameliorated.

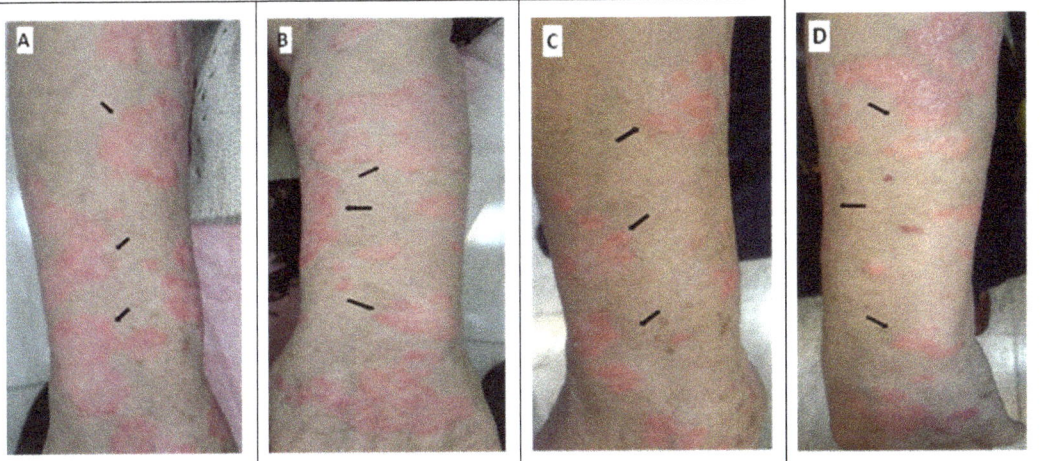

Figure 4. Clinical manifestations of skin psoriasis of a selected patient before and after the application of CUR-NIO gel 0.1% versus placebo. Before application of CUR-NIO gel 0.1% (**A**). Before application of placebo (**B**). After treated with CUR-NIO gel 0.1% (**C**). After treated with placebo (**D**). The skin of a PS patient was examined before and after treatment with CUR-NIO gel compared to a placebo. The results indicated that using the CUR-NIO gel had positive effects on the patients' lesions, such as a reduction in redness, PS plaque levels, and scaling. Additionally, the uncomfortable symptoms of itching and skin dryness also decreased in lesions following treatment with CUR-NIO gel compared to placebo. Moreover, the redness and inflammation surrounding the skin lesions significantly improved. Representative photographs show localized improvement of psoriasis on the patient's skin with reduced redness, scaling. The presence of hyaluronic acid and marine-collagen compounds in both pharmaceutical and placebo gels reduced inflammation in both symmetrical lesions. Black arrows indicate intended lesions before (**A,B**) and after (**C,D**) treatment.

4. Discussion

As an autoimmune disease, PS affects a small population globally but negatively impacts patients' quality of life. To date, conventional treatments such as topical corticosteroids, phototherapy, and several systemic anti-inflammatory drugs have not been entirely successful in patient treatment and can have various adverse effects [59]. Therefore, achieving effective formulations with the most negligible side effects should be developed for the treatment of PS. Various animal investigations and clinical trials have been conducted to understand the molecular mechanisms of PS pathogenesis better and to introduce novel therapeutic agents. A vast number of medications can effectively control PS; approximately 75% of patients with mild-to-moderate PS respond positively to local treatments [60]. Of note, CUR, the major derivative of curcuma longa, may have anti-inflammatory effects on psoriasis patients [61]. Curcumin has been introduced as a beneficial compound for the management of various inflammatory skin diseases [62]. Kang et al. evaluated the inhibitory effects of CUR on Kv1.3 potassium channels on T cells, and demonstrated the anti-inflammatory roles of CUR by showing that the application of 10 µM of CUR significantly inhibited the secretion of inflammatory factors, such as interleukin (IL)-17, IL-22, IFN-γ, IL-2, IL-8, and TNF-α in T cells. However, their study also revealed that the proliferation of T cells was inhibited by more than 50% when exposed to 100 µM curcumin. It is important to recognize that their study was conducted using a mouse model, which may not be entirely representative of human skin [63]. There have been other studies evaluating the effects of curcumin on psoriasis patients; Kurd et al. administered it orally but did not evaluate inflammatory or immunologic factors [64]. Sarafian et al. did not mention or quantify the exact concentration of the curcumin used in their study [65]. Thus, further research was needed to determine the optimal dose and mode of administration for curcumin in treating psoriasis in humans. Consequently, an examination was conducted to determine the potential toxicity of curcumin on PBMCs at various concentrations. The concentration of 15 µM was identified as having the least toxic effects, and was therefore chosen as the concentration for testing.

Our study found that the positive effects observed on PS patients' skin lesions after treatment with CUR-NIO gel were supported by a decrease in the expressions of IL17, IL23, IL22, and TNFα in the skin lesions. These results align with previous findings, indicating that CUR-NIO gel has anti-inflammatory properties that can effectively alleviate the symptoms associated with PS. Varma et al. demonstrated that the proliferation of psoriatic-like cells was inhibited, while the apoptosis induction was increased by CUR via downregulation of pro-inflammatory cytokines, such as IL-17, TNFα, IFNγ, IL-6 [66]. Jain et al. showed that the phenotypic and histopathological features of PS skin treated with tacrolimus and CUR-loaded liposphere gel, were enhanced and, the level of TNF-α, IL-17 and IL-22 were reduced compared to imiquimod group [67]. Antiga et al. demonstrated that CUR could be effective as an adjuvant therapy for the treatment of psoriasis vulgaris by reducing serum levels of IL-22 [39]. Sun et al. demonstrated that topical application of CUR encapsulated in nanoparticles in a mice model of PS might help reduce inflammatory cytokines including IL17/IL23, IL22 and TNFα [68].

CUR with its anti-inflammatory and antioxidant properties can reduce inflammation. The anti-inflammatory properties of CUR on PS, in addition to its low toxicity, have been defined in various studies [69]. However, the main problem of CUR is its relatively low solubility and low capacity for skin penetration which leads to its rapid disappearance in the epidermis [70]. Algahtani et al. showed that the CUR nanoemugel could be a promising candidate for the long-term management of PS in mice [71]. However, no study, to the best of our knowledge, has studied the effects of CUR-NIO in a clinical fashion on PS patients. Permeation of CUR increases 7–8-fold when formulated with permeation enhancers like nanoparticles and gel form [72]. In the present study, niosome nanoparticles were used to increase the efficiency and absorption of CUR in the psoriatic skin lesions. Niosomes have the capability of modifying the structure of the stratum corneum with the assistance of their surfactant properties and enhancing the smoothness by the substitution of lost skin lipids. They play an important role in drug delivery for a wide variety of dermally active compounds and aid as a safe penetration enhancer [73]. Some studies have shown that the application of niosomes increases the absorption of topical drugs for the treatment of skin diseases, including PS and dermatitis [74,75]. It was found that the niosomes prepared for this study had a mean diameter of about 14 nm, indicating they were nanoparticles of the right size, thus making them easily pass through the stratum corneum and causing DCs to uptake CUR-NIO, thus modulating an immune response [76]. Moreover, hyaluronic acid's ideal solubility has been considered one of the most important carriers for topical drug delivery to the skin [77]. Therefore, this study considered hyaluronic acid and marine-collagen as the CUR-NIO matrix.

Contrary to our hypothesis, CUR-treated PBMCs of PS patients and healthy donors demonstrated no significant decrease in IL17 gene expression in any of the studied combinations (Figure 2). Brück et al. also showed that the effects of CUR on T cell polarization were not mediated by direct action. Instead, the particular population of immune cells affected by CUR is the DC population [78]. This evidence could support the insignificant decrease in IL17 gene expression observed in our samples. However, another study showed a substantial effect of CUR (at higher concentrations) on inhibition of IFNγ and IL17A-producing cells [79].

As observed by Sun et al., CUR could affect the IL23/IL17 axis in mice by inhibiting IL1β/IL6 and indirectly regulating IL17/IL22 expression [80]. In this regard, CUR-NIO gel significantly decreases the expression of all tested genes related to IL23/IL17 axis (including IL23, IL22, TNFα and IL17) in the psoriatic lesions, compared to the placebo arm (Figure 3). Furthermore, ki67 downregulation following CUR administration in our patients (Figure 3B) could indicate the control of abnormal keratinocyte proliferation in PS skin tissues, which was also observed previously in an in vitro study [81].

We discovered that there were notable reductions in the expression of S100A7, S100A12, and ki67 genes in skin lesions of PS patients treated with CUR-NIO gel, as compared to lesions that were treated with the placebo. The IL17/IL22 could upregulate the S100A7 and S100A12 expression in keratinocytes reciprocally. The keratinocyte-secreted S100A7 may stimulate the production of pro-inflammatory cytokines and recruit immune cells into the skin, which indicates a distinct feature of psoriatic skin lesion [22,23,82]. According to the previous studies, S100A7 and S100A12 are the most promising markers of PS disease activity, and increased expression of both are typical features shown in PS [26,83] and CUR could reduce their expression, as observed in HaCaT keratinocyte cell line [84]. Substantial downregulation of these peptides by CUR-NIO gel in our patients (vs. placebo, Figure 3B) signify the therapeutic capacity of our treatment.

No adverse effects, such as allergic reactions, skin irritations, staining, or photosensitivity were observed during the studied treatments. The most important limitation of our study was related to the criteria for patient selection, which resulted in a low number of patients with mild/moderate disease severity, no corticosteroid treatment, and at least two symmetrical/similar skin lesions for drug and placebo treatments. However, the last criterion meant that each patient was his/her own control and this was the most important advantage of our study. Consequently, any interference regarding genetic and environmental variations was eliminated which makes the comparisons between treatment and placebo very valuable and reliable in our clinical study.

5. Conclusions

In conclusion, the administration of our CUR-NIO gel as a topical drug could stimulate therapeutic effects on the psoriatic skin lesions and lead to healing processes. This could be induced by expression regulation in the main pathogenic inflammatory genes in PS patients. CUR-NIO gel possibly will be a promising drug for improving the quality of life of PS patients.

Supplementary Materials: The following supporting information can be downloaded at: https://www.mdpi.com/article/10.3390/life13051076/s1, Table S1: Key demographic and clinical characteristics of the psoriasis patients.

Author Contributions: Conceptualization, H.K., S.M. and A.M.; Methodology, H.K., A.M., V.K., V.E.-M., F.L. and S.M.; Software, H.K. and S.M.; Validation, S.M. and A.M.; Formal analysis, H.K., S.M. and A.M.; Investigation, H.K.; Resources, A.M.; Data curation, S.M. and A.M.; Writing—original draft preparation, H.K.; Writing—review and editing, S.M. and A.M.; Supervision, A.M., V.K., V.E.-M., F.L. and S.M.; Project administration, A.M.; Funding acquisition, A.M. All authors have read and agreed to the published version of the manuscript.

Funding: This research was funded by Department of Research and Technology at Golestan University of Medical Sciences, Gorgan, Iran, grant number: 110631.

Institutional Review Board Statement: The study was conducted according to the guidelines of the Declaration of Helsinki, and approved by the Ethics Committee of Golestan University of Medical Sciences (Code of ethics: IR.GOUMS.REC.1397.275). This study was also registered and approved by the Iranian Registry of Clinical Trials (IRCT) (IRCT20181217042030N1).

Informed Consent Statement: Informed consent was obtained from all subjects involved in the study.

Data Availability Statement: Data would be available by the corresponding authors upon request.

Acknowledgments: We would like to appreciate the comprehensive scientific assistance from Batul Yousefi in helping with the preparation of nanoparticles.

Conflicts of Interest: The authors declare no conflict of interest.

References

1. Raychaudhuri, S.K.; Maverakis, E.; Raychaudhuri, S.P. Diagnosis and classification of psoriasis. *Autoimmun. Rev.* **2014**, *13*, 490–495. [CrossRef] [PubMed]
2. Rendon, A.; Schäkel, K. Psoriasis pathogenesis and treatment. *Int. J. Mol. Sci.* **2019**, *20*, 1475. [CrossRef] [PubMed]
3. Bu, J.; Ding, R.; Zhou, L.; Chen, X.; Shen, E. Epidemiology of psoriasis and comorbid diseases: A narrative review. *Front. Immunol.* **2022**, *13*, 2484. [CrossRef] [PubMed]
4. Gialouri, C.G.; Evangelatos, G.; Iliopoulos, A.; Tektonidou, M.G.; Sfikakis, P.P.; Fragoulis, G.E.; Nikiphorou, E. Late-Onset Psoriatic Arthritis: Are There Any Distinct Characteristics? A Retrospective Cohort Data Analysis. *Life* **2023**, *13*, 792. [CrossRef]
5. Springate, D.; Parisi, R.; Kontopantelis, E.; Reeves, D.; Griffiths, C.; Ashcroft, D. Incidence, prevalence and mortality of patients with psoriasis: A UK population-based cohort study. *Br. J. Dermatol.* **2017**, *176*, 650–658. [CrossRef]
6. Parisi, R.; Iskandar, I.Y.; Kontopantelis, E.; Augustin, M.; Griffiths, C.E.; Ashcroft, D.M. National, regional, and worldwide epidemiology of psoriasis: Systematic analysis and modelling study. *BMJ* **2020**, *369*, m1590. [CrossRef] [PubMed]
7. Ayala-Fontánez, N.; Soler, D.C.; McCormick, T.S. Current knowledge on psoriasis and autoimmune diseases. *Psoriasis* **2016**, *6*, 7.
8. Kim, S.; Ryu, Y.W.; Kwon, J.I.; Choe, M.S.; Jung, J.W.; Cho, J.W. Differential expression of cyclin D1, Ki-67, pRb, and p53 in psoriatic skin lesions and normal skin. *Mol. Med. Rep.* **2018**, *17*, 735–742. [CrossRef]
9. Nicolescu, A.C.; Ionescu, M.-A.; Constantin, M.M.; Ancuta, I.; Ionescu, S.; Niculet, E.; Tatu, A.L.; Zirpel, H.; Thaçi, D. Psoriasis Management Challenges Regarding Difficult-to-Treat Areas: Therapeutic Decision and Effectiveness. *Life* **2022**, *12*, 2050. [CrossRef] [PubMed]
10. Balato, A.; Zink, A.; Babino, G.; Buononato, D.; Kiani, C.; Eyerich, K.; Ziehfreund, S.; Scala, E. The Impact of Psoriasis and Atopic Dermatitis on Quality of Life: A Literature Research on Biomarkers. *Life* **2022**, *12*, 2026. [CrossRef]
11. Lin, A.M.; Rubin, C.J.; Khandpur, R.; Wang, J.Y.; Riblett, M.; Yalavarthi, S.; Villanueva, E.C.; Shah, P.; Kaplan, M.J.; Bruce, A.T. Mast cells and neutrophils release IL-17 through extracellular trap formation in psoriasis. *J. Immunol.* **2011**, *187*, 490–500. [CrossRef] [PubMed]
12. Stritesky, G.L.; Yeh, N.; Kaplan, M.H. IL-23 promotes maintenance but not commitment to the Th17 lineage. *J. Immunol.* **2008**, *181*, 5948–5955. [CrossRef] [PubMed]
13. Bugaut, H.; Aractingi, S. Major role of the IL17/23 axis in psoriasis supports the development of new targeted therapies. *Front. Immunol.* **2021**, *12*, 621956. [CrossRef]
14. Li, H.; Yao, Q.; Mariscal, A.G.; Wu, X.; Hülse, J.; Pedersen, E.; Helin, K.; Waisman, A.; Vinkel, C.; Thomsen, S.F. Epigenetic control of IL-23 expression in keratinocytes is important for chronic skin inflammation. *Nat. Commun.* **2018**, *9*, 1420. [CrossRef] [PubMed]
15. Zhou, X.; Chen, Y.; Cui, L.; Shi, Y.; Guo, C. Advances in the pathogenesis of psoriasis: From keratinocyte perspective. *Cell Death Dis.* **2022**, *13*, 81. [CrossRef]
16. Dyring-Andersen, B.; Honoré, T.V.; Madelung, A.; Bzorek, M.; Simonsen, S.; Clemmensen, S.N.; Clark, R.A.; Borregaard, N.; Skov, L. IL-17A and IL-22 producing neutrophils in psoriatic skin. *Br. J. Dermatol.* **2017**, *177*, e321. [CrossRef]
17. Volpe, E.; Servant, N.; Zollinger, R.; Bogiatzi, S.I.; Hupé, P.; Barillot, E.; Soumelis, V. A critical function for transforming growth factor-β, interleukin 23 and proinflammatory cytokines in driving and modulating human TH-17 responses. *Nat. Immunol.* **2008**, *9*, 650–657. [CrossRef]
18. Boniface, K.; Guignouard, E.; Pedretti, N.; Garcia, M.; Delwail, A.; Bernard, F.X.; Nau, F.; Guillet, G.; Dagregorio, G.; Yssel, H. A role for T cell-derived interleukin 22 in psoriatic skin inflammation. *Clin. Exp. Immunol.* **2007**, *150*, 407–415. [CrossRef]
19. Moots, R.J.; Curiale, C.; Petersel, D.; Rolland, C.; Jones, H.; Mysler, E. Efficacy and safety outcomes for originator TNF inhibitors and biosimilars in rheumatoid arthritis and psoriasis trials: A systematic literature review. *BioDrugs* **2018**, *32*, 193–199. [CrossRef]
20. Furue, M.; Furue, M. Interleukin-22 and keratinocytes; pathogenic implications in skin inflammation. *Explor. Immunol.* **2021**, *1*, 37–47. [CrossRef]
21. Broome, A.-M.; Ryan, D.; Eckert, R.L. S100 protein subcellular localization during epidermal differentiation and psoriasis. *J. Histochem. Cytochem.* **2003**, *51*, 675–685. [CrossRef] [PubMed]
22. Hegyi, Z.; Zwicker, S.; Bureik, D.; Peric, M.; Koglin, S.; Batycka-Baran, A.; Prinz, J.C.; Ruzicka, T.; Schauber, J.; Wolf, R. Vitamin D analog calcipotriol suppresses the Th17 cytokine–induced proinflammatory S100 "alarmins" psoriasin (S100A7) and koebnerisin (S100A15) in psoriasis. *J. Investig. Dermatol.* **2012**, *132*, 1416–1424. [CrossRef] [PubMed]
23. Chiricozzi, A.; Nograles, K.E.; Johnson-Huang, L.M.; Fuentes-Duculan, J.; Cardinale, I.; Bonifacio, K.M.; Gulati, N.; Mitsui, H.; Guttman-Yassky, E.; Suárez-Fariñas, M. IL-17 induces an expanded range of downstream genes in reconstituted human epidermis model. *PLoS ONE* **2014**, *9*, e90284. [CrossRef]
24. Yang, D.; Han, Z.; Oppenheim, J.J. Alarmins and immunity. *Immunol. Rev.* **2017**, *280*, 41–56. [CrossRef]
25. Furue, M.; Furue, K.; Tsuji, G.; Nakahara, T. Interleukin-17A and keratinocytes in psoriasis. *Int. J. Mol. Sci.* **2020**, *21*, 1275. [CrossRef] [PubMed]
26. Wilsmann-Theis, D.; Wagenpfeil, J.; Holzinger, D.; Roth, J.; Koch, S.; Schnautz, S.; Bieber, T.; Wenzel, J. Among the S100 proteins, S100A12 is the most significant marker for psoriasis disease activity. *J. Eur. Acad. Dermatol. Venereol.* **2016**, *30*, 1165–1170. [CrossRef] [PubMed]
27. Kim, W.B.; Jerome, D.; Yeung, J. Diagnosis and management of psoriasis. *Can. Fam. Physician* **2017**, *63*, 278–285.
28. Carrascosa, J.M.; Theng, C.; Thaçi, D. Spotlight on Topical Long-Term Management of Plaque Psoriasis. *Clin. Cosmet. Investig. Dermatol.* **2020**, *13*, 495. [CrossRef]

29. Barnes, L.; Kaya, G.; Rollason, V. Topical corticosteroid-induced skin atrophy: A comprehensive review. *Drug Saf.* **2015**, *38*, 493–509. [CrossRef]
30. Brunner, K.; Oláh, P.; Moezzi, M.; Pár, G.; Vincze, Á.; Breitenbach, Z.; Gyulai, R. Association of nonalcoholic hepatic fibrosis with body composition in female and male psoriasis patients. *Life* **2021**, *11*, 763. [CrossRef]
31. Dodero-Anillo, J.M.; Lozano-Cuadra, I.C.; Rios-Sanchez, E.; Pedrosa-Martinez, M.J.; Ruiz-Carrascosa, J.C.; Galan-Gutierrez, M.; Armario-Hita, J.C. Optimising the Therapeutic Interval for Biologics in Patients with Psoriasis. *Life* **2022**, *12*, 2075. [CrossRef] [PubMed]
32. Hoffmann, J.; Gendrisch, F.; Schempp, C.M.; Wölfle, U. New herbal biomedicines for the topical treatment of dermatological disorders. *Biomedicines* **2020**, *8*, 27. [CrossRef]
33. Olveira, A.; Augustin, S.; Benlloch, S.; Ampuero, J.; Suárez-Pérez, J.A.; Armesto, S.; Vilarrasa, E.; Belinchón-Romero, I.; Herranz, P.; Crespo, J. The Essential Role of IL-17 as the Pathogenetic Link between Psoriasis and Metabolic-Associated Fatty Liver Disease. *Life* **2023**, *13*, 419. [CrossRef] [PubMed]
34. Yang, C.; Su, X.; Liu, A.; Zhang, L.; Yu, A.; Xi, Y.; Zhai, G. Advances in clinical study of curcumin. *Curr. Pharm. Des.* **2013**, *19*, 1966–1973. [PubMed]
35. Mahammedi, H.; Planchat, E.; Pouget, M.; Durando, X.; Curé, H.; Guy, L.; Van-Praagh, I.; Savareux, L.; Atger, M.; Bayet-Robert, M. The new combination docetaxel, prednisone and curcumin in patients with castration-resistant prostate cancer: A pilot phase II study. *Oncology* **2016**, *90*, 69–78. [CrossRef]
36. Basu, P.; Dutta, S.; Begum, R.; Mittal, S.; Dutta, P.D.; Bharti, A.C.; Panda, C.K.; Biswas, J.; Dey, B.; Talwar, G.P. Clearance of cervical human papillomavirus infection by topical application of curcumin and curcumin containing polyherbal cream: A phase II randomized controlled study. *Asian Pac. J. Cancer Prev.* **2013**, *14*, 5753–5759. [CrossRef]
37. Wongcharoen, W.; Jai-Aue, S.; Phrommintikul, A.; Nawarawong, W.; Woragidpoonpol, S.; Tepsuwan, T.; Sukonthasarn, A.; Apaijai, N.; Chattipakorn, N. Effects of curcuminoids on frequency of acute myocardial infarction after coronary artery bypass grafting. *Am. J. Cardiol.* **2012**, *110*, 40–44. [CrossRef]
38. Cruz–Correa, M.; Shoskes, D.A.; Sanchez, P.; Zhao, R.; Hylind, L.M.; Wexner, S.D.; Giardiello, F.M. Combination treatment with curcumin and quercetin of adenomas in familial adenomatous polyposis. *Clin. Gastroenterol. Hepatol.* **2006**, *4*, 1035–1038. [CrossRef]
39. Antiga, E.; Bonciolini, V.; Volpi, W.; Del Bianco, E.; Caproni, M. Oral curcumin (Meriva) is effective as an adjuvant treatment and is able to reduce IL-22 serum levels in patients with psoriasis vulgaris. *BioMed Res. Int.* **2015**, *2015*, 283634. [CrossRef]
40. Kumar, A.; Harsha, C.; Parama, D.; Girisa, S.; Daimary, U.D.; Mao, X.; Kunnumakkara, A.B. Current clinical developments in curcumin-based therapeutics for cancer and chronic diseases. *Phytother. Res.* **2021**, *35*, 6768–6801. [CrossRef]
41. Bahraini, P.; Rajabi, M.; Mansouri, P.; Sarafian, G.; Chalangari, R.; Azizian, Z. Turmeric tonic as a treatment in scalp psoriasis: A randomized placebo-control clinical trial. *J. Cosmet. Dermatol.* **2018**, *17*, 461–466. [CrossRef] [PubMed]
42. Bilia, A.R.; Bergonzi, M.C.; Isacchi, B.; Antiga, E.; Caproni, M. Curcumin nanoparticles potentiate therapeutic effectiveness of acitrein in moderate-to-severe psoriasis patients and control serum cholesterol levels. *J. Pharm. Pharmacol.* **2018**, *70*, 919–928. [CrossRef]
43. Lee, G.; Chung, H.-S.; Lee, K.; Lee, H.; Kim, M.; Bae, H. Curcumin attenuates the scurfy-induced immune disorder, a model of IPEX syndrome, with inhibiting Th1/Th2/Th17 responses in mice. *Phytomedicine* **2017**, *33*, 1–6. [CrossRef]
44. Umerska, A.; Gaucher, C.; Oyarzun-Ampuero, F.; Fries-Raeth, I.; Colin, F.; Villamizar-Sarmiento, M.G.; Maincent, P.; Sapin-Minet, A. Polymeric nanoparticles for increasing oral bioavailability of curcumin. *Antioxidants* **2018**, *7*, 46. [CrossRef]
45. Shome, S.; Talukdar, A.D.; Choudhury, M.D.; Bhattacharya, M.K.; Upadhyaya, H. Curcumin as potential therapeutic natural product: A nanobiotechnological perspective. *J. Pharm. Pharmacol.* **2016**, *68*, 1481–1500. [CrossRef] [PubMed]
46. Abd, E.; Namjoshi, S.; Mohammed, Y.H.; Roberts, M.S.; Grice, J.E. Synergistic skin penetration enhancer and nanoemulsion formulations promote the human epidermal permeation of caffeine and naproxen. *J. Pharm. Sci.* **2016**, *105*, 212–220. [CrossRef] [PubMed]
47. Hua, S. Lipid-based nano-delivery systems for skin delivery of drugs and bioactives. *Front. Pharmacol.* **2015**, *6*, 219. [CrossRef]
48. Sohrabi, S.; Haeri, A.; Mahboubi, A.; Mortazavi, A.; Dadashzadeh, S. Chitosan gel-embedded moxifloxacin niosomes: An efficient antimicrobial hybrid system for burn infection. *Int. J. Biol. Macromol.* **2016**, *85*, 625–633. [CrossRef]
49. Kumar, N.; Goindi, S. Statistically designed nonionic surfactant vesicles for dermal delivery of itraconazole: Characterization and in vivo evaluation using a standardized Tinea pedis infection model. *Int. J. Pharm.* **2014**, *472*, 224–240. [CrossRef]
50. Handjani-Vila, R.; Ribier, A.; Rondot, B.; Vanlerberghie, G. Dispersions of lamellar phases of non-ionic lipids in cosmetic products. *Int. J. Cosmet. Sci.* **1979**, *1*, 303–314. [CrossRef]
51. Brown, M.B.; Jones, S.A. Hyaluronic acid: A unique topical vehicle for the localized delivery of drugs to the skin. *J. Eur. Acad. Dermatol. Venereol.* **2005**, *19*, 308–318. [CrossRef] [PubMed]
52. Lv, Y.; Xu, C.; Zhao, X.; Lin, C.; Yang, X.; Xin, X.; Zhang, L.; Qin, C.; Han, X.; Yang, L. Nanoplatform assembled from a CD44-targeted prodrug and smart liposomes for dual targeting of tumor microenvironment and cancer cells. *ACS Nano* **2018**, *12*, 1519–1536. [CrossRef]
53. Yeo, L.K.; Chaw, C.S.; Elkordy, A.A. The effects of hydration parameters and co-surfactants on methylene blue-loaded niosomes prepared by the thin film hydration method. *Pharmaceuticals* **2019**, *12*, 46. [CrossRef] [PubMed]

54. Hasani, M.; Sani, N.A.; Khodabakhshi, B.; Arabi, M.S.; Mohammadi, S.; Yazdani, Y. Encapsulation of Leflunomide (LFD) in a novel niosomal formulation facilitated its delivery to THP-1 monocytic cells and enhanced Aryl hydrocarbon receptor (AhR) nuclear translocation and activation. *DARU J. Pharm. Sci.* **2019**, *27*, 635–644. [CrossRef] [PubMed]
55. Langley, R.G.; Ellis, C.N. Evaluating psoriasis with psoriasis area and severity index, psoriasis global assessment, and lattice system physician's global assessment. *J. Am. Acad. Dermatol.* **2004**, *51*, 563–569. [CrossRef]
56. Mohammadi, S.; Sedighi, S.; Memarian, A. IL-17 is aberrantly overexpressed among under-treatment systemic lupus erythematosus patients. *Iran. J. Pathol.* **2019**, *14*, 236. [CrossRef]
57. Campbell, N.K.; Fitzgerald, H.K.; Malara, A.; Hambly, R.; Sweeney, C.M.; Kirby, B.; Fletcher, J.M.; Dunne, A. Naturally derived Heme-Oxygenase 1 inducers attenuate inflammatory responses in human dendritic cells and T cells: Relevance for psoriasis treatment. *Sci. Rep.* **2018**, *8*, 10287. [CrossRef]
58. Mohammadi, S.; Sedighi, S.; Memarian, A.; Yazdani, Y. Overexpression of interferon-γ and indoleamine 2, 3-dioxygenase in systemic lupus erythematosus: Relationship with the disease activity. *LaboratoriumsMedizin* **2017**, *41*, 41–47. [CrossRef]
59. Jhaj, R.; Asati, D.P.; Chaudhary, D.; Sadasivam, B. Topical steroid containing combinations: Burden of adverse effects and why the recent regulatory action may not be enough. *Indian J. Pharmacol.* **2021**, *53*, 371.
60. Seminara, N.; Abuabara, K.; Shin, D.; Langan, S.; Kimmel, S.; Margolis, D.; Troxel, A.; Gelfand, J. Validity of The Health Improvement Network (THIN) for the study of psoriasis. *Br. J. Dermatol.* **2011**, *164*, 602–609. [CrossRef]
61. Mollazadeh, H.; Cicero, A.F.; Blesso, C.N.; Pirro, M.; Majeed, M.; Sahebkar, A. Immune modulation by curcumin: The role of interleukin-10. *Crit. Rev. Food Sci. Nutr.* **2019**, *59*, 89–101. [CrossRef] [PubMed]
62. Thangapazham, R.L.; Sharma, A.; Maheshwari, R.K. Beneficial role of curcumin in skin diseases. In *Molecular Targets and Therapeutic Uses of Curcumin in Health and Disease*; Springer: Boston, MA, USA, 2007; pp. 343–357.
63. Kang, D.; Li, B.; Luo, L.; Jiang, W.; Lu, Q.; Rong, M.; Lai, R. Curcumin shows excellent therapeutic effect on psoriasis in mouse model. *Biochimie* **2016**, *123*, 73–80. [CrossRef] [PubMed]
64. Kurd, S.K.; Smith, N.; VanVoorhees, A.; Troxel, A.B.; Badmaev, V.; Seykora, J.T.; Gelfand, J.M. Oral curcumin in the treatment of moderate to severe psoriasis vulgaris: A prospective clinical trial. *J. Am. Acad. Dermatol.* **2008**, *58*, 625–631. [CrossRef] [PubMed]
65. Sarafian, G.; Afshar, M.; Mansouri, P.; Asgarpanah, J.; Raoufinejad, K.; Rajabi, M. Topical Turmeric Microemulgel in the Management of Plaque Psoriasis; A Clinical Evaluation. *Iran. J. Pharm. Res.* **2015**, *14*, 865–876. [PubMed]
66. Varma, S.R.; Sivaprakasam, T.O.; Mishra, A.; Prabhu, S.; Rafiq, M.; Rangesh, P. Imiquimod-induced psoriasis-like inflammation in differentiated Human keratinocytes: Its evaluation using curcumin. *Eur. J. Pharmacol.* **2017**, *813*, 33–41. [CrossRef]
67. Jain, A.; Doppalapudi, S.; Domb, A.J.; Khan, W. Tacrolimus and curcumin co-loaded liposphere gel: Synergistic combination towards management of psoriasis. *J. Control. Release* **2016**, *243*, 132–145. [CrossRef]
68. Sun, L.; Liu, Z.; Wang, L.; Cun, D.; Tong, H.H.; Yan, R.; Chen, X.; Wang, R.; Zheng, Y. Enhanced topical penetration, system exposure and anti-psoriasis activity of two particle-sized, curcumin-loaded PLGA nanoparticles in hydrogel. *J. Control. Release* **2017**, *254*, 44–54. [CrossRef]
69. Reena, K.; Singh, L.; Sharma, S. Curcumin: A Review of its' Efficacy in the Management of Psoriasis. *Drug Deliv. Lett.* **2022**, *12*, 163–183. [CrossRef]
70. Raja, M.A.; Zeenat, S.; Arif, M.; Liu, C. Self-assembled nanoparticles based on amphiphilic chitosan derivative and arginine for oral curcumin delivery. *Int. J. Nanomed.* **2016**, *11*, 4397. [CrossRef]
71. Algahtani, M.S.; Ahmad, M.Z.; Ahmad, J. Nanoemulsion loaded polymeric hydrogel for topical delivery of curcumin in psoriasis. *J. Drug Deliv. Sci. Technol.* **2020**, *59*, 101847. [CrossRef]
72. Patel, N.A.; Patel, N.J.; Patel, R.P. Formulation and evaluation of curcumin gel for topical application. *Pharm. Dev. Technol.* **2009**, *14*, 83–92. [CrossRef]
73. Sharma, R.; Dua, J.; Parsad, D. An overview on Niosomes: Novel Pharmaceutical drug delivery system. *J. Drug Deliv. Ther.* **2022**, *12*, 171–177. [CrossRef]
74. Shah, A.; Boldhane, S.; Pawar, A.; Bothiraja, C. Advanced development of a non-ionic surfactant and cholesterol material based niosomal gel formulation for the topical delivery of anti-acne drugs. *Mater. Adv.* **2020**, *1*, 1763–1774. [CrossRef]
75. Abdelbary, A.A.; AbouGhaly, M.H. Design and optimization of topical methotrexate loaded niosomes for enhanced management of psoriasis: Application of Box–Behnken design, in-vitro evaluation and in-vivo skin deposition study. *Int. J. Pharm.* **2015**, *485*, 235–243. [CrossRef]
76. Fernández, T.D.; Pearson, J.R.; Leal, M.P.; Torres, M.J.; Blanca, M.; Mayorga, C.; Le Guével, X. Intracellular accumulation and immunological properties of fluorescent gold nanoclusters in human dendritic cells. *Biomaterials* **2015**, *43*, 1–12. [CrossRef] [PubMed]
77. Kong, M.; Park, H.; Feng, C.; Hou, L.; Cheng, X.; Chen, X. Construction of hyaluronic acid noisome as functional transdermal nanocarrier for tumor therapy. *Carbohydr. Polym.* **2013**, *94*, 634–641. [CrossRef]
78. Brück, J.; Holstein, J.; Glocova, I.; Seidel, U.; Geisel, J.; Kanno, T.; Kumagai, J.; Mato, N.; Sudowe, S.; Widmaier, K. Nutritional control of IL-23/Th17-mediated autoimmune disease through HO-1/STAT3 activation. *Sci. Rep.* **2017**, *7*, 44482. [CrossRef]
79. Skyvalidas, D.N.; Mavropoulos, A.; Tsiogkas, S.; Dardiotis, E.; Liaskos, C.; Mamuris, Z.; Roussaki-Schulze, A.; Sakkas, L.I.; Zafiriou, E.; Bogdanos, D.P. Curcumin mediates attenuation of pro-inflammatory interferon γ and interleukin 17 cytokine responses in psoriatic disease, strengthening its role as a dietary immunosuppressant. *Nutr. Res.* **2020**, *75*, 95–108. [CrossRef]

80. Sun, J.; Zhao, Y.; Hu, J. Curcumin inhibits imiquimod-induced psoriasis-like inflammation by inhibiting IL-1beta and IL-6 production in mice. *PLoS ONE* **2013**, *8*, e67078. [CrossRef]
81. Pol, A.; Bergers, M.; Schalkwijk, J. Comparison of antiproliferative effects of experimental and established antipsoriatic drugs on human kerationocytes, using a simple 96-well-plate assay. *Vitr. Cell. Dev. Biol.-Anim.* **2003**, *39*, 36–42. [CrossRef]
82. Guilloteau, K.; Paris, I.; Pedretti, N.; Boniface, K.; Juchaux, F.; Huguier, V.; Guillet, G.; Bernard, F.-X.; Lecron, J.-C.; Morel, F. Skin inflammation induced by the synergistic action of IL-17A, IL-22, oncostatin M, IL-1α, and TNF-α recapitulates some features of psoriasis. *J. Immunol.* **2010**, *184*, 5263–5270. [CrossRef] [PubMed]
83. Granata, M.; Skarmoutsou, E.; Mazzarino, M.C.; D'Amico, F. S100A7 in psoriasis: Immunodetection and activation by CRISPR technology. In *Calcium-Binding Proteins of the EF-Hand Superfamily*; Springer: Berlin/Heidelberg, Germany, 2019; pp. 729–738.
84. Lin, J.; Tang, Y.; Kang, Q.; Feng, Y.; Chen, A. Curcumin inhibits gene expression of receptor for advanced glycation end-products (RAGE) in hepatic stellate cells in vitro by elevating PPARγ activity and attenuating oxidative stress. *Br. J. Pharmacol.* **2012**, *166*, 2212–2227. [CrossRef] [PubMed]

Disclaimer/Publisher's Note: The statements, opinions and data contained in all publications are solely those of the individual author(s) and contributor(s) and not of MDPI and/or the editor(s). MDPI and/or the editor(s) disclaim responsibility for any injury to people or property resulting from any ideas, methods, instructions or products referred to in the content.

Review
Annular Erythemas and Purpuras

Nicolas Kluger

Department of Dermatology, Allergology and Venereology, Helsinki University Hospital & University of Helsinki, 00250 Helsinki, Finland; nicolas.kluger@hus.fi

Abstract: Annular dermatoses are a heterogeneous and extremely diverse group of skin diseases, which share in common annular, ring-like patterns with centrifugal spreading. Numerous skin diseases can sometimes display annular lesions, but some specific skin conditions are originally annular. We take the opportunity to review here mainly the causes of primary annular erythemas and their differential diagnoses, but also the rare causes of annular purpuras.

Keywords: annular dermatosis; erythema annulare; erythema marginatum; erythema migrans; erythema centrifugum; figurate erythema; annular purpura

Citation: Kluger, N. Annular Erythemas and Purpuras. *Life* **2023**, *13*, 1245. https://doi.org/10.3390/life13061245

Academic Editor: Jacek C. Szepietowski

Received: 1 March 2023
Revised: 13 May 2023
Accepted: 23 May 2023
Published: 24 May 2023

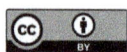

Copyright: © 2023 by the author. Licensee MDPI, Basel, Switzerland. This article is an open access article distributed under the terms and conditions of the Creative Commons Attribution (CC BY) license (https://creativecommons.org/licenses/by/4.0/).

1. Introduction

Annular dermatoses (AD) are a heterogeneous group of skin diseases, whose common feature is essentially the annular or circular arrangement of the lesions with centrifugal spreading [1]. They belong to the group of figurate dermatoses, to which can be added linear or serpiginous dermatoses, for example. They are a fascinating curiosity for the dermatologist, as they form patterns and arabesques on the patient's body.

Clinically, AD rarely present as a flat erythematous macule or spot. The active border is often redder and palpable, and the initial lesion is a papule or plaque that will spread as a ring. The confluence of nearby lesions gives a polycyclic appearance. Finally, the rings may be closed circles or ovals, or well opened, arciform or crescent-shaped. In its recent update of the glossary of descriptive terms for skin lesions, the International League of Dermatological Societies (ILDS) suggested the use of the following terms to describe the lesions: annular, arciform, polycyclic and oval [2].

AD are most often annular erythema. Careful examination of the surface of the rash can also determine whether the process arises from the epidermis (dermatophyte) or from the dermis (erythema migrans, etc.). However, purpuras can also display a ring-like pattern in cases of cutaneous vasculitis, pigmented purpura or infection. In this review, we mainly discuss AD from the perspective of erythema annulare, and at the end, we review some cases of purpura annulare. Pediatric erythema annulare is a broad group of dermatoses whose differentiation is often based on subtle clinical and histologic nuances [3]. We discuss only some of these pediatric entities.

2. Classification of Annular Dermatoses

AD can be classified in different ways. (i) AD can be either primarily or secondarily annular. In the first case, the annular pattern is an intrinsic characteristic of the dermatoses and defines them (erythema annulare migrans, centrifugal erythema annulare of Darier, tinea, granuloma annulare, subacute lupus, etc.). In the second case, a large number of skin conditions can display any annular pattern among their possible clinical presentation. Most likely, any dermatologic disease may display an annular pattern, so the list is long, as follows: mycosis fungoides, syphilis, roseola, seborrheic dermatosis, sarcoidosis, herpetic dermatitis, linear IgA dermatosis, etc. (Table 1, Figure 1). (ii) AD can be classified according to their causes (infectious, para-infectious, inflammatory, paraneoplastic, drug-induced) [4], (iii) according to the age of onset (infant/adult, Table 2) [3], (iv) according to the type of histological infiltrate (Table 3) [4], or finally, (v) according to the acute or chronic onset. This last classification [1] seems to us to be the simplest in daily practice. Indeed, classification by group of causes [4] lead to a large laundry list mixing common and rare conditions, as well as acute and chronic conditions. Histopathological classification [5] is of interest when a biopsy is taken to allow a clinical confrontation; however, this is not always necessary.

Table 1. Main dermatoses that can *sometimes* display an annular presentation (non-exhaustive list).

Seborrheic dermatosis
Urticaria and urticarial vasculitis
Sweet syndrome
Eosinophilic dermatosis, Wells cellulitis
Psoriasis: annulare psoriasis, psoriasis gyrata
Eczema
Leprosy
Granuloma faciale
Sarcoidosis
Mycosis fungoides

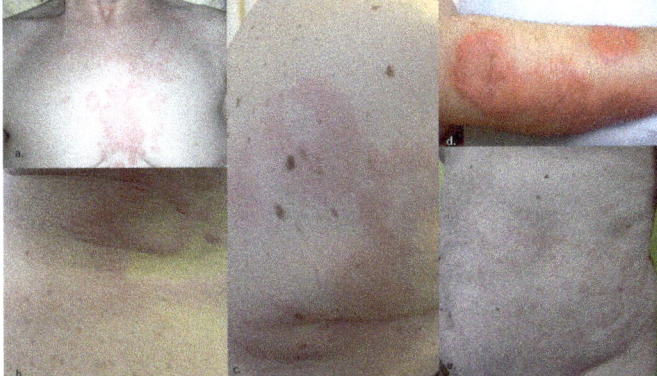

Figure 1. Examples of dermatoses with possible presentation as annular lesions. (**a**) Seborrheic dermatitis of the trunk, (**b**) acute urticaria, (**c**) urticarial vasculitis, (**d**) Sweet syndrome, (**e**) chronic eczema.

Table 2. Annular erythema of infancy [a] (modified from Patrizi et al. [3]).

Neonatal lupus erythematosus
• variant: erythema gyratum atrophicans transiens neonatale
Erythema annulare with anti-Ro/SSa antibodies (Sjögren)
Erythema marginatum rheumaticum
Erythema marginatum associated with hereditary angioedema
Erythema migrans
Erythema annulare centrifugum
• variant: familial annular erythema
Annulare erythema of infancy
• variant: neutrophilic figurated erythema
Eosinophilic annular erythema

[a] Common dermatoses are not included (psoriasis, tinea, etc.).

Table 3. Annular erythema according to the main inflammatory infiltrate (modified from Ríos-Martín et al. [5]).

Lymphocytes	Neutrophils, Eosinophils	Granulomas	Plasmocytes
Erythema annulare with anti-Ro/SSa antibodies	CRAND		
Erythema annulare centrifugum	Eosinophilic dermatosis		
Erythema gyratum repens	Eosinophilic erythema annulare		
Erythema migrans	Erythema marginatum	Granuloma annulare	Erythema migrans
Erythema multiformis	Neutrophic dermatosis	Leprosy	Syphilis
Erythrokeratodermia variabilis	IgA pemphigus	Sarcoïdose	
Leprosy	Linear IgA dermatosis		
Lupus	Neutrophilic erythema annulare of infancy		
Mycosis fungoides	Psoriasis		
	Sneddon–Wilkinson syndrome		
	Urticarial vasculitis		

CRAND: Chronic recurrent annular neutrophilic dermatosis.

3. Acute Annulare Dermatoses

3.1. Pityriasis Rosea

Pityriasis rosea is a benign squamous eruptive exanthema due to HHV-6 and HHV-7 that mainly affects the young. The classic initial erythemato-squamous, round or oval, annular "medallion" or herald patch with raised edges and a clear center, and of variable size, precedes the generalized eruption [6]. Its identification allows the diagnosis (Figure 2). On the other hand, if the primary lesion is seen alone before the rash, tinea infection may be wrongly suspected. Differential diagnoses include secondary syphilis and psoriasis.

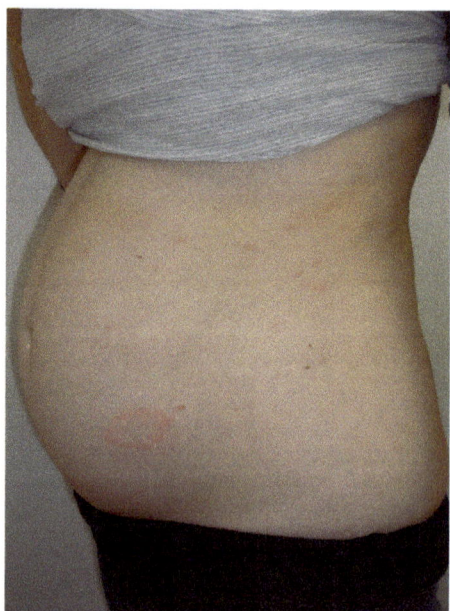

Figure 2. Pityriasis rosea in a pregnant woman with its typical initial ring medallion.

3.2. Erythema Marginatum

Erythema marginatum was first described in 1831 by Bright and has been referred to by several names (érythème marginé discoïde de Besnier, Lehndorff–Leiner's erythema annulare rheumaticum, Keil's erythema marginatum rheumaticum). Although a rare manifestation (<6% of cases), erythema marginatum is still considered a specific lesion of post-streptococcal rheumatic fever (RF) and a major criterion in the new 2015 revision of the Jones criteria [7]. RF and erythema marginatum usually affect children, and more rarely, adults [8]. Erythema marginatum is characterized by a painless and non-pruritic, annular, polycyclic, raised or non-raised border rash that is red to purplish in color and usually rapidly evolving [9] with an occasional disappearance and reappearance of lesions. Centrifugal evolution is not systematic [8]. Erythema marginatum affects the trunk, extremities and sometimes the face. It occurs after untreated angina with fever in association with migratory inflammatory joint pain and an inflammatory syndrome. In case of a heart murmur, an ultrasound must be performed to eliminate a valvulopathy. A skin biopsy shows a perivascular neutrophilic inflammatory infiltrate [9], that is sometimes lymphocytic [8] in the dermis, without vasculitis and without alteration of the epidermis [8,9]. Direct immunofluorescence is negative. The evolution is favorable under antibiotic therapy with penicillin A in the following weeks. A rapid angina test is positive [8], and antistreptolysins can be positive [9]. The infection is not immunizing, and the rash may recur in case of a new infection [8]. RF has become rare in developed countries due to the use of antibiotics for streptococcal infections. Given the decrease in the prevalence of RF, it is important to be aware of this diagnosis in case of fever and joint pain after angina, especially in patients from developing countries.

3.3. Erythema Marginatum with Hereditary Angioedema

The occurrence of a non-pruritic erythema annulare, reticular or serpiginous would concern 56% of patients with hereditary angioedema [10]. This "erythema marginatum" has been observed since the end of the 19th century. It affects the upper part of the trunk and the limbs. It may precede or accompany angioedema attacks [10,11]. If it is mistaken for urticaria, the diagnosis of hereditary angioedema is delayed. Its pathophysiology is unclear but may involve bradykinin [10].

3.4. African Trypanosomiasis

The lymphatic blood phase of trypanosome dissemination occurs 1 to 3 weeks after the infesting tsetse fly bite. It associates fever, hepatosplenomegaly, cervical adenopathies and trypanides. These are erythematopapular lesions of variable size which may take on the appearance of a polycytic centrifugal annular erythema with a marked erythematous active border, most often on the trunk or the roots of the limbs. In a suggestive context (expatriate living in black Africa), these trypanids are characteristic but rare (10 to 50% of cases), fleeting, recurrent, leave no sequelae and may naturally go unnoticed on dark skin [12–14].

4. Chronic Annular Dermatoses
4.1. Tinea Corporis

Infection of the glabrous skin by *Trichophyton rubrum* or *T mentagrophytes* constitutes the prototype of ring dermatosis. It initially presents as a small pinkish macule of a progressive centrifugal extension forming a circle or a closed oval, with an active vesicular border, sometimes scaly, more or less pruritic, until it ends up in a large placard, sometimes polycyclic, in case of confluence with other lesions. The center of the lesion takes on a brown hue (Figure 3). Fold dermatophyte has a similar appearance as an extensive, unilateral, ring-shaped placard with an active border and a brown center. The application of local corticosteroids can significantly delay the diagnosis by masking the initial appearance (tinea incognito). However, the annular appearance may remain visible and suggestive (Figure 4). Finally, tinea imbricata or tokelau is a chronic superficial dermatophyte due to *T concentricum* (anthropophilic germ) endemic to the South Pacific islands, but also to South Asia and South America. It is responsible for particularly impressive concentric or annular figured skin lesions [15,16].

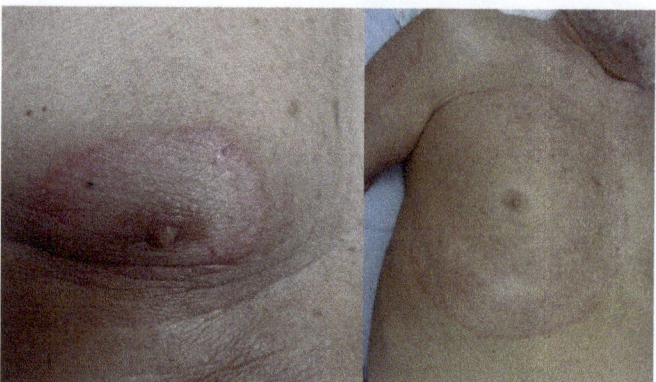

Figure 3. Dermatophytosis of the glabrous skin with *T. rubrum* centered on the right nipple (**left**). Extension and progression over 9 months due to poor compliance with home treatment (**right**).

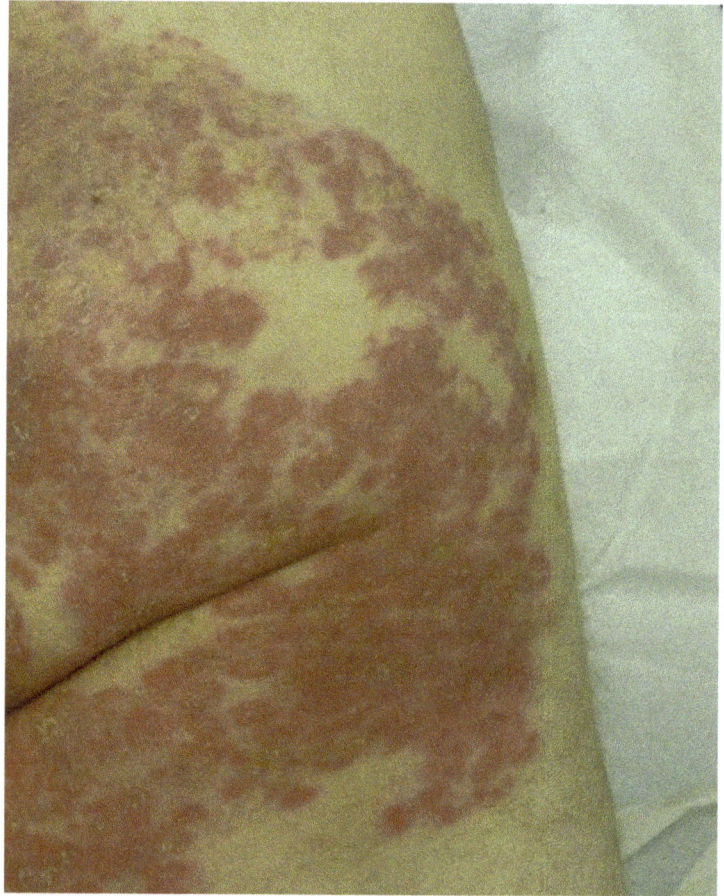

Figure 4. Close-up view of tinea corporis incognito initially treated with very high potency dermocorticoids.

4.2. Erythema Migrans

Erythema migrans (EM) is the first manifestation of *Borrelia burgdorferi* infection and indicates Lyme disease. It occurs in 90% of patients between 2 days and 3 months after a tick bite; on average, it occurs 2 weeks after the bite [17]. The bite of an Ixodes nymph may go unnoticed. The typical form of EM is an erythematous macule or papule with a centrifugal annular extension and central clearing. It is highly variable in size [18]. It may be asymptomatic, pruritic or painful. If the central site of the inoculation is still visible, the EM displays the typical bull's eye appearance (Figure 5).

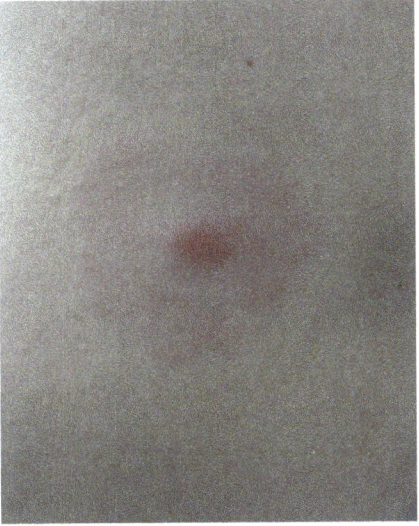

Figure 5. Erythema migrans with a bull's eye sign.

However, in practice, EM can be highly polymorphous, making borreliosis a major simulacrum in the same way that syphilis is in endemic areas (Figure 6) [18,19].

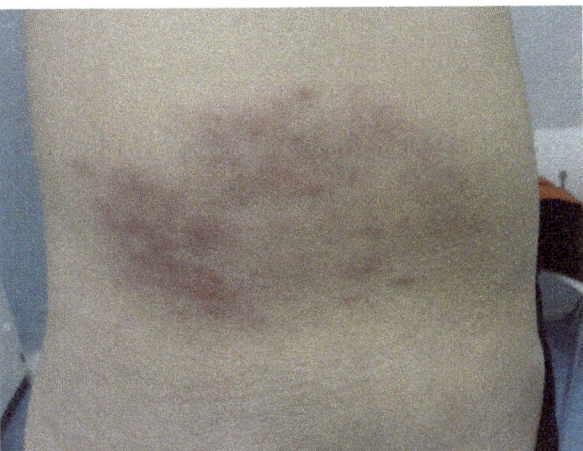

Figure 6. Atypical erythema migrans presenting an annular hematoma.

General signs are sometimes present. Serology is neither useful nor recommended at that stage of the disease. In the case of an atypical form, a biopsy reveals a deep and superficial perivascular and interstitial lymphocytic infiltrate with low neutrophil counts. The presence of plasma cells is suggestive of the diagnosis. Warthin–Starry staining may reveal the spirochete in the papillary dermis, but currently, PCR techniques confirm the presence of Borrelia in the skin [20]. Empirical treatment is based on amoxicillin or doxycycline per os for two weeks. In the absence of treatment, EM lesions disappear rapidly with a risk of secondary dissemination. The presence of multiple, smaller, non-expanding annular lesions at a distance from the site of the inoculation indicates a hematogenous and lymphatic dissemination of the disease and is common in the European form of borreliosis [17,18].

4.3. Granuloma Annulare

Granuloma annulare (GA) is a benign non-infectious granulomatous skin disorder of unknown origin. GA has been associated with a wide number of conditions such as diabetes, HIV infection, malignancy or medications [21]. There are various clinical variants of GA. The most common form of GA presents as a pink or flesh-colored non-squamous annular erythematous plaque with an active border with a palisading or interstitial granulomatous inflammatory infiltrate (Figure 7). It can be localized to the extremities or generalized [22]. GA is often self-limited and does not require treatment. The generalized form displays a protracted evolution and is more difficult to treat. The list of treatments that have been given for GA is exceedingly long [21].

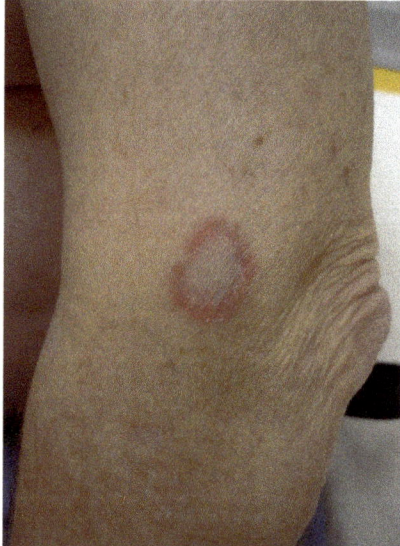

Figure 7. Granuloma annulare of the elbow.

4.4. Subacute Cutaneous Lupus Erythematosus

Subacute cutaneous lupus erythematosus (SCLE) most commonly affects white women over 50 years of age. The lesions are polycyclic, with an erythemato-squamous or vesiculous and crusty border and a greyish hypopigmented center that is sometimes covered with telangiectasias. They regress, leaving post-inflammatory hypo- or hyperpigmentation and telangiectasia, but without atrophy. The lesions predominantly occur on photoexposed areas (face, neck, décolleté, shoulders, extension side of the arms and back of the hands) and on the trunk (Figure 8).

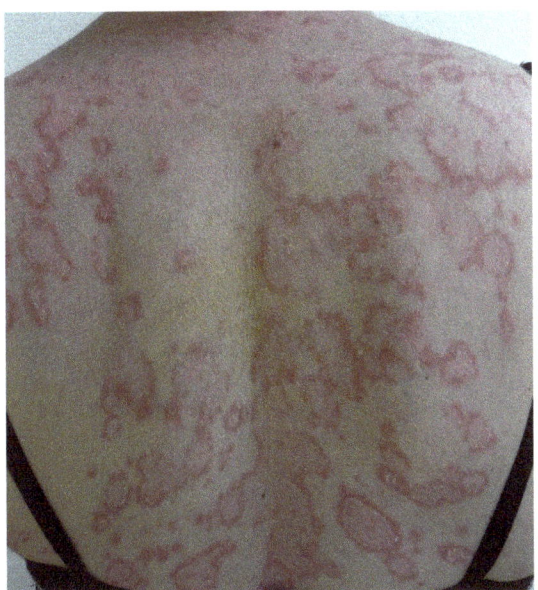

Figure 8. Subacute cutaneous lupus erythematosus of the back.

Hyperkeratosis, mucosal body atrophy, extensive basal keratinocyte degeneration, thickening of the basement membrane and the presence of a dermal CD4 lymphocytic infiltrate are suggestive of the diagnosis. Direct immunofluorescence is inconsistently positive [23]. SCLE is the most frequently reported form of cutaneous drug-induced lupus erythematosus. It should always be considered in case of onset among the elderly patients. The clinical presentation, patterns and distribution of the cutaneous lesions are not distinguishable from idiopathic SCLE. Culprit drugs include terbinafine, anti-TNF alpha, antieplieptics and proton pump inhibitors [24]. Treatment includes photoprotection, the application of dermocorticoids and the initiation of hydroxycholoroquine. Systemic involvement should be ruled out [23].

4.5. Neonatal Lupus

The transplacental passage of maternal anti-Ro/SSa and/or anti-La/SSb or anti-U1-RNP antibodies may be accompanied by skin lesions that occur early in the first three months of life and resolve during the first year after the elimination of maternal antibodies. The rash is similar to adult subacute lupus with polycyclic annular lesions. Residual pigmentation may occur. Atrophy or scarring is rare. Erythema gyratum atrophicans transiens neonatale of Giannotti and Ermacora [25] is probably a variant with central whitish atrophy [26].

4.6. Erythema Annulare with Ro-SSA Antibodies and Sjögren's Syndrome

Lesions of erythema annulare, similar to those seen in SCLE, were also reported in patients with Sjögren's syndrome [27]. In addition, a "borderline" sub-entity was reported by Japanese authors in the form of a deep annular erythema with thick borders and a clear doughnut center, mainly affecting the face, and sometimes the upper limbs. The histology shows a perivascular CD4 lymphocytic infiltrate and edema of the dermis without vasculitis or epidermal involvement. The appearance is evocative of lupus tumidus. Patients always present with Ro/SSa antibodies, but the diagnosis may be uncertain between lupus and Sjögren's syndrome [28].

4.7. Neutrophilic Dermatoses

Neutrophilic dermatoses are a group of rare skin conditions characterized by the presence of an abnormally high number of neutrophils in the epidermis and/or the dermis and/or the subcutis. These conditions can present with a variety of clinical features such as painful erythematous (red) papules, plaques, pustules and vesicles. Some of the most common neutrophilic dermatoses are Sweet syndrome and pyoderma gangrenosum [29]. Lesions of Sweet syndrome can sometimes evolve secondarily into polycyclic annular lesions (Table 3). However, there are also some conditions among the neutrophilic dermatoses (ND) group, during which the lesions are primarily annular.

Neutrophilic erythema multiforme of infancy is an exceptional inflammatory dermatosis affecting healthy newborns or small children with no other underlying pathology. It is characterized by asymptomatic, annular erythematous lesions, sometimes polycyclic, without vesicles or scaling. The histology shows a neutrophilic infiltrate and leukocytoclasia, without vasculitis. The dermatosis may progress to remission or chronicity [3].

Chronic recurrent annular neutrophilic dermatosis (CRAND) was first described in 1989. CRAND is a peculiar and rarely described form of neutrophilic dermatosis marked by an annular and chronic course, and a histological involvement like Sweet syndrome, but without any general signs, biological abnormalities or underlying systemic pathology [30]. It seems to affect adult women after 40 years of age. Oral steroids, colchicine and dapsone are the treatments of choice [31]. Croci-Torti et al. discuss some clinical cases in the literature that do not yet fit into specific nosological entity [31] cases as erythema annulare with a neutrophilic infiltrate on histology [32].

4.8. (Darier's) Erythema Annulare Centrifugum

Erythema annulare centrifugum (EAC) is characterized by mildly symptomatic annular plaques on the trunk, buttocks and proximal parts of the limbs, while it spares the face and extremities. EAC can occur at any age, with a predominance in people who are in their 50s [33]. The number of lesions is also variable, averaging from two to five. In his original description, Darier stated that pink rings consist of a peripheral bump, a 3–5 mm cord, with a gentle slope to the skin on the inner side of the ring and a sharp edge toward the healthy skin [1]. Scaling of the inner edge of the ring is sometimes noted, while the central area takes on a bister or buff color (Figure 9).

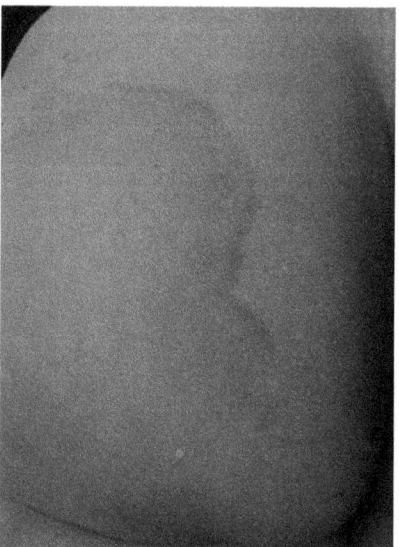

Figure 9. Erythema annulare centrifugum.

The lesions may coalesce into polycyclic rings and evolve over several days, weeks or months. The following two forms are currently considered: the superficial form and a deep form (that has been described by Darier). A biopsy of recent lesions of superficial CAE shows a superficial spongiform dermatitis with an eosinophilic infiltrate and sometimes neutrophils. In older lesions, the infiltrate is lymphocytic without spongiosis. In the deep form, there is a superficial and deep perivascular lymphocytic infiltrate. In this case, various differential diagnoses arise, such as lupus tumidus or erythema migrans. The etiology and pathophysiology of EAC are not known. Treatment is only proposed in the case of discomfort. The disease resolves spontaneously within a year, although prolonged courses are possible.

4.9. Eosinophilic Annular Erythema

Eosinophilic annular erythema (EAE) is a rare entity in the literature. It was first described in 1981 by Peterson and Jarrat [34]. The first cases were described in children as annular erythema of infancy [34,35], but later, similar cases were observed in adults [35]. It is a chronic dermatosis, characterized by arciform annular plaques with a dark red center, which may affect the trunk, limbs or face. The edges are raised, smooth, non-scaly, pruritic [35] or not pruritic [36]. The lesions disappear without atrophy or scarring [35], but new lesions may reappear on the top of regressing lesions [36]. The general condition is preserved. Arthralgias may occur. Usually, no systemic disease is reported, although we found one case associated with a chronic hypereosinophilic syndrome [37] and one associated with metastatic prostate cancer [38]. The evolution is variable, ranging from spontaneous resolution in a few weeks without recurrence [39], to chronic forms over several years. The biopsy discloses an interstitial, perivascular and perisudoral dermal infiltrate, predominantly lymphocytic and eosinophilic, but poor in neutrophils and without plasma cells. There is no evidence of flame figure, granuloma or vasculitis. Mucin deposits may be present. Vacuolation of the basement membrane and spongiosis and exocytosis in the epidermis are also noted [36]. Circulating hypereosinophilia is inconsistent. Treatment is difficult. Anti-inflammatory drugs such as indomethacin, anti-malarial drugs and even Disulone seem to be the most effective [40]. The question of the link between EAE and Wells syndrome remains open. The distinction is based on clinico-biological differences (no pseudo-cellulitis appearance, absence of hypereosinophilia), histological features (absence of flame figure, granuloma and eosinophilic degranulation) and possibly therapeutic nuances (corticosteroid therapy versus hydroxychloroquine and NSAIDs).

4.10. Erythema Gyratum Repens

Described in 1952, erythema gyratum repens is a rare (70–80% of cases) paraneoplastic syndrome whose diagnosis is clinical. It affects the trunk and extremities with characteristic erythematous, raised, scaly, serpiginous, concentric or annular bands arranged in parallel giving a "wood-ribbed" appearance and centrifugal extension. It is mainly associated with bronchial, breast and esophageal cancers. The histology is non-specific with a superficial lymphocytic perivascular infiltrate. The main purpose of the histology is to eliminate differential diagnoses [41]. Cases have been recently associated with COVID-19 infection [42,43] and SARS-CoV-2 vaccination [44].

5. Annular Purpura

5.1. Majocchi's Purpura Annularis Telangiectodes

Pigmented purpuric dermatoses are a group of skin disorders characterized by a chronic or persistent course, varied clinical picture (macules, papules and plaques) and unknown origin (e.g., contact allergy, pressure, physical training, medication) [45]. Among this group of pigmented purpuric dermatoses, Majocchi's purpura annulare (purpura annularis telangiectodes) presents as purpuric patches of a centrifugal extension with a bright red border and a yellowish central area that is sometimes atrophic, located on the lower limbs (Figure 10). It tends to affect young people of both sexes. The rings are a few millimeters thick and covered with telangiectasias and punctiform purpura. The rings are closed or open, isolated or confluent and polycyclic. The size of the lesions is variable. The lesions regress in a few months or years without scarring. Histologically, there is lymphocytic capillaritis with an extravasation of red blood cells and lymphocytic infiltrate without vasculitis [46,47].

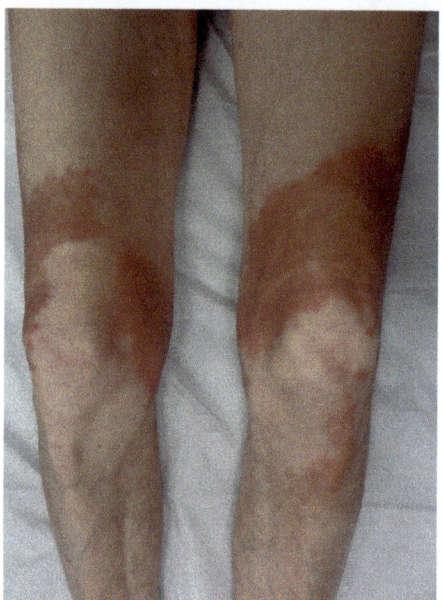

Figure 10. Majocchi's purpura annulare.

5.2. Annular Leucocytoclastic Cutaneous Vasculitis

It is not unusual to see an annular pattern within purpuric lesions in cutaneous vasculitis (Figure 11). However, a singular entity was described in 1996 [48] as the skin lesions were purpuric annular plaques of a centrifugal extension with a polycyclic extension to the limbs and trunk, leaving a residual pigmentation. There are no extracutaneous symptoms or impairment of general condition. The histology was consistent with leucocytoclastic vasculitis with inflammatory infiltrate. The lesions regress with dapsone [48], but spontaneous regression is possible [49].

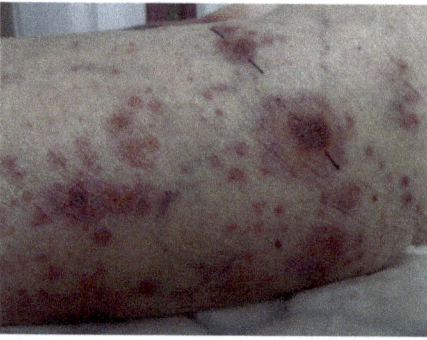

Figure 11. Cutaneous vasculitis disclosing annulare features.

5.3. Post-Infectious Purpura

A few curiosities have been reported, such as pityriasis rosea in a purpuric and annular variant [50] or annular hemorrhagic purpura in hantavirus, as we reported in a case of Puumala virus infection in Finland [51].

6. Conclusions

Annular dermatoses encompass a large number of various and heterogenous conditions that make it difficult to define decisional algorithms. Diagnoses can be only achieved via proper history intake, past dermatological diseases, proper analysis of the clinical presentation (acute/chronic, isolated/multiple lesions, erythema/purpura, etc.) and microscopic findings. Annularity is a dynamic process, and the lesions may change with time and between observations. Physicians should also enquire whether the patient has taken pictures of the skin lesions at the very beginning of their occurrence or at various stages of their evolution. Differential diagnoses of annular dermatoses encompass, by definition, the other annular dermatoses.

Funding: This research received no external funding.

Institutional Review Board Statement: Not applicable.

Informed Consent Statement: No informed consent was obtained. The pictures were cropped to ensure the anonymity of the patients.

Data Availability Statement: Data are unavailable; no new data were generated due to privacy.

Conflicts of Interest: The author declares no conflict of interest.

References

1. Degos, R. (Ed.) *Dermatologie*; Médecine-Sciences: Paris, France, 1974.
2. Nast, A.; Griffiths, C.E.; Hay, R.; Sterry, W.; Bologna, J.L. The 2016 International League of Dermatological Societies' Revised Glossary for the Description of Cutaneous Lesions. *Br. J. Dermatol.* **2016**, *174*, 1351–1358. [CrossRef] [PubMed]
3. Patrizi, A.; Savoia, F.; Varotti, E.; Gaspari, V.; Passarini, B.; Neri, I. Neutrophilic figurate erythema of infancy. *Pediatr. Dermatol.* **2008**, *25*, 255–260. [CrossRef] [PubMed]
4. Narayanasetty, N.K.; Pai, V.V.; Athanikar, S.B. Annular lesions in dermatology. *Indian J. Dermatol.* **2013**, *58*, 157. [CrossRef] [PubMed]
5. Ríos-Martín, J.J.; Ferrándiz-Pulido, L.; Moreno-Ramírez, D. Aproximación al diagnóstico dermatopatológico de las lesiones figuradas. *Actas Dermo-Sifiliogr.* **2011**, *102*, 316–324. [CrossRef]
6. Leung, A.K.C.; Lam, J.M.; Leong, K.F.; Hon, K.L. Pityriasis Rosea: An Updated Review. *Curr. Pediatr. Rev.* **2021**, *17*, 201–211. [CrossRef]
7. Gewitz, M.H.; Baltimore, R.S.; Tani, L.Y.; Sable, C.A.; Shulman, S.T.; Carapetis, J. Revision of the Jones Criteria for the Diagnosis of Acute Rheumatic Fever in the Era of Doppler Echocardiography: A Scientific Statement from the American Heart Association. *Circulation* **2015**, *131*, 1806–1818. [CrossRef]
8. Alimova, E.; Le Roux-Villet, C.; Neuville, S.; Dubertret, L.; Petit, A. Erythème annulaire récidivant après angine streptococcique: Érythème marginé rhumatismal de l'adulte. *Ann. Dermatol. Venereol.* **2008**, *135*, 496–498. [CrossRef]
9. Troyer, C.; Grossman, M.E.; Silvers, D.N. Erythema Marginatum in Rheumatic Fever: Early Diagnosis by Skin Biopsy. *J. Am. Acad. Dermatol.* **1983**, *8*, 724–728. [CrossRef]
10. Rasmussen, E.R.; Freitas, P.V.; Bygum, A. Urticaria and Prodromal Symptoms Including Erythema Marginatum in Danish Patients with Hereditary Angioedema. *Acta Derm.-Venereol.* **2016**, *96*, 373–376. [CrossRef]
11. Hubiche, T.; Boralevi, F.; Jouvencel, P.; Taïeb, A.; Leaute-Labreze, C. Érythème annulaire réticulé annonciateur de crises d'œdème angioneurotique héréditaire chez un enfant. *Ann. Dermatol. Venereol.* **2005**, *132*, 249–251. [CrossRef]
12. McGovern, T.W.; Williams, W.; Fitzpatrick, J.E.; Cetron, M.S.; Hepburn, B.C.; Gentry, R.H. Cutaneous Manifestations of African Trypanosomiasis. *Arch. Dermatol.* **1995**, *131*, 1178–1182. [CrossRef]
13. Ezzedine, K.; Darie, H.; Le Bras, M.; Malvy, D. Skin Features Accompanying Imported Human African Trypanosomiasis: Hemolymphatic Trypanosoma Gambiense Infection among Two French Expatriates with Dermatologic Manifestations. *J. Travel Med.* **2007**, *14*, 192–196. [CrossRef]
14. Hope-Rapp, E.; Moussa Coulibaly, O.; Klement, E.; Danis, M.; Bricaire, F.; Caumes, E. Chancres cutanés révélant une trypanosomose africaine à Trypanosoma brucei gambiense chez un résident français au Gabon. *Ann. Dermatol. Venereol.* **2009**, *136*, 341–345. [CrossRef]
15. Burns, C.; Valentine, J. Tinea Imbricata. *N. Engl. J. Med.* **2016**, *375*, 2272. [CrossRef]

16. Veraldi, S.; Giorgi, R.; Pontini, P.; Tadini, G.; Nazzaro, G. Tinea Imbricata in an Italian Child and Review of the Literature. *Mycopathologia* **2015**, *180*, 353–357. [CrossRef]
17. Couilliet, D.; Guillaume, J.C. Manifestations cutanées de la borréliose de Lyme. *Ann. Dermatol.* **2000**, *127*, 523–527.
18. Eriksson, P.; Schröder, M.T.; Niiranen, K.; Nevanlinna, A.; Panelius, J.; Ranki, A. The Many Faces of Solitary and Multiple Erythema Migrans. *Acta Derm. Venereol.* **2013**, *93*, 693–700. [CrossRef]
19. Kluger, N.; Habib, F.; Joujoux, J.; Dandurand, M.; Meunier, L. Atypical Presentation of Erythema Migrans with Multiple Lesions. *J Eur. Acad. Dermatol. Venereol.* **2007**, *21*, 283–284.
20. Wechsler, J. Infiltrats dermiques sans vascularite. In *305–385 in Pathologie Cutanée Non Tumorale*; Wechsler, J., Ed.; Elsevier SAS: Paris, France, 2005.
21. Wang, J.; Khachemoune, A. Granuloma Annulare: A Focused Review of Therapeutic Options. *Am. J. Clin. Dermatol.* **2018**, *19*, 333–344. [CrossRef]
22. Piette, E.W.; Rosenbach, M. Granuloma annulare: Clinical and histologic variants, epidemiology, and genetics. *J. Am. Acad. Dermatol.* **2016**, *75*, 457–465. [CrossRef]
23. Francès, C.; Barète, S.; Piette, J.C. Manifestations dermatologiques du lupus. *Rev. Med. Interne* **2008**, *29*, 701–709. [CrossRef] [PubMed]
24. Bataille, P.; Chasset, F.; Monfort, J.B.; De Risi-Pugliese, T.; Soria, A.; Francès, C.; Barbaud, A.; Senet, P. Cutaneous drug-induced lupus erythematosus: Clinical and immunological characteristics and update on new associated drugs. *Ann. Dermatol. Venereol.* **2021**, *148*, 211–220. [CrossRef] [PubMed]
25. Gianotti, F.; Ermacora, E. Erythema gyratum atrophicans transiens neonatale. *Arch. Dermatol.* **1975**, *111*, 615–616. [CrossRef] [PubMed]
26. Puig, L.; Moreno, A.; Alomar, A.; Moragas, J.M. Erythema gyratum atrophicans transiens neonatale: A variant of cutaneous neonatal lupus erythematosus. *Pediatr. Dermatol.* **1988**, *5*, 112–116. [CrossRef]
27. Brito-Zerón, P.; Retamozo, S.; Akasbi, M.; Gandía, M.; Perez-De-Lis, M.; Soto-Cardenas, M.J. Annular Erythema in Primary Sjogren's Syndrome: Description of 43 Non-Asian Cases. *Lupus* **2014**, *23*, 166–175. [CrossRef]
28. Kawakami, T.; Saito, R. The Relationship between Facial Annular Erythema and Anti-SS-A/Ro Antibodies in Three East Asian Women. *Br. J. Dermatol.* **1999**, *140*, 136–140. [CrossRef]
29. Wallach, D.; Vignon-Pennamen, M.D. Pyoderma gangrenosum and Sweet syndrome: The prototypic neutrophilic dermatoses. *Br. J. Dermatol.* **2018**, *178*, 595–602. [CrossRef]
30. Christensen, O.B.; Holst, R.; Svensson, A. Chronic recurrent annular neutrophilic dermatosis. An entity? *Acta Derm. Venereol.* **1989**, *69*, 415–418.
31. Croci-Torti, A.; Guillot, B.; Rigau, V.; Bessis, D. Dermatose neutrophilique annulaire récurrente chronique. *Ann. Dermatol. Venereol.* **2016**, *144*, 362–367. [CrossRef]
32. Ozdemir, M.; Engin, B.; Toy, H.; Demirkesen, C. Neutrophilic Figurate Erythema. *Int. J. Dermatol.* **2008**, *47*, 262–264. [CrossRef]
33. Weyers, W.; Diaz-Cascajo, C.; Weyers, I. Erythema annulare centrifugum: Results of a clinicopathologic study of 73 patients. *Am. J. Dermatopathol.* **2003**, *25*, 451–462. [CrossRef]
34. Peterson, A.O., Jr.; Jarratt, M. Annular Erythema of Infancy. *Arch Dermatol.* **1981**, *117*, 145–148. [CrossRef]
35. Sempau, L.; Larralde, M.; Luna, P.C.; Casas, J.; Staiger, H. Eosinophilic Annular Erythema. *Dermatol. Online J.* **2012**, *18*, 8. [CrossRef]
36. Howes, R.; Girgis, L.; Kossard, S. Eosinophilic Annular Erythema: A Subset of Wells' Syndrome or a Distinct Entity? *Australas. J. Dermatol.* **2008**, *49*, 159–163. [CrossRef]
37. Miljković, J.; Bartenjev, I. Hypereosinophilic Dermatitis-like Erythema Annulare Centrifugum in a Patient with Chronic Lymphocytic Leukaemia. *J. Eur. Acad. Dermatol. Venereol.* **2005**, *19*, 228–231. [CrossRef]
38. González-López, M.A.; López-Escobar, M.; Fernández-Llaca, H.; González-Vela, M.C.; López-Brea, M. Eosinophilic Annular Erythema in a Patient with Metastatic Prostate Adenocarcinoma. *Int. J. Dermatol.* **2015**, *54*, e80–e82. [CrossRef]
39. Prajapati, V.; Cheung-Lee, M.; Schloss, E.; Salopek, T.G. Spontaneously Resolving Eosinophilic Annular Erythema. *J. Am. Acad. Dermatol.* **2012**, *67*, e75–e77. [CrossRef]
40. Manriquez, J.; Berroeta-Mauriziano, D.; Andino-Navarrete, R.; Vera-Kellet, C. Eosinophilic Annular Erythema: Complete Clinical Response with Dapsone. *Int. J. Dermatol.* **2015**, *54*, e96–e98. [CrossRef]
41. Rongioletti, F.; Fausti, V.; Parodi, A. Erythema Gyratum Repens Is Not an Obligate Paraneoplastic Disease: A Systematic Review of the Literature and Personal Experience. *J. Eur. Acad. Dermatol. Venereol.* **2014**, *28*, 112–115. [CrossRef]
42. Peres, G.; Miot, H.A. Erythema gyratum repens following COVID-19 infection. *Int. J. Dermatol.* **2021**, *60*, 1435–1436. [CrossRef]
43. Castro Silva, R.; Castro Silva, G.; Castro Silva, M.C.; Lupi, O. Erythema gyratum repens after COVID-19. *J. Eur. Acad. Dermatol. Venereol.* **2021**, *35*, e859–e861. [CrossRef] [PubMed]
44. Chiquito, D.; Xavier-Junior, J.C.C.; Peres, G.; Lupi, O. Erythema gyratum repens after COVID vaccination. *J. Eur. Acad. Dermatol. Venereol.* **2022**, *36*, e520–e522. [CrossRef] [PubMed]
45. Spigariolo, C.B.; Giacalone, S.; Nazzaro, G. Pigmented Purpuric Dermatoses: A Complete Narrative Review. *J. Clin. Med.* **2021**, *10*, 2283. [CrossRef] [PubMed]
46. Hoesly, F.J.; Huerter, C.J.; Shehan, J.M. Purpura Annularis Telangiectodes of Majocchi: Case Report and Review of the Literature. *Int. J. Dermatol.* **2009**, *48*, 1129–1133. [CrossRef]

47. Miller, K.; Fischer, M.; Kamino, H.; Meehan, S.; Cohen, D. Purpura annularis telangiectoides. *Dermatol. Online J.* **2012**, *18*, 5. [CrossRef]
48. Cribier, B.; Cuny, J.F.; Schubert, B.; Colson, A.; Truchetet, F.; Grosshans, E. Recurrent Annular Erythema with Purpura: A New Variant of Leucocytoclastic Vasculitis Responsive to Dapsone. *Br. J. Dermatol.* **1996**, *135*, 972–975. [CrossRef]
49. Moawad, S.; Bursztejn, A.C.; Schmutz, J.L.; Barbaud, A. Vasculite leucocytoclasique annulaire: Une forme particulière de vasculite des petits vaisseaux? *Ann. Dermatol. Venereol.* **2016**, *143*, 364–368. [CrossRef]
50. Sonthalia, S.; Singal, A.; Pandhi, D.; Singh, U.R. Annular purpuric eruption in an adult male. *Indian J. Dermatol. Venereol. Leprol.* **2011**, *77*, 731.
51. Salava, A.; Kluger, N. Le purpura du campagnol. *Images Dermatol.* **2014**, *7*, 61–66.

Disclaimer/Publisher's Note: The statements, opinions and data contained in all publications are solely those of the individual author(s) and contributor(s) and not of MDPI and/or the editor(s). MDPI and/or the editor(s) disclaim responsibility for any injury to people or property resulting from any ideas, methods, instructions or products referred to in the content.

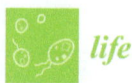

Article

Clinical, Dermoscopic, and Histological Characteristics of Melanoma Patients According to the Age Groups: A Retrospective Observational Study

Monika Słowińska [1,2,*], Iwona Czarnecka [1], Robert Czarnecki [3], Paulina Tatara [1], Anna Nasierowska-Guttmejer [4,5], Małgorzata Lorent [6], Szczepan Cierniak [6] and Witold Owczarek [1]

[1] Department of Dermatology, Central Clinical Hospital Ministry of Defense, Military Institute of Medicine—National Research Institute, Szaserow 128, 04-141 Warsaw, Poland; iczarnecka@wim.mil.pl (I.C.); ptatara@wim.mil.pl (P.T.); wowczarek@wim.mil.pl (W.O.)
[2] Evimed Medical Centre Ltd., Private Dermatologic Practice, JP Woronicza 16, 02-625 Warsaw, Poland
[3] Department of Cardiology, LUX MED Oncology, Limited Liability Company, St. Elizabeth Hospital, Goszczynskiego 1, 02-616 Warsaw, Poland; robert.czarnecki@luxmed.pl
[4] Department of Pathomorphology, Central Clinical Hospital of Ministry of Interior and Administration—National Medical Institute, Woloska 137, 02-507 Warsaw, Poland; anna.nasierowska@cskmswia.pl
[5] Faculty of Medicine, Lazarski University, Swieradowska 43, 02-662 Warsaw, Poland
[6] Department of Pathomorphology, Central Clinical Hospital Ministry of Defense, Military Institute of Medicine—National Research Institute, Szaserow 128, 04-141 Warsaw, Poland; mlorent@wim.mil.pl (M.L.); scierniak@wim.mil.pl (S.C.)
* Correspondence: mslowinska@wim.mil.pl

Citation: Słowińska, M.; Czarnecka, I.; Czarnecki, R.; Tatara, P.; Nasierowska-Guttmejer, A.; Lorent, M.; Cierniak, S.; Owczarek, W. Clinical, Dermoscopic, and Histological Characteristics of Melanoma Patients According to the Age Groups: A Retrospective Observational Study. *Life* **2023**, *13*, 1369. https://doi.org/10.3390/life13061369

Academic Editor: Alin Laurentiu Tatu

Received: 16 April 2023
Revised: 27 May 2023
Accepted: 7 June 2023
Published: 12 June 2023

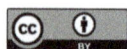

Copyright: © 2023 by the authors. Licensee MDPI, Basel, Switzerland. This article is an open access article distributed under the terms and conditions of the Creative Commons Attribution (CC BY) license (https://creativecommons.org/licenses/by/4.0/).

Abstract: Background: Although the role of melanoma risk factors is well documented, their correlation with patients' age is less frequently analyzed. Method: The analysis was performed among 189 melanoma patients in different age groups, including <30 years, 31–60 years, and >60 years, to investigate the risk factors, topography, and coexistence of morphological features of 209 melanomas (dermoscopic and histopathological). Results: Among the youngest age group, no correlation with the presence of estimated risk factors was found. The most common dermoscopic pattern was spitzoid and multicomponent asymmetric. The group of middle-aged patients was the most diverse in terms of the occurrence of risk factors, solar lentiginosis, dermoscopic patterns, topography, histological subtypes, and invasiveness of melanomas. The oldest group characterized a strong correlation between solar lentiginosis, NMSC comorbidity, the prevalence of facial melanomas, the dermoscopic pattern of melanoma arising on chronic sun-damaged skin, and regression. Conclusion: The findings regarding the presence of age-specific features in melanoma patients, especially in the youngest and middle-aged groups, might be helpful for clinicians and to target secondary prevention efforts.

Keywords: melanoma; dermoscopy; nevi; age factors; comorbidity

1. Introduction

Over the past few decades, there has been a large increase in the incidence of melanoma and non-melanoma skin cancers (NMSC), especially among the white population [1,2]. A worldwide total of 325,000 new melanoma cases and 57,000 melanoma-related deaths were estimated for 2020 with wide geographic variations [1]. With the continuation of the current rates, it is estimated that there will be a 50% increase in melanoma incidence and a 68% increase in melanoma deaths by the year 2040 [1]. Since reducing melanoma mortality is an unmet need, secondary prevention can be reconsidered to increase the effectiveness of the early detection of patients in a situation of limited health care capacity.

Numerous association studies have confirmed the correlation of known patient-related risk factors, multiple genetic factors, and lifestyle or iatrogenic factors [3–7]. Estimates of their effects indicate that high intermittent or intentional UV exposure increases the risk by about 60%; indoor tanning increases the risk by about 20%; a history of sunburns doubles the risk; similarly to skin prototype I, skin prototype II increases the risk by 80%; multiple acquired (common) nevi increase the risk sevenfold; and having at least five atypical nevi increases the risk sixfold [4]. Among patients undergoing dermoscopic screening, the above-mentioned risk factors occur with different frequencies, but their higher co-occurrence should be expected with age.

Independently, epidemiological data indicate an increase in the incidence of melanoma in all age groups. Based on epidemiological data from the National Cancer Institute and the SEER Registry regarding the cutaneous melanoma incidence rates by age at diagnosis within the years 2016 and 2020 (Supplement S1) [8] and from the Polish National Cancer Registry regarding the crude incidence rates in the period 2016–2020 for the adult population (Supplement S2) [9], two increases in incidence were found—for the population over 30 years of age and for the population over 60 years of age. Therefore, the aim of the study was to analyze adult melanoma patients in three age groups in terms of the coexistence of morphological features of melanomas (dermoscopic and histological) and patient-related risk factors that manifested clinically.

2. Materials and Methods

Retrospective analysis included consecutive adult patients referred to a dermoscopic skin examination at Dermatology Department, Central Clinical Hospital Ministry of Defense, Military Institute of Medicine—National Research Institute or private dermatological practice (Evimed Medical Centre Ltd., Warsaw, Poland) in Warsaw between 1 January 2015 and 31 October 2022. The study protocol was approved by the Local Ethics Committee (#21/WIM/2021, 19 May 2021).

Patients' medical records were evaluated based on the following:

- Epidemiologic data (gender, age at the moment of melanoma diagnosis, and location of melanoma), family or personal history of melanoma, and previous non-melanoma skin cancer (NMSC).
- The topography of melanoma was described as head and neck, trunk, upper limb and lower limb (including acral melanomas), and special locations (nail apparatus, mucous membrane of the oral or genital area, and eye).
- Melanoma risk factors that manifested clinically, including multiple acquired melanocytic nevi (above 50 melanocytic nevi), atypical nevus syndrome, skin phototype I or II, solar lentiginosis (as a marker for sun burn episodes), previous/coexisting non-melanoma skin cancer (NMSC), and genetic syndromes.
- Presence of histopathological report of melanoma. The histopathological subtypes of melanoma were evaluated as lentigo maligna (facial and extrafacial), lentigo maligna melanoma (facial), superficial spreading melanoma, nodular melanoma, spitzoid melanoma, nevoid melanoma, and desmoplastic melanoma. The melanoma invasiveness was described according to the TNM staging system/8th AJCC classification as pTis, pT1, pT2, pT3, and pT4 [10].
- Videodermoscopic documentation of melanoma. The dermoscopic pattern of melanoma was allocated to one of the following subtypes: multicomponent asymmetric, spitzoid, melanoma on sun damaged skin, hypomelanotic/amelanotic, homogenous, nodular, melanoma on face, and melanoma in special location (nail apparatus/acral/mucous membranes). The dermoscopic regression structures were regarded as present or absent.

The dermoscopic documentation was performed with the use of Fotofinder HD 800 or Medicam 1000 (FotoFinder Systems GmbH, Bad Birnbach, Germany) or Mole Max (Derma Medical Systems Handels u. Entwicklungs GmbH Vienna, Austria) and captured in polarized light and at the same 20-fold magnification.

Patients were enrolled in the study based on the inclusion and exclusion criteria listed below. Inclusion criteria: at least 18 years old at time of melanoma diagnosis; the full pathological report documented primary melanoma diagnosis according to the TNM staging system/8th AJCC classification including topography and melanoma subtype; pathological reports documented NMSC diagnosis; full videodermoscopic documentation enabling the classification of a dermoscopic pattern of melanoma; presence of melanocytic nevi; concomitant NMSC; solar lentiginosis; a skin phototype; information about the melanoma diagnosis among close relatives present in patient's medical chart. Exclusion criteria: a lack of videodermoscopic documentation; lack of pathological report of primary melanoma; recurrent melanoma; melanoma of unknown primary location; metastatic melanoma after the excision of the primary lesion; melanoma in a location that prevents the dermoscopic/videodermoscopic examination; lack of data enabling the assessment of melanoma risk factors.

Statistical Analysis

Statistical analysis was performed using R software environment (version 4.2.2 "Innocent and Trusting"; R Foundation for Statistical Computing, Vienna, Austria); https://www.R-project.org accessed on 7 November 2022; RStudio (Integrated Development Environment for R, version 2022.07.2+567 "Spotted Wakerobin" Release; Boston, MA, USA); http://www.rstudio.com accessed on 7 November 2022; and R packages including tidyverse, knitr, summarytools, kableExtra, crosstables, broom, scales, FSA, and epitools [11].

Frequencies of count data were calculated with cross tables. Differences in frequencies were estimated with Fisher's exact test (expected counts in some groups were lower than 5). Differences in means of continuous numerical data were calculated with Kruskal–Wallis rank test (numerical data in whole data and groups were not normally distributed). Differences in means between multiple groups were calculated with Dunn's test with Bonferroni's p-value correction. Crude odds ratios with 95% confidence intervals for pairs of binomial variables in age groups were calculated using conditional maximum likelihood estimation. Odds ratios adjusted for age and gender with 95% confidence intervals were calculated using multivariable logistic regression.

3. Results

The data from the dermoscopic visits of 7367 patients (aged 2 months–92 years) admitted in the period 1 January 2015–31 October 2022 to two dermatological sites were analyzed, identifying 269 melanomas in 248 patients (aged 20–90 years; median 45 years; mean 49.3 years). As the videodermoscopic documentation of 209 melanomas was available in 189 patients (63.5% female and 36.5% men), this group was further analyzed. The summary of the epidemiological, clinicopathological, and dermoscopic data are presented in Table 1.

3.1. The Characteristics of the Melanoma Patients

Among the 189 patients (aged 20–90 years) enrolled in the study, the mean age at the diagnosis of melanoma was 51.6, and the median age was 47 years. Among 209 melanomas 61.7% (129/209) were detected during the first dermoscopic visit, and 38.3% (80/209) were detected during the monitoring visits. There was no statistical difference in the invasiveness of melanomas, although most small–size melanomas were detected during the monitoring visits as new lesions. Eighteen patients (9.5%) were diagnosed with at least 2 melanomas, and one (0.5%) was diagnosed with 3 melanomas. Among the 18 (8.6%) patients, melanoma had occurred in an immediate family member.

The melanoma risk factors manifested clinically by atypical nevus syndrome or by numerous acquired nevi (ANS/NAN) were found in 121 (64%) patients, solar lentiginosis was found in 87 (41.6%) patients, and 41 (21.7%) patients had previous or coexisting NMSCs (nearly all had basal cell carcinoma—BCC). No genetic syndromes were detected among the patients. The group of 189 patients was very homogeneous in terms of skin phototype, as only 6 (3.2%) patients had phototype I or III, while the remaining 177 (93.6%) patients had phototype II. In 29 cases, melanoma occurred in a special location: 22 (10.5%) on the face, 3 (1.4%) on the scalp, 4 (1.9%) acral, 2 (1%) on mucous membranes (oral mucosa and vulva), and 1 (0.5%) within the nail apparatus.

Table 1. Epidemiological, clinical, histopathological, topographical, and dermoscopic data of patients diagnosed with melanoma divided into three age groups and calculated based on Fisher's exact test for count data with simulated p-value ($p < 0.05$ was considered statistically significant). NS—not statistically significant.

	Total n (%)	Age < 31 y n (%) Within the Group	Age 31–60 y n (%) Within the Group	Age > 60 y n (%) Within the Group	p Value
Gender		12	113	64	
Female	120 (63.5%)	6 (50.0%)	71 (62.8%)	43 (67.2%)	NS
Male	69 (36.5%)	6 (50.0%)	42 (37.2%)	21 (32.8%)	
History of personal/familial melanoma					
Yes	24 (12.5%)	0 (0%)	18 (15.9%)	6 (9.4%)	NS
No	165 (87.3%)	12 (100.00%)	95 (84.1%)	58 (90.6%)	
Multiple acquired nevi/Atypical nevus syndrome					
Yes	121 (64.0%)	8 (66.7%)	86 (76.1%)	27 (42.2%)	<0.0005
No	68 (36%)	4 (33.3%)	27 (23.9%)	37 (57.8%)	
Skin phototype					
I	6 (3.2%)	3 (25.0%)	2 (1.7%)	1 (1.5%)	
II	177 (93.6%)	9 (75.0%)	107 (94.7%)	61 (95.3%)	NS
III	6 (3.2%)	0 (0%)	4 (3.5%)	2 (3.1%)	
IV–V	0 (0%)	0 (0%)	0 (0%)	0 (0%)	
Solar lentiginosis					
Yes	81 (42.9%)	2 (16.7%)	32 (28.3%)	47 (73.4%)	<0.0005
No	108 (57.1%)	10 (83.3%)	81 (71.7%)	17 (26.6%)	
Histopathological report:					
- LM	25 (12.0%)	0 (0%)	10 (8.0%)	15 (20.8%)	
- LMM	4 (1.9%)	0 (0%)	0 (0%)	4 (5.5%)	
Melanoma:					
- pTis	47 (22.5%)	2 (16.6%)	28 (22.4%)	17 (23.6%)	<0.01
- pT1	101 (48.3%)	7 (58.3%)	69 (55.2%)	25 (34.7%)	
- pT2	24 (11.5%)	2 (16.6%)	13 (10.4%)	9 (12.5%)	
- pT3	3 (1.4%)	1 (8.3%)	1 (0.8%)	1 (1.4%)	
- pT4	5 (2.4%)	0 (0%)	4 (3.2%)	1 (1.4%)	

Table 1. Cont.

	Total n (%)	Age < 31 y n (%) Within the Group	Age 31–60 y n (%) Within the Group	Age > 60 y n (%) Within the Group	p Value
Dermoscopic pattern of melanoma					
Multicomponent asymmetric	91 (43.5%)	4 (33.3%)	63 (50.4%)	24 (33.3%)	
Spitzoid	37 (17.7%)	6 (50.0%)	28 (22.4%)	3 (4.2%)	
Melanoma on sun damaged skin	25 (12.0%)	0 (0%)	9 (7.2%)	16 (22.2%)	
Hypomelanotic/amelanotic	10 (4.8%)	0 (0%)	7 (5.6%)	3 (4.2%)	<0.0005
Homogenous	5 (2.4%)	0 (0%)	4 (3.2%)	1 (1.4%)	
Nodular	12 (5.7%)	1 (8.3%)	6 (4.8%)	5 (6.9%)	
Melanoma on face	22 (10.5%)	0 (0%)	3 (2.4%)	19 (26.4%)	
Melanoma in special location (nail apparatus/acral/mucous membranes)	7 (3.3%)	1 (8.3%)	5 (4.0%)	1 (1.4%)	
Dermoscopic structures of regression					
Yes	61 (29.2%)	1 (8.3%)	27 (21.6%)	33 (45.8%)	<0.001
No	148 (70.8%)	11 (91.7%)	98 (78.4%)	39 (54.2%)	
Melanoma location:					
- Head and neck	25 (11.9%)	0 (0%)	6 (4.8%)	19 (26.%)	
- Trunk	70 (33.5%)	4 (33.3.%)	46 (36.8%)	20 (27.8%)	
- Upper limb	40 (19.1%)	3 (25.0%)	22 (17.6%)	15 (20.8%)	<0.0005
- Lower limb	71 (34.0%)	4 (33.3%)	49 (39.2%)	18 (25.0%)	
- Nail apparatus	1 (0.5%)	1 (8.3%)	0 (0%)	0 (0%)	
- Mucous membrane	2 (1%)	0 (0%)	2 (1.6%)	0 (0%)	
Previous/concomitant NMSC					
Yes	41 (21.7%)	0 (0%)	10 (8.9%)	31 (48.4%)	<0.0005
No	148 (78.3%)	12 (100%)	103 (91.1%)	33 (51.6%)	

The majority of melanomas (84.7%) were diagnosed as thin melanoma (lentigo maligna, melanoma in situ, or pT1 stage), and the superficial spreading histological type was predominant (77%). Nodular melanoma (NM) was rarely detected and consisted of 5.7% of cases. Spitzoid, desmoplastic, or nevoid melanomas were not found in pathological reports. The predominant dermoscopic melanoma pattern was multicomponent asymmetric, with 91 patients (43.5%); followed by spitzoid, with 37 patients (17.7%); melanoma on chronically sun damaged skin, with 25 patients (12%); and melanoma on the face, with 22 patients (10.5%).

3.2. The Analysis between the Individual Age Groups

The analysis between the individual age groups revealed statistically significant differences in the frequencies of multiple melanocytic nevi ($p < 0.0005$), previous/concomitant NMSC ($p < 0.0005$), solar lentiginosis ($p < 0.0005$), melanoma location ($p < 0.001$), melanoma histopathology ($p < 0.01$), melanoma dermoscopic pattern ($p < 0.0005$), and regression structures ($p < 0.001$) (Table 1). Figure 1 presents detailed data regarding the statistically significant differences among the individual age groups with regard to melanoma location, histopathological diagnosis, and the dermoscopic melanoma pattern.

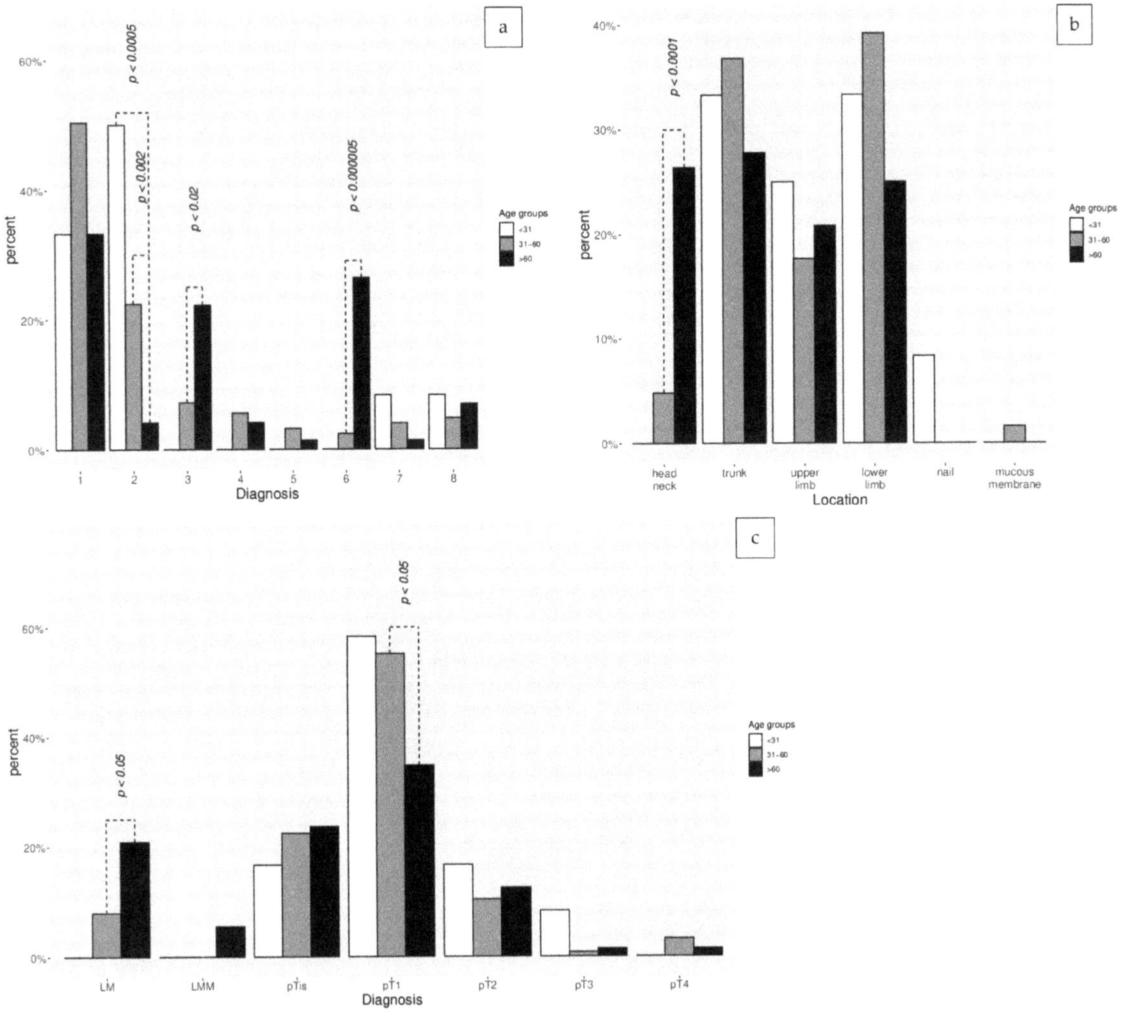

Figure 1. The Fisher's exact tests for count data with simulated p-value analysis regarding the differences in melanoma location (**a**). The histopathological diagnosis (**b**) and the dermoscopic melanoma patterns (**c**) between the individual age groups (below 31 years, 31–60 years, and over 60 years). Legend for dermoscopic patterns on axis (x) for Figure 1c: 1—multicomponent asymmetric; 2—spitzoid; 3—melanoma on sun damaged skin; 4—hypomelanotic/amelanotic; 5—homogenous; 6—melanoma on face; 7—melanoma in special location (nail/acral/mucous membranes); 8—nodular.

The group of patients younger than 31 years old had low statistical power due to the small number of melanomas (12 cases). In comparison to other age groups, striking differences were observed for the dermoscopic pattern of melanoma. The most common melanomas were spitzoid (16.2% of all/50% in the age group) and multicomponent asymmetric (4.4% of all/33.3% in the age group), and the age group also had the lowest incidence of regression structures (1.6% of all/8.3% in the age group) and solar lentiginosis (2.3% of all/16.7% in the age group). No cases of previous/coexisting NMSCs, melanoma located on the head/neck, and mucous membrane area were detected in the group.

The group of patients aged 31–60 years was characterized by the presence of personal or familial melanoma incidence (74.3% of all/20.8% in the age group) and a high number of melanocytic nevi (70.3% of all/77.6% in the age group). Another feature was the wide diversity of dermoscopic melanoma patterns. The most common dermoscopic patterns were multicomponent asymmetric (69.2% of all/50.4% in the age group), spitzoid (75.7% of all/22.4% in the age group), hypomelanotic/amelanotic (70% of all/5.6% in the age group), and homogenous (80% of all/3.2% in the age group). The group of patients aged 31–60 years was also characterized by a higher incidence of thick melanomas (pT2—54.1% of total/10.4% in the age group; pT3—33.3% of all/0.8% in the age group; pT4—80% of all/3.2% in the age group). The topography of melanomas revealed the predominance of melanoma location on the lower limbs (69% of all/39.2% in the age group) and a general high diversity of melanoma locations, including extrafacial melanomas in special areas (66.6% of all/1.6% in the age group) (Figure 1).

The oldest group of melanoma patients is characterized by the common presence of solar lentiginosis (60.9% of all/73.6% in the age group), the highest incidence of facial melanoma (86.3% of all/26.4% in the age group), and lentigo maligna (60% of all/20.8% in the age group). The predominant dermoscopic melanoma patterns were melanoma on the face (86.3% of all/26.4% in the age group), melanoma on chronically sun damaged skin (64% of all/22.2% in the age group), and multicomponent asymmetric (26.4% of all/33.3% in the age group). Commonly present were features of regression under dermoscopy (54.1% of all/45.8% in the age group) and the co-occurrence of NMSC (64.29% of all/45.57% in the age group) (Figure 1).

3.3. Crude (Unadjusted) Odds Ratios for the Age Groups (Table 2)

The summary of the odds ratios, 95% confidence intervals, and p-value results for the clinical, dermoscopic, and epidemiologic characteristics of the melanoma patients in the individual age groups are presented in Table 2.

The analysis of the group of patients younger than 31 years old revealed an absence of NMSC; thus, odds ratios were not calculated. In comparison to other age groups, there was a significantly lower prevalence of solar lentiginosis (OR 0.26, 95% CI: 0.04–1.06, $p > 0.05$). None of the other evaluated factors differed significantly from those of the other age groups (Figure 2a).

In the group of patients aged 31–60 years, the statistical significance of odds difference was reached for ANS/NAN (OR 3.69, 95% CI: 1.99–6.99, $p < 0.00001$). The incidences of NMSC (OR 0.14, 95% CI 0.06–0.31, $p < 0.000001$), dermoscopic regression (OR 0.41, 95% CI: 0.22–0.75, $p < 0.005$), and solar lentiginosis (OR 0.22, 95% CI: 0.12–0.41, $p < 0.000001$) were lower than in other age groups (Figure 2b).

The statistical significance of incidences of multiple factors in the group of patients over 60 years old was revealed: previous/concomitant NMSC (OR 10.53, 95% CI: 4.81–24.94, $p < 0.000001$), the presence of solar lentiginosis (OR 7.27, 95% CI: 3.74–14.74, $p < 0.000001$), regression under dermoscopy (OR 3.27, 95% CI 1.76–6.15, $p < 0.0001$), and ANS/NAN (OR 0.24, 95% CI: 0.13–0.46, $p < 0.00001$) (Figure 2c).

The limitation of the study was the retrospective analysis and the low statistical power of the group of patients below 31 years old due to the small sample size. The analysis of melanoma risk factors was entirely based on empirical data collected from medical procedures.

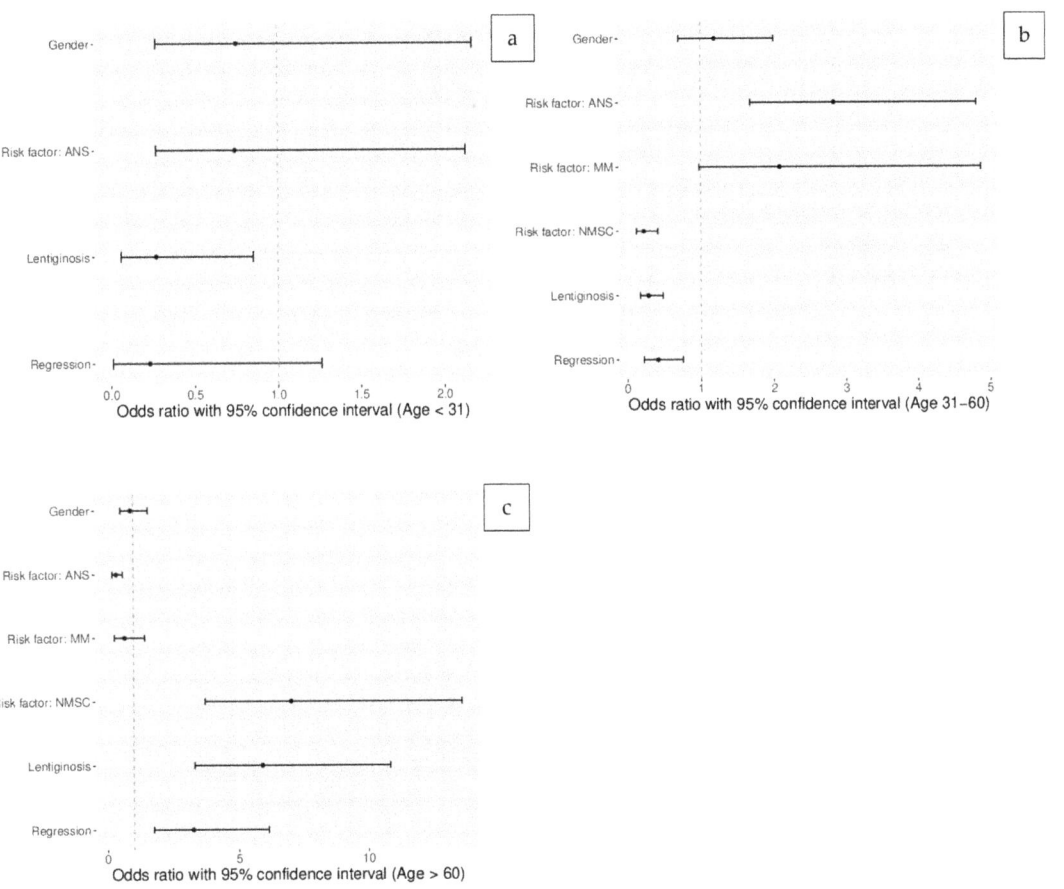

Figure 2. The characteristics of individual age groups of melanoma patients presenting unadjusted odds ratios with 95% confidence interval ($p < 0.05$ was considered statistically significant): (**a**) age group below 31 years old; (**b**) age group 31–60 years old; (**c**) age group over 60 years old.

Table 2. Summary of odds ratios, 95% confidence intervals, and p-value results for clinical, dermoscopic, and epidemiologic characteristics of melanoma patients in individual age groups. $p < 0.05$ was considered statistically significant; NS—not statistically significant; ND—no data

Factor	OR	95%CI	p-Value
Characteristics of melanoma patients below 31 years of age (unadjusted)			
Gender (male)	1.8	0.53–6.15	NS
Melanoma (previous/concomitant or in family history)	ND	ND	ND
Atypical nevus syndrome or multiple acquired nevi	1.11	0.33–4.46	NS
NMSC (previous/concomitant)	ND	ND	ND
Regression under dermoscopy	0.23	0.01–1.26	NS
Solar lentiginosis	0.26	0.04–1.06	NS

Table 2. *Cont.*

Factor	OR	95%CI	*p*-Value
Characteristics of melanoma patients between 31 and 60 years of age (unadjusted)			
Gender (male)	0.7	0.59–1.98	NS
Melanoma (previous/concomitant or in family history)	2.17	0.85–6.34	NS
Atypical nevus syndrome or multiple acquired nevi	3.69	1.99–6.99	<0.00001
NMSC (previous/concomitant)	0.14	0.06–0.31	<0.000001
Regression under dermoscopy	0.41	0.22–0.75	<0.005
Solar lentiginosis	0.22	0.12–0.41	<0.000001
Characteristics of melanoma patients 60 years old (unadjusted)			
Gender (male)	0.79	0.41–1.48	NS
Melanoma (previous/concomitant or in family history)	0.63	0.21–1.6	NS
Atypical nevus syndrome or multiple acquired nevi	0.24	0.13–0.46	0.00001
NMSC (previous/concomitant)	10.53	4.81–24.94	<0.000001
Regression under dermoscopy	3.27	1.76–6.15	<0.0001
Solar lentiginosis	7.27	3.74–14.74	<0.000001

4. Discussion

Morbidity from melanoma is increasing worldwide, especially in fair-skinned populations in all age groups [1,3]. Cutaneous melanoma mostly occurs in patients between 40 and 60 years old but is the most common form of cancer in young adults between 25 and 29 years old [1,7,12–14]. Currently, melanoma secondary prevention programs cover a small percentage of the adult population due to the lack of data supported or refuted by survival analyses from large randomized controlled trials, the high workloads of specialists, and the high economic costs [7,13–15]. As a result, they are mainly implemented via the opportunistic screening and surveillance of high-risk patients, as well as recommendations for self-examination and skin awareness to the general population [14]. The effectiveness of opportunistic screening was covered in studies by Argenziano et al. and Omara et al. [16,17].

Dermoscopy is one of the most important pillars of the secondary prevention of melanomas [18–21]. It enables their diagnosis at an early stage and thus contributes to a reduction in melanoma mortality [18–21]. Recently, Kalloniati et al., in a comparative study, showed 78.2% sensitivity and 71.4% specificity in identifying the clinical atypia based on naked eye examinations versus 89.1% sensitivity and 93.7% specificity based on dermoscopy [22]. Nazzaro et al. discussed the reasons for the increased incidence and diagnosis of thin melanomas (especially in situ and in small-sized melanomas) observed within the years 2006–2020 [23]. The authors pointed out the possible coexistence of two potential causes of this trend. The first resulted in the rapidly growing global incidence of melanoma, especially in white populations, and the second resulted in overdiagnosis. The latter could be derivative of the increasingly common use of dermoscopy, the use of new diagnostic methods (such as reflectance confocal microscopy), greater patient awareness, and healthcare-seeking behavior for skin cancer screening. In our opinion, all the above aspects should be taken into account, considering the fact that melanomas with a nodular component (spizoid and non-spitzoid) are characterized by a different histogenetic subtype, which was the subject of recent publications by Dessinioti et al., Raghavan et al., and Pusiol et al. [24–26]. BRAF mutations are more likely to be detected in SSM, while NM is associated more strongly with the 'non-nevus' melanoma pathway development model and NRAS mutations [24]. A SEER registry study reported that median Breslow thickness decreased for SSM over the period 1989–2009, whereas median Breslow thickness increased for nodular melanoma (NM) over time [27]. NM has been reported more frequently in older patients (>50 years), specifically in older men compared to SSM, and with low nevus counts [24]. Lower total-body nevus counts have been associated with thicker melanoma. These findings highlight a subset of melanoma patients that do not have well-established risk factors, i.e., high nevus count, and that could be at a higher risk for thicker aggressive melanomas [24]. The incidence of NM in our study was low (5.7%) and similarly frequent in the middle-aged and the oldest patients. Due to the small sample size of NM, no statistical correlation with the incidence of the risk factors could be performed. Although all the international melanoma screening guidelines stated the effectiveness of conducting skin examinations in patients harboring melanoma risk, specific recommendations on the age at which this screening should begin and the optimal visit intervals are lacking [1,7,14,28–30]. Moreover, no unique scoring system has been developed to discriminate high-risk versus low-risk individuals with respect to melanoma development [14]. As the elderly population presents the highest morbidity and mortality rates of melanoma, Nagore et al. investigated the impact of 17 risk factors for the development of melanoma in this population [4]. The authors found the strongest impact for fair eyes, severe sunburns, years of occupational sun exposure, smoking, over 50 melanocytic nevi, and a personal history of NMSC or other non-cutaneous neoplasms [5]. Tobacco smoking was an independent risk factor for cutaneous melanoma in this group.

Patients with melanoma are at increased risk of developing melanoma and NMSC, but also patients with NMSC have increased risk of melanoma and NMSC development [1–3,30–33]. Given the high global incidence of NMSCs, their comorbidity with melanomas is not that common. The overall prevalence of NMSCs was 7% among melanoma cases in the study by Neale et al. and 21.7% in our study [31]. In contrast, many melanoma patients never experience NMSCs, even BCCs, which share a similar pattern of UV exposure [14,32,33].

Our publication describes a population of adult patients both self-referring to a skin screening and those who were referred to this examination by other specialists who considered them to be at a high risk. The two sites participating in this study are both dermatological centers specialized in non-invasive skin cancer diagnostics providing dermoscopy, digital monitoring under videodermoscopy, and reflectance confocal microscopy (RCM) examinations in selected cases. The importance of secondary prevention in such a population might be proved by our findings: 84.7% of melanomas were preinvasive, 61.7% were detected during the first dermoscopic visit, and 38.3% were detected during the monitoring visits. Furthermore, 10% (19/189) of patients were diagnosed with more than one melanoma, among whom five patients presented with two concomitant melanomas during the first skin examination. In other patients, secondary melanomas were diagnosed between 6 months and 40 years following the primary diagnosis. In the context of educational campaigns encouraging periodic dermoscopic examinations, the repeated correlation of the higher frequency of early melanomas (including small melanomas) in middle-aged women is also noteworthy [7,13,24,34–37]. This is probably due to the fact that this population of patients is the most willing to come for screening [34]. Given the huge increase in the incidence of melanoma, it seems particularly important to direct the media's message to groups of middle-aged men. Perhaps the delay in the diagnosis of this group of patients is the reason for the observed change in the proportions between the sexes in the group of middle-aged (predominance of women) and elderly (predominance of men or similar frequency for both sexes) patients [Supplement S2]; Refs. [1,13,24]. This might also be the reason for the more frequent diagnosis of advanced melanomas in elderly men [13,24,37].

The analysis of the three age groups of patients revealed differences in the presence of patient-related risk factors, topographical, and dermoscopic and histological aspects of detected melanomas. The incidence of melanoma in the youngest age group was rare (5.7% of our study population). What we found very interesting was that the statistical analysis excluded the correlation with common melanoma risk factors. Furthermore, the youngest group of adult patients (18–30 years) showed a dermoscopic similarity of melanomas with the patients described by Carrera et al. regarding the pediatric population—a spitzoid (pigmented or non-pigmented) and non-spitzoid (predominant multicomponent asymmetric) pattern [38]. Recently, De Giorgi et al. indicated a new finding—that pediatric melanomas were predominantly pigmented (95% of their cases) and characterized by at least two melanoma-specific structures in dermoscopy, among which the streaks and pseudopods (typical for the spitzoid pattern) were the most commonly found [39]. This could be explained by recent data, which indicated that genetic, rather than UV-induced, factors are responsible for the evolution of spitzoid lesions (Spitz/Reed nevi, spitzoid melanoma, and atypical spitzoid tumours) [25]. Based on the above data, younger populations should be educated to pay special attention to newly emerging and fast-growing lesions that are pink or dark brown and black in color and nodular in palpation, matching the features of spitzoid lesions [40–42]. In a study by Costa et al., 25.8% of those lesions were melanomas in the age group of 20–31 years [42]. Therefore, young patients with multiple growing nevi require close digital dermoscopy monitoring and the excision of Reed/Spitz-looking lesions [40–42]. The remaining frequently detected dermoscopic pattern in patients aged below 31 years was the multicomponent asymmetric one. It should be easily detected even based on the clinical ABCDE melanoma criteria, although with the risk of early invasive melanoma detection [43].

The incidence of patient-related risk factors showed their higher occurrence among patients between 31 and 60 years of age. In our study, this population was characterized by multiple acquired melanocytic nevi/ANS, the individual or familial occurrence of melanoma, the co-occurrence of NMSC, and solar lentiginosis. Moreover, we found the greatest clinicopathological and dermoscopic diversity of melanomas. All five cases of nevus-associated melanomas, most of the small-sized melanomas, and melanomas in special locations were found (although facial melanoma was more common in the older population). Summarizing the above results, the middle-aged population may require extensive dermoscopic examinations, precision in total-body skin examinations, the digital monitoring of selected lesions, and, perhaps, total-body photography and reflectance confocal microscopy (RCM) in order to reduce the number of unnecessary excisions and increase diagnostic accuracy.

The characteristics of melanoma patients aged over 60 years in our study confirmed earlier findings regarding the common presence of solar lentiginosis; comorbidity with NMSC; regression structures under dermoscopy; and the location of melanomas in the face, trunk, and upper limbs [4,37,44]. Contrary to the study by Nagore et al., the incidence of common risk factors—multiple melanocytic nevi/ANSs and a personal/family history of melanoma—were not statistically significant in our group. Generally, among those patients, we found two subgroups of melanomas. The first, with striking signs of melanomas, presented as facial or superficial spreading melanomas. The second—with great difficult in detection—presented as simulators of solar lentigines or regressed seborrheic keratoses, which present as light brown, pink, and grey in color. This is why the most common dermoscopic patterns found in this age group were the melanoma pattern on chronic sun-damaged skin (including extrafacial lentigo maligna), the multicomponent asymmetric pattern, and the homogenous pattern, which was consistent with previous observations [45,46]. Although many studies reported a higher incidence of nodular melanoma resulting in lower 10-year disease-specific survival among men over 65, we have not found a higher incidence of primary nodular melanomas (the advanced superficial spreading melanomas with a nodular component are not included in this category) in this age group [4,14,37,47,48]. Regarding the common detection of melanoma on the head in elderly patients, it is extremely important to focus on scalp melanomas (SM) due to their poor prognosis and difficult dermoscopic diagnostics. In a recent publication, Porto et al. showed that SM presents differently depending on the comorbidity with androgenetic alopecia and that patients without alopecia had higher Breslow thickness due to late diagnosis (because of hair concealment) [49]. Furthermore, SM has a distinct molecular profile with a high frequency of BRAF V600K, NF1 mutations, and a high frequency of detrimental mutations, which might explain their poor prognosis.

Our additional investigation aimed to describe the correlation between NMSC, as a melanoma risk factor, with the clinical and dermoscopic features of melanoma patients and showed higher odds ratios with statistical significance in the age group above 60 years and in patients with solar lentiginosis symptoms. Those findings have a practical impact as, by revealing the presence of NMSC and solar lentiginosis in elderly or middle-aged patients during skin examination, we might expect certain types of melanoma—characteristic for chronic sun-damaged skin—which should increase dermoscopists attention to regressed and difficult-to-find lesions.

The results of our study proved the necessity for closer surveillance of middle-aged patients, among whom melanomas are diagnosed most. These patients not only frequently harbor different risk factors but also may present a wide diversity of difficult-to-diagnose melanomas. Therefore, middle-aged patients will benefit to the greatest extent from the advantages of systematic diagnostic workflows, including RCM [21]. Lastly, this group also has a poor projected prognosis regarding mortality caused by melanoma in 2040 among patients over 60 years of age as those data describe the current middle-aged population [1].

5. Conclusions

The striking differences in the prevalence of common melanoma risk factors, melanoma-specific dermoscopic patterns, and topography were found among the three age groups.

Among the youngest and the oldest patients, no correlation with common melanoma risk factors was found. Patients aged 18–30 years present pediatric dermoscopic patterns of melanoma—the spitzoid and multicomponent asymmetric ones. The patients aged over 60 years presented consequences of the effects of sun exposure over a lifetime (both intermittent and cumulative solar damage or sunburns), which were represented by solar lentiginosis, comorbidity with NMSC, LM/LMM, and the SSM histological subtype, as well as the regression structures characteristic for the multicomponent asymmetric pattern and melanoma on sun-damaged skin dermoscopic patterns.

The incidence of patient-related risk factors showed a higher occurrence among patients between 31 and 60 years of age, which showed the highest general melanoma detection rate. Moreover, we found the greatest clinicopathological and dermoscopic diversity of melanomas (including the highest incidence of small-size melanomas). This makes the middle-aged group the most in need of precise examinations and digital monitoring.

Knowledge of age group differentiation factors may increase the precision of dermoscopic and dermatological surveillance and might influence the content and targeting of melanoma secondary prevention campaigns.

Supplementary Materials: The following supporting information can be downloaded at https://www.mdpi.com/article/10.3390/life13061369/s1. Supplement S1 [8]; Supplement S2 [9].

Author Contributions: Conceptualization, M.S.; methodology, M.S. and R.C.; software, R.C.; validation, M.S., I.C., R.C., P.T., A.N.-G., M.L. and S.C.; formal analysis, M.S., I.C., R.C. and P.T; investigation, M.S., I.C., P.T., A.N.-G., M.L. and S.C.; resources M.S.; I.C., P.T. and W.O.; data curation, M.S., I.C. and R.C.; writing—original draft preparation, M.S., I.C., and R.C.; writing—review and editing, M.S., I.C., R.C., A.N.-G., M.L., S.C. and W.O.; visualization M.S. and R.C.; supervision, M.S. and W.O.; project administration, M.S.; funding acquisition M.S. and W.O. All authors have read and agreed to the published version of the manuscript.

Funding: This research received no external funding.

Institutional Review Board Statement: The study protocol was approved by the Local Ethics Committee (#21/WIM/2021, 19 May 2021).

Informed Consent Statement: Patient consent was waived due to the retrospective analysis and the possible distress or confusion of participants.

Data Availability Statement: The data presented in this study are available on request from the corresponding author. The data are not publicly available due to privacy and ethical restrictions.

Acknowledgments: The authors would like to thank the patients and their families.

Conflicts of Interest: The authors have no relevant conflict of interest to declare regarding this article.

References

1. Arnold, M.; Singh, D.; Laversanne, M.; Vignat, J.; Vaccarella, S.; Meheus, F.; Cust, A.E.; de Vries, E.; Whiteman, D.C.; Bray, F. Global Burden of Cutaneous Melanoma in 2020 and Projections to 2040. *JAMA Dermatol.* **2022**, *158*, 495–503. [CrossRef]
2. Hu, W.; Fang, L.; Ni, R.; Zhang, H.; Pan, G. Changing trends in the disease burden of non-melanoma skin cancer globally from 1990 to 2019 and its predicted level in 25 years. *BMC Cancer* **2022**, *22*, 836. [CrossRef]
3. Raimondi, S.; Suppa, M.; Gandini, S. Melanoma Epidemiology and Sun Exposure. *Acta Dermato-Venereol.* **2020**, *100*, adv00136. [CrossRef]
4. Nagore, E.; Hueso, L.; Botella Estrada, R.; Alfaro Rubio, A.; Serna, I.; Guallar, J.; González, I.; Ribes, I.; Guillen, C. Smoking, sun ex-posure, number of nevi and previous neoplasias are risk factors for melanoma in older patients (60 years and over). *J. Eur. Acad. Dermatol. Venereol.* **2010**, *24*, 50–57. [CrossRef]
5. Massone, C.; Hofman-Wellenhof, R.; Chiodi, S.; Sola, S. Dermoscopic Criteria, Histopathological Correlates and Genetic Findings of Thin Melanoma on Non-Volar Skin. *Genes* **2021**, *12*, 1288. [CrossRef]
6. Zhang, T.; Dutton-Regester, K.; Brown, K.M.; Hayward, N.K. The genomic landscape of cutaneous melanoma. *Pigment. Cell Melanoma Res.* **2016**, *29*, 266–283. [CrossRef]
7. Djavid, A.R.; Stonesifer, C.; Fullerton, B.T.; Wang, S.W.; Tartaro, M.A.; Kwinta, B.D.; Grimes, J.M.; Geskin, L.J.; Saenger, Y.M. Etiologies of Melanoma Development and Prevention Measures: A Review of the Current Evidence. *Cancers* **2021**, *13*, 4914. [CrossRef]
8. Available online: https://seer.cancer.gov/statistics-network/explorer/application.html?site=53&data_type=1&graph_type=3&compareBy=race&chk_race_1=1&chk_race_6=6&chk_race_5=5&chk_race_4=4&chk_race_9=9&chk_race_8=8&chk_race_3=3&chk_race_2=2&rate_type=2&sex=1&advopt_precision=1&advopt_show_ci=on&hdn_view=0&advopt_show_apc=on&advopt_display=2#resultsRegion0 (accessed on 22 May 2023).
9. Available online: https://onkologia.org.pl/pl/raporty (accessed on 22 May 2023).
10. Gershenwald, J.E.; Scolyer, R.A.; Hess, K.R.; Sondak, V.K.; Long, G.V.; Ross, M.I.; Lazar, A.J.; Faries, M.B.; Kirkwood, J.M.; McArthur, G.A.; et al. Melanoma of the skin. In *AJCC Cancer Staging Manual*, 8th ed.; Amin, M.B., Edge, S.B., Greene, F.L., Byrd, D.R., Brookland, R.K., Washington, M.K., Gershenwald, J.E., Compton, C.C., Hess, K.R., Sullivan, D.C., et al., Eds.; Springer International Publishing: New York, NY, USA, 2017; pp. 563–585.
11. Wickham, H.; Averick, M.; Bryan, J.; Chang, W.; McGowan, L.D.A.; François, R.; Grolemund, G.; Hayes, A.; Henry, L.; Hester, J.; et al. Welcome to the tidyverse. *J. Open Source Softw.* **2019**, *4*, 1686. [CrossRef]
12. Sacchetto, L.; Zanetti, R.; Comber, H.; Bouchardy, C.; Brewster, D.H.; Broganelli, P.; Chirlaque, M.D.; Coza, D.; Galceran, J.; Gavin, A.; et al. Trends in incidence of thick, thin and in situ melanoma in Europe. *Eur. J. Cancer* **2018**, *92*, 108–118. [CrossRef]
13. Boada, A.; Tejera-Vaquerizo, A.; Requena, C.; Manrique-Silva, E.; Traves, V.; Nagore, E. Association between melanoma thickness and clinical and demographic characteristics. *Eur. J. Dermatol.* **2021**, *31*, 514–520. [CrossRef]
14. Dubbini, N.; Puddu, A.; Salimbeni, G.; Malloggi, S.; Gandini, D.; Massei, P.; Ferraùto, G.; Rubino, T.; Ricci, L.; Menchini, G.; et al. Melanoma Prevention: Comparison of Different Screening Methods for the Selection of a High Risk Population. *Int. J. Environ. Res. Public Health* **2021**, *18*, 1953. [CrossRef]
15. Johansson, M.; Brodersen, J.; Gøtzsche, P.C.; Jørgensen, K.J. Screening for reducing morbidity and mortality in malignant melanoma. *Cochrane Database Syst. Rev.* **2019**, *6*, CD012352. [CrossRef]
16. Argenziano, G.; Zalaudek, I.; Hofmann-Wellenhof, R.; Bakos, R.M.; Bergman, W.; Blum, A.; Broganelli, P.; Cabo, H.; Caltagirone, F.; Catricalà, C.; et al. Total body skin examination for skin cancer screening in patients with focused symptoms. *J. Am. Acad. Dermatol.* **2012**, *66*, 212–219. [CrossRef]
17. Omara, S.; Wen, D.; Ng, B.; Anand, R.; Matin, R.N.; Taghipour, K.; Esdaile, B. Identification of Incidental Skin Cancers Among Adults Referred to Dermatologists for Suspicious Skin Lesions. *JAMA Netw. Open* **2020**, *3*, e2030107. [CrossRef]
18. Guitera, P.; Menzies, S.W.; Coates, E.; Azzi, A.; Fernandez-Penas, P.; Lilleyman, A.; Badcock, C.; Schmid, H.; Watts, C.G.; Collgros, H.; et al. Efficiency of Detecting New Primary Melanoma among Individuals Treated in a High-Risk Clinic for Skin Surveillance. *JAMA Dermatol.* **2021**, *157*, 521–530. [CrossRef]
19. Argenziano, G.; Albertini, G.; Castagnetti, F.; De Pace, B.; Di Lernia, V.; Longo, C.; Pellacani, G.; Piana, S.; Ricci, C.; Zalaudek, I. Early diagnosis of melanoma: What is the impact of dermoscopy? *Dermatol. Ther.* **2012**, *25*, 403–409. [CrossRef]
20. Pizarro, A.; Arranz, D.; Villeta, M.; Valencia, J. Absence of thick, nodular melanomas during long-term surveillance with total body photography and digital dermatoscopy. *J. Eur. Acad. Dermatol. Venereol.* **2019**, *33*, e341–e342. [CrossRef]
21. Pellacani, G.; Farnetani, F.; Chester, J.; Kaleci, S.; Ciardo, S.; Bassoli, S.; Casari, A.; Longo, C.; Manfredini, M.; Cesinaro, A.M.; et al. Cutaneous Melanoma Systematic Diagnostic Workflows and Integrated Reflectance Confocal Microscopy Assessed with a Retrospective, Comparative Longitudinal (2009–2018) Study. *Cancers* **2022**, *14*, 838. [CrossRef]

22. Kalloniati, E.; Cavouras, D.; Plachouri, K.M.; Geropoulou, E.; Sakellaropoulos, G.; Georgiou, S. Clinical, dermoscopic and histological assessment of melanocytic lesions: A comparative study of the accuracy of the diagnostic methods. *Hippokratia* **2021**, *25*, 156–161.
23. Nazzaro, G.; Passoni, E.; Pozzessere, F.; Maronese, C.A.; Marzano, A.V. Dermoscopy Use Leads to Earlier Cutaneous Melanoma Diagnosis in Terms of Invasiveness and Size? A Single-Center, Retrospective Experience. *J. Clin. Med.* **2022**, *11*, 4912. [CrossRef]
24. Dessinioti, C.; Geller, A.; Whiteman, D.; Garbe, C.; Grob, J.; Kelly, J.; Scolyer, R.; Rawson, R.; Lallas, A.; Pellacani, G.; et al. Not all melanomas are created equal: A review and call for more research into nodular melanoma. *Br. J. Dermatol.* **2021**, *185*, 700–710. [CrossRef]
25. Raghavan, S.S.; Peternel, S.; Mully, T.W.; North, J.P.; Pincus, L.B.; LeBoit, P.E.; McCalmont, T.H.; Bastian, B.C.; Yeh, I. Faculty Opinions recommendation of Spitz melanoma is a distinct subset of spitzoid melanoma. *Mod. Pathol.* **2020**, *33*, 1122–1134. [CrossRef]
26. Pusiol, T.; Piscioli, F.; Speziali, L.; Zorzi, M.G.; Morichetti, D.; Roncati, L. Clinical Features, Dermoscopic Patterns, and Histological Diagnostic Model for Melanocytic Tumors of Uncertain Malignant Potential (MELTUMP). *J. Natl. Cancer Inst.* **2015**, *23*, 185–194.
27. Shaikh, W.R.; Dusza, S.W.; Weinstock, M.A.; Oliveria, S.A.; Geller, A.C.; Halpern, A.C. Melanoma Thickness and Survival Trends in the United States, 1989 to 2009. *J. Natl. Cancer Inst.* **2016**, *108*, djv294. [CrossRef]
28. Hübner, J.; Waldmann, A.; Eisemann, N.; Noftz, M.; Geller, A.C.; Weinstock, M.A.; Volkmer, B.; Greinert, R.; Breitbart, E.W.; Katalinic, A. Association between risk factors and detection of cutaneous melanoma in the setting of a population-based skin cancer screening. *Eur. J. Cancer Prev.* **2018**, *27*, 563–569. [CrossRef]
29. Gimotty, P.A.; Elder, D.E.; Fraker, D.L.; Botbyl, J.; Sellers, K.; Elenitsas, R.; Ming, M.E.; Schuchter, L.; Spitz, F.R.; Czerniecki, B.J.; et al. Identification of High-Risk Patients Among Those Diagnosed With Thin Cutaneous Melanomas. *J. Clin. Oncol.* **2007**, *25*, 1129–1134. [CrossRef]
30. Stracci, F.; Fabrizi, V.; D'alò, D.; La Rosa, F.; Papini, M. Risk of multiple primary cancers following melanoma and non-melanoma skin cancer. *J. Eur. Acad. Dermatol. Venereol.* **2012**, *26*, 1384–1388. [CrossRef]
31. Neale, R.E.; Forman, D.; Murphy, M.F.G.; Whiteman, D.C. Site-specific occurrence of nonmelanoma skin cancers in patients with cutaneous melanoma. *Br. J. Cancer* **2005**, *93*, 597–601. [CrossRef]
32. Ghiasvand, R.; Robsahm, T.E.; Green, A.C.; Rueegg, C.S.; Weiderpass, E.; Lund, E.; Veierød, M.B. Association of Phenotypic Characteristics and UV Radiation Exposure With Risk of Melanoma on Different Body Sites. *JAMA Dermatol.* **2019**, *155*, 39–49. [CrossRef]
33. Kim, D.P.; Kus, K.J.; Ruiz, E. Basal Cell Carcinoma Review. *Hematol. Oncol. Clin. N. Am.* **2019**, *33*, 13–24. [CrossRef]
34. Slowinska, M.; Kaminska-Winciorek, G.; Kowalska-Oledzka, E.; Czarnecka, I.; Czarnecki, R.; Nasierowska-Guttmejer, A.; Paluchowska, E.; Owczarek, W. Dermoscopy of Small Diameter Melanomas with the Diagnostic Feasibility of Selected Algorithms—A Clinical Retrospective Multicenter Study. *Cancers* **2021**, *13*, 6095. [CrossRef]
35. Nazzaro, G.; Maronese, C.A.; Casazza, G.; Giacalone, S.; Spigariolo, C.B.; Roccuzzo, G.; Avallone, G.; Guida, S.; Brancaccio, G.; Broganelli, P.; et al. Dermoscopic predictors of melanoma in small diameter melanocytic lesions (mini-melanoma): A retrospective multicentric study of 269 cases. *Int. J. Dermatol.* **2023**. [CrossRef]
36. Pereira, A.R.; Corral-Forteza, M.; Collgros, H.; El Sharouni, M.; Ferguson, P.M.; Scolyer, R.A.; Guitera, P. Dermoscopic features and screening strategies for the detection of small-diameter melanomas. *Clin. Exp. Dermatol.* **2022**, *47*, 932–941. [CrossRef]
37. Demierre, M.-F. Thin melanomas and regression, thick melanomas and older men: Prognostic implications and perspectives on secondary prevention. *Arch. Dermatol.* **2002**, *138*, 678–682. [CrossRef]
38. Carrera, C.; Scope, A.; Dusza, S.W.; Argenziano, G.; Nazzaro, G.; Phan, A.; Tromme, I.; Rubegni, P.; Malvehy, J.; Puig, S.; et al. Clinical and dermoscopic characterization of pediatric and adolescent melanomas: Multicenter study of 52 cases. *J. Am. Acad. Dermatol.* **2018**, *78*, 278–288. [CrossRef]
39. De Giorgi, V.; Magnaterra, E.; Zuccaro, B.; Magi, S.; Magliulo, M.; Medri, M.; Mazzoni, L.; Venturi, F.; Silvestri, F.; Tomassini, G.M.; et al. Is Pediatric Melanoma Really That Different from Adult Melanoma? A Multicenter Epidemiological, Clinical and Dermoscopic Study. *Cancers* **2023**, *15*, 1835. [CrossRef]
40. Lallas, A.; Moscarella, E.; Longo, C.; Kyrgidis, A.; de Mestier, Y.; Vale, G.; Guida, S.; Pellacani, G.; Argenziano, G. Likelihood of finding melanoma when removing a Spitzoid-looking lesion in patients aged 12 years or older. *J. Am. Acad. Dermatol.* **2015**, *72*, 47–53. [CrossRef]
41. Lallas, A.; Apalla, Z.; Ioannides, D.; Lazaridou, E.; Kyrgidis, A.; Broganelli, P.; Alfano, R.; Zalaudek, I.; Argenziano, G.; International Dermoscopy Society; et al. Update on dermoscopy of Spitz/Reed naevi and management guidelines by the International Dermoscopy Society. *Br. J. Dermatol.* **2017**, *177*, 645–655. [CrossRef]
42. Costa, C.; Megna, M.; Cappello, M.; Napolitano, M.; Monfrecola, G.; Scalvenzi, M. Melanoma frequency among symmetrical Spitzoid-looking lesions: A retrospective study. *G. Ital. Dermatol. Venereol.* **2019**, *154*, 26–31. [CrossRef]
43. Duarte, A.F.; Sousa-Pinto, B.; Azevedo, L.F.; Barros, A.M.; Puig, S.; Malvehy, J.; Haneke, E.; Correia, O. Clinical ABCDE rule for early melanoma detection. *Eur. J. Dermatol.* **2021**, *31*, 771–778. [CrossRef]
44. Tiodorovic-Zivkovic, D.; Argenziano, G.; Lallas, A.; Thomas, L.; Ignjatovic, A.; Rabinovitz, H.; Moscarella, E.; Longo, C.; Hofmann-Wellenhof, R.; Zalaudek, I. Age, gender, and topography influence the clinical and dermoscopic appearance of lentigo maligna. *J. Am. Acad. Dermatol.* **2015**, *72*, 801–808. [CrossRef]

45. Jaimes, N.; Marghoob, A.A.; Rabinovitz, H.; Braun, R.P.; Cameron, A.; Rosendahl, C.; Canning, G.; Keir, J. Clinical and dermoscopic characteristics of melanomas on nonfacial chronically sun-damaged skin. *J. Am. Acad. Dermatol.* **2015**, *72*, 1027–1035. [CrossRef]
46. DeWane, M.E.; Kelsey, A.; Oliviero, M.; Rabinovitz, H.; Grant-Kels, J.M. Melanoma on chronically sun-damaged skin: Lentigo maligna and desmoplastic melanoma. *J. Am. Acad. Dermatol.* **2019**, *81*, 823–833. [CrossRef]
47. Lasithiotakis, K.; Leiter, U.; Meier, F.; Eigentler, T.; Metzler, G.; Moehrle, M.; Breuninger, H.; Garbe, C. Age and gender are significant independent predictors of survival in primary cutaneous melanoma. *Cancer* **2008**, *112*, 1795–1804. [CrossRef]
48. Gutiérrez-González, E.; López-Abente, G.; Aragones, N.; Pollán, M.; Pastor-Barriuso, R.; Sánchez, M.; Pérez-Gómez, B. Trends in mortality from cutaneous malignant melanoma in Spain (1982–2016): Sex-specific age-cohort-period effects. *J. Eur. Acad. Dermatol. Venereol.* **2019**, *33*, 1522–1528. [CrossRef]
49. Porto, A.C.; Blumetti, T.P.; Calsavara, V.F.; Torrezan, G.T.; de Paula, C.A.A.; Lellis, R.; Neto, J.P.D.; Carraro, D.M.; Braga, J.C.T. A cross-sectional study of clinical, dermoscopic, histopathological, and molecular patterns of scalp melanoma in patients with or without androgenetic alopecia. *Sci. Rep.* **2022**, *12*, 15096. [CrossRef]

Disclaimer/Publisher's Note: The statements, opinions and data contained in all publications are solely those of the individual author(s) and contributor(s) and not of MDPI and/or the editor(s). MDPI and/or the editor(s) disclaim responsibility for any injury to people or property resulting from any ideas, methods, instructions or products referred to in the content.

MDPI
St. Alban-Anlage 66
4052 Basel
Switzerland
www.mdpi.com

Life Editorial Office
E-mail: life@mdpi.com
www.mdpi.com/journal/life

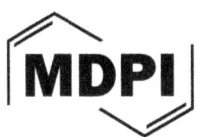

Disclaimer/Publisher's Note: The statements, opinions and data contained in all publications are solely those of the individual author(s) and contributor(s) and not of MDPI and/or the editor(s). MDPI and/or the editor(s) disclaim responsibility for any injury to people or property resulting from any ideas, methods, instructions or products referred to in the content.